The Troubled Mind

The Troubled Mind
Published by The Conrad Press Ltd. in the United Kingdom 2024

Tel: +44(0)1227 472 874

www.theconradpress.com
info@theconradpress.com

ISBN 978-1-916966-29-1

Typesetting and cover design by Michelle Emerson
www.michelleemerson.co.uk

The Conrad Press logo was designed by Maria Priestley

Printed and bound in Great Britain by Clays Ltd, Elcograf S.p.A.

The Troubled Mind

Stories of Uncertainty and Hope

Sean Baumann

Illustrated by Fiona Moodie

Canst thou not minister to a mind diseased,
Pluck from the memory a rooted sorrow,
Raze out the written troubles of the brain,
And with some sweet oblivious antidote
Cleanse the fraught bosom of the perilous stuff
Which weighs upon the heart?

Macbeth
Act 5 Scene 5
William Shakespeare

This book was initially published by Jonathan Ball Publishers in South Africa under the title
Madness: stories of uncertainty and hope.

I wish to thank James Essinger of The Conrad Press for publishing this revised version of *Madness*, and for his support and encouragement throughout the process.

In this edition, chapters have been added and the text has been revised.
SB

Contents

Introduction

This book is an attempt to make some sense of the experiences I have gained working as a psychiatrist in an admission unit of a public hospital for over twenty-five years.

Through a description of clinical encounters, I have sought to address issues that I hope to be of interest but that are also problematic or contentious in the contemporary practice of clinical psychiatry. Many of the questions that arise from these stories I believe extend beyond the confines of whatever might be defined as mental illness and pose concerns regarding the tenuous nature of the self, of consciousness, and of free will and community that have relevance to us all.

A further motivation has been a wish and a need to describe these encounters in a respectful and authentic way, troubled as I am by the often careless misrepresentations of madness and the harmful effects these distortions have in causing further suffering and exclusion. These misrepresentations arise to some extent from misconceptions − including, among many, the notion of mental illness as lacking the gravity of general medical conditions, or being merely a reflection of social ills, or being due to some sort of moral weakness or failure. An association with violence persists, mental illness is considered untreatable, and a conflation of vaguely construed notions of neurosis, psychopathy and psychosis prevails in an uncritical way. In the absence of biological markers, madness is considered as being oddly unreal.

These notions are hurtful and damaging.

This is a determinedly non-academic text. Given the concerns regarding the detrimental effects of misunderstanding or a lack of information, the book is intended for a general readership. I have sought to avoid all technical language or professional jargon and to make the issues as accessible as possible without oversimplification. This is not an introduction to general psychiatry; it is more a set of questions and arguments. It is an attempt to outline some of the difficulties in this uncertain domain.

The book comprises forty-four chapters, each of which is independent. There is no linear structure or narrative, but there are certain interwoven themes. These include the problem of stigma and a discussion of the various factors that might contribute to its vexing persistence, the enduring problem of a dualism that confuses our thinking about psychiatry, and the need to reconsider mental illness in more general terms, beyond the confines of medical pathology as a form of human suffering, whether expressed in the idiom of the mind or the body.

A strictly biomedical approach has led to significant advances, but is limited by a reductive position. Consciousness is inherently subjective, and central to any discussion of the mind and its maladies. A complementary subjective or first-person perspective therefore needs to be addressed to account for the lived experience of illness and ways of coping and finding meaning. An argument is made that meanings, however elusive, might be found in these strange stories – and, furthermore, that these meanings might be intrinsic to the process of recovery.

The categories of mental illness or psychiatric diagnoses have a limited scientific basis, and by restricting expressions of human suffering in this way we allow exclusion and limit our understanding and our capacity to be helpful.

A concern also arises in regard to the misuse of diagnoses and the inappropriate medicalisation of human suffering, thereby undermining the ability to cope with adversity. Thresholds for the diagnoses of psychiatric disorders are uncertain. Overextending the boundaries of what might be considered an illness is not helpful and can cause further harm in creating inappropriate expectations and leading to unnecessary and potentially harmful treatment.

The encounters described and the stories that are told to develop these themes are all authentic, and arise directly from my work as a clinical psychiatrist in the male admission service of Valkenberg Hospital in Cape Town. Names have been invented and certain details changed to respect the privacy of our patients and their families, and to respect confidentiality.

In the difficult circumstances described, I have been deeply moved and inspired and filled with hope by my engagement with our patients and their families. They demonstrate great courage and resilience in struggling with extreme and profoundly ill-understood forms of distress.

This book is an attempt to change our harmful ways of thinking about mental illness. It also seeks to pay tribute to those who live with these mysteriously altered states of mind and ways of being in our shared world.

Sean Baumann

Prologue

The hospital on the other side of the river

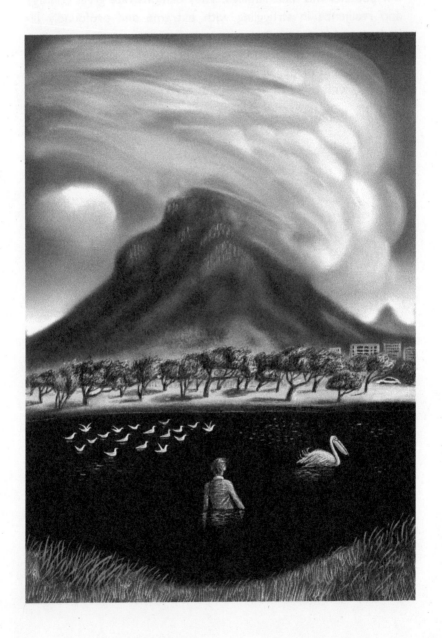

A patient is standing in the middle of the river. He is gazing across the water to the city and the mountain above where the sun is setting. His back is turned to the hospital. The nurses are waiting for him patiently on the river bank. He seems uncertain whether to cross the river or to return. There is no danger. He is on the edge, in an in-between space, as is the hospital where I have worked as a specialist psychiatrist for over twenty five years.

It is time to get away. The corridor is quiet. My colleagues have left. I close the computer, as if that could shut out the clamour. I take nothing with me, hoping that this will enable me to turn my back on the events of the day. At the door of the Education Centre a voice calls out from behind the fence of the male high care unit. "Goodbye Doctor. Safe trip home." The simple gesture seems to me to be an act of surprising kindness. This man has been admitted to the hospital as an involuntary patient. I am as the treating psychiatrist partly responsible for keeping him here. Yet he shows a generosity of spirit, not anger. On the other female side of the unit, the women are ululating as if it is a party. Then silence. The shadows of the mountain are stretching across the river and across the fence and into the grounds of the hospital. At the gate the security guard cursorily glances in the back of the car and smiles and waves, as if she herself is bemused by the arbitrariness of the process of crossing the threshold.

Leaving the hospital, on the right is the entrance to the Observatory. Here adjacent to the hospital, on the same side of the river and at the edge of the city our colleagues are gazing at the edge of the universe. I imagine a great stillness, an immense calm out there in contrast to the tumult of the hospital. I dream of a great overarching cosmic order putting into a consoling perspective the microscopic disarray of the human brain, the personal and private anguish of madness. This is illusory I am informed, and there is a swirling chaos out there that is in parallel to the frenzy of the mind in a state of extreme distress. A photograph I find in an astronomy journal of the outer edges of the universe is virtually indistinguishable from an image of the central nervous system.

The road leads away from the hospital and the observatory to a bridge across the river. The flamingos have left and so has the man standing in the river but there are flocks of gulls and ibises. The birds are motionless, their bright reflections in the evening light mirrored in the shallow water, another threshold to cross, away from the sadness and mysteries of the unit where I work.

Xolani is not responding to treatment. He is terrified, insisting that he is bewitched and that he must get away to save his life. The hospital is part of the conspiracy. Attempting to help we are contributing to the horror of his psychosis. Rico is doing well and we would like to discharge him soon but his family say they will kill him if he comes home. They say they will hold the hospital responsible. They are exhausted and angry. Previously, on many occasions after he is discharged he stops the treatment and he abuses drugs. His violent behaviour then becomes extreme and the family has become ostracized by the outraged and fearful community. What is to be gained by admitting him again, they demand exasperated, if we discharge him as soon as he is well. The hospital cannot help. Nobody can help.

Nico was discharged from the unit a month ago and now the parents have told me he has disappeared, they think up into the mountain. They are desperately worried and angry. He was well at the time of his discharge but they demand to know why we had allowed him to leave. This had happened before but now they feared for his life. They held the hospital responsible for his disappearance. What were we going to do now they wanted to know. How were we going to find him? "Where is he doctor? Tell us where Nico is?" they cried, as if I could know, as if I could undo what had happened.

There are two pastors fighting with each other on the ward. Both believe the other to be the devil incarnate. The other gods, allahs, angels and masters of the universe seem to get along with each other relatively well. Even the king of Africa and the king of Cape Town seem to have developed an amicable relationship, and it is something of a mystery as to why the pastors seem to be locked together in this hateful enmity.

Fear, rage, kindness, and a strange grace ebb and flow in the confined spaces of the acute unit. We seem almost constantly to be on the edge. Kobus insists that he does not want to die but he has no choice. The incessant voices are telling him that he must kill himself. He must do this to save his family. There is no option. He must die. Our staff numbers are worryingly low, particularly at night, and despite the suicide watch the situation is dangerous. Everybody is anxious.

Moletsi simply stares at me. I cannot read him. It is something beyond fear, something profoundly indecipherable, a deeply disconcerting state of catatonia. He appears to be baffled, but that is what I merely observe, an interpretation. Another person's mental state is ultimately unknowable. That is accepted, although something which we are not inclined to dwell upon in our customary interactions with others. But this unnerves me. He is unreachable.

Last week a pelican appeared on the river, alone. It was majestic, disproportionate, gliding in the shallow water amongst the smaller birds as if unsure whether it belonged on this drab stretch of a polluted river, running in its sluggish course between the hospital and squalor of the suburbs. Seemingly disdainful, it stretched its vast wings and lumbered into the sky, and turned westward towards the setting sun.

It was Cassiem who was standing almost in the same place in this river some months earlier, knee deep in the water, uncertain whether he should go forward or turn back.

A group of nurses watch him from the grass verge. It is not clear whether he intends to drown himself. He is shaking. This could be the cold, or his apprehension, but it is also due to the Huntington's disease, a progressive neurodegenerative disorder that he knows will kill him. He is staring away from the hospital, his gaze directed up towards the eastern buttress of the mountain. Everybody is waiting. There is a patient expectation that he will return to the hospital side of the riverbank. He makes an enormously sad shrugging movement, as if defeated. The water is too shallow to be drowned in, and the attempted suicide was absurd and futile, a mere gesture of despair.

Perhaps he had imagined the river symbolically, and that by immersing himself in its spiritually healing torrents he would be carried away from the misery of his body, to the oblivion of heaven. He stands in the water, motionless, his back to the hospital, until one of the nurses cautiously enters the water and takes his hand and without a word leads him back to the verge, back to the ward, to momentary safety and a cup of tea.

Crossing the river, crossing the road, entering into the suburb of Observatory now in shadows, I find myself in fatigue wishing and hoping that these predicaments might with distance and time begin to seem less insurmountable. This is not a particularly helpful or resourceful attitude, and equally without reason I imagine that in the morning I will return with a renewed vigour and hopefulness.

The suburb of Observatory itself seems to be on the margins, between the hospital and the more ordered city, many of its inhabitants living precariously, just holding on, the south easterly wind now blasting through the forlorn streets, papers dancing in frenzy, blank faces trapped in cars, people huddled in doorways, some of whom I recognize as previous patients.

Rising away from the suburb the road joins the highway and turns westward, across the shoulder of Devils Peak towards the city. Buffeted from the south by the increasingly furious wind the city hovers at the edge of a churning green sea, and beyond the bay at the edge of a vast continent.

The cloud has become a towering wave of silver in the evening light, pouring over the mountain and obscuring the ravines. The cables rising from the lower station disappear in the distance like frail threads into this swirling chaos. Absurdly an image comes to me. I have taken control of the winches in the lower station. I pull the levers, release the brakes. The cables tremble and the great wheels turn. We all look upward into the churning cloud. At first nothing. The cables strain and pull, and then gradually, emerging from the howling tumult a figure emerges suspended from the cable, being brought down carefully, slowly to safety. We draw him down to us. It is Nico, restored at last to his waiting family who embrace him in joyful relief. I am annoyed with myself: surely things cannot be that desperate that one resorts to this sort of wistful fantasy. And even were Nico to recover, as he in all likelihood should, it will only be a matter of time before he disappears again, lost in the mountains somewhere, back into the darkness, his parents calling in anguish, "What have you done, doctor, how could you let him go? Bring him back, bring back our son".

There is a constant pressure to discharge. The male acute service where I am a consultant comprises one hundred beds. There are about eighty to one hundred admissions a month, which means we need to maintain a constant throughput, to discharge in order to admit. Earlier in the day I had been informed that there were over forty people on the waiting list. These are patients who have undergone a seventy two hour assessment and are considered to need further hospital care, usually on the basis of a psychotic illness and some degree of dangerousness, either to themselves or others. Usually these patients are accommodated in units unfit for the purpose, awaiting transfer to our hospital. This causes much distress, and is a source of great anxiety and exasperation to the harried nursing and medical staff who in this casualty setting also need to attend to medical emergencies. Thus in order to admit these very disturbed mostly young men we are obliged to discharge patents, often before we would have considered them ready.

The parents of Oscar want me to discharge him. He clearly remains unwell but they insist they can manage. They know him, they have been through this before, and they say that the other patients in the ward are making him fearful. I need the bed. Hurriedly I give instructions for the paperwork to be done so that he can be discharged late on the Friday afternoon. On Sunday evening he is readmitted as an emergency. Everything had gone well on the Friday evening and on the Saturday. On the Sunday morning he had brought his parents breakfast in bed. They thanked him and the mother asked if she could have some honey with the tea. He had then pulled out a large knife from behind his back and lunged at his father. Somehow the parents had managed to wrestle the knife way from him and nobody was injured. The father later said there was some uncertainty in his movements, as if he was unsure of what he was doing.

Oscar said to us: "I wanted to feel what it was like to kill somebody", then later, "I had to do it...I was following instructions". Now he is back, and we will have to keep him for longer, but for how long? "Doctor we are living in fear of our lives. What is the guarantee that when you discharge him he is not going to attack us again?" No, no of course, there is no guarantee I am afraid.

The sun has passed behind the mountain and the city is in shadow. The wind has picked up ferociously. The cloud, steaming over the mountain disappears at the upper edges of the city and turns into a invisible torrent of wind, chasing through the empty streets and generating in many of us hurrying homeward a restless and disconcerting sense of desolation. Nothing seems substantial: all is movement and uncertainty. Everything seems precarious. After days of this relentless south easterly gale people say: "I can't stand it anymore. The wind is making me mad".

Stephen whom I saw this afternoon in the outpatient clinic has become unwell. He gazes through me, vague, perplexed. His mother had phoned me a day before to express her deep concern. He had been so well for so long perhaps both of us, and Stephen, had begun to imagine that this was over and that his recovery would endure. He had been assaulted close to his home a week earlier but even before this traumatic event his mother said that he had become increasingly withdrawn and had isolated himself in his bedroom. "What is it Stephen, what's happening?" A long silence ensues while he seems to be struggling to form a response. Then, making a great effort he mumbles, "I don't know". He stares out of the window but he does not seem to see the birds on the river. His mind is elsewhere. There is another long pause and he mutters, almost to himself, distractedly: "No, no. go away. It's too late. It is too late. You can't help me".

I don't know if this is some insight on his part. I don't know whether we will be able to help him. In this profound altered state of absence recovery seems improbable. We will need to be patient. We need to be have hope, but that in itself often seems elusive. The city turns away from the hospital on the other side of the river, turning against the darkness and uncertainty and sadness as night falls, bringing with it a dream of respite, as if madness might rest.

The notion of madness

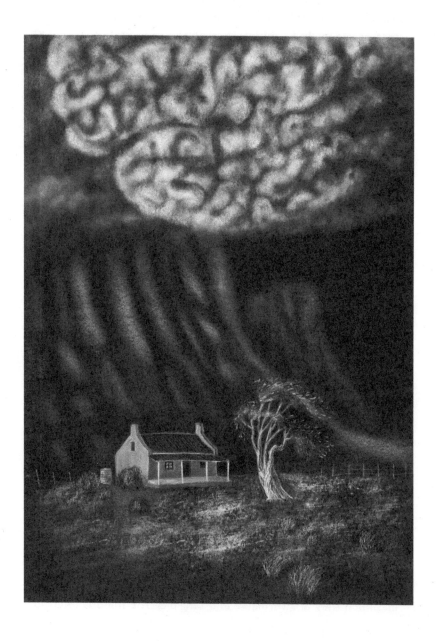

The notion of madness is problematic and controversial. Part of the problem is terminology. Madness is a folk term, it is outside the conservative domain of medicine, it is fraught with metaphors. It can seem casual and flippant, and so cause hurt. The word is used here deliberately but cautiously, and with a degree of anxiety that its use might be misinterpreted as provocative.

I most certainly do not want to cause offense and I would be dismayed if the use of the term became a source of distress to those suffering from various forms of mental illness and their families. I have discussed this with the patients in my care. None have objected. Claude did express some concern that the term might be misinterpreted. There was in this a sense of wariness, of fatalism. It seemed to me understandable that he was sceptical, and that the use of the word "madness" by a doctor would merely entrench its misuse, and grant an insulting and spurious authority to the dismissal and exclusion of those struggling with mental illnesses.

Perhaps it is inappropriate. Perhaps it is naïve and too ambitious, at this time, in this place. The intention is in a way to reclaim madness, to change the way we think about madness, and without being romantic or simply ignorant, to restore a degree of dignity and respect for these extreme states of mind.

If there is a problem with the term, and it is acknowledged that there is, the issue then arises as to what alternatives are available. What might be more positive, or helpful, and less negative or pejorative? "Mentally ill", or "severely mentally ill" in this context seems squeamish, and restricts madness to the medical domain. The wish is to take the term outside the powerfully defining and confining control of medicine, to rethink madness, in the hope of diminishing its otherness.

The tension or conflict in the use of the term madness also applies to the terminology of mental illness. "Mental" infers a mind-body dualism that arguably, albeit in an abstract or philosophical way reinforces stigma and exclusion. In a prevailing materialist culture, and within the unexamined assumptions of a biomedical language the mind is not a real thing. Things are real inasmuch they are verifiable and tangible. The mind is intangible and therefore mysterious or ephemeral. Our fears and our joys are thus considered mere epiphenomena of the structures and functions of the brain. The search for meaning is meaningless. Loss and yearning, the love for another, the fear of death are of no consequence, mere emanations arising from fifteen hundred millilitres of a grey putty-like substance confined within our skulls.

When confronted by the complex phenomenon of chronic pain a question that seems to arise for most doctors is whether the pain is physical or psychological. "Physical" is real, requiring the attention and respect of the medical profession. "Psychological" is not real, and it is therefore not clear what should be done with it. Perhaps the problem could be diverted to a psychiatrist or a psychologist. If it is psychological and not real in not having an ostensible, physical cause where does it come from? The most obvious answer, and I don't think that this is examined critically, is that it comes from the patient, that it is made up, that it is manufactured.

The concern is not merely of terminology but of the notion of madness itself, and a large part of this, and the burden of this, is the otherness of madness. To say something is mad is to dismiss it. To say somebody is mad is to suggest a difference of a fundamental nature, deserving, or requiring exclusion. Madness defines our reasonableness, our sanity. It reassures us of our normality. Inclusion requires exclusion, fences are necessary, boundaries need to be defined to keep at bay the roaming threats of unease and uncertainty. The notion of madness is a useful strategy to compartmentalize and displace these difficult parts of ourselves, these unfortunate concomitants of human consciousness.

In these respects, madness is a vague, amorphous concept, a necessary, virtually inevitable abstraction. At a more pragmatic level, and veering more towards the less emotionally charged language of medicine and psychiatry the term psychosis is often used. This itself is open to debate, and defined in various ways. It might indicate severity, suggesting a continuum, or a spectrum ranging from a mild disruption of the soothing tide of events to the calamity of psychosis, or madness. It might also indicate specific phenomena, most characteristically delusions and hallucinations. Of concern, and particularly with regard to the notion of otherness is the extent to which these phenomena are considered qualitatively different. Is madness a matter of degree, a merely quantitative issue, or is it a more fundamentally, qualitatively different affliction? Conceptualizing madness as a matter of degree, on a continuum with what we would regard as consolingly normal would surely undermine if not dispel the notion of the other, the terror of madness, and its deplorable consequences.

This is not merely rhetorical. It is a question that can be answered by considering the evidence. This shows that a significant proportion of particularly young people, during the period when schizophrenia is most likely to manifest for the first time describe psychotic symptoms in the absence of any sign of illness. Symptoms therefore need to be delinked from syndromes, but this does not happen. Hearing voices or being deluded is perceived as equalling psychosis, or madness. A young person perhaps in stressful circumstances complains of hearing a voice when nobody else is present. An assumption of psychosis is made, or of a severe mental illness, and the person becomes a patient. This can be the beginning of a long, fraught and contested process. Long because mental illnesses are considered chronic disorders, fraught because the young person has become identified as being ill, and contested because of course this identity is rejected. In the turbulent environment of an out-patient clinic, and more probably in the public sector the necessary caution and patience is rarely exercised. Simply being watchful is not considered an option, or deemed negligent as in recent years a persuasive argument has been made for early intervention, with the claim made that the duration of an untreated psychosis is associated with poorer outcomes.

Another fairly similar argument for regarding psychotic symptoms on a continuum, and not necessarily inevitably or intrinsically indicative of pathology is the recognition that we all, in certain circumstances have the capacity to experience psychotic symptoms. Sensory deprivation, certain illnesses, particularly febrile states and metabolic disorders, and a wide range of medications and psychoactive substances can trigger psychotic symptoms. Surely many of us have had the painful experience in bereavement of hearing the voice, or feeling the presence of somebody who is no longer with us.

It might be useful to interpret these curious phenomena in the light of current neuroscientific thinking in an attempt to diminish the otherness, the stigmatizing pathology of these altered states. Light is without colour. The redness of the apple is not inherent in the apple. The colour of red is generated in my mind as an outcome of series of complex processes beginning with light waves of various frequencies, but without colour, impinging of the rods and cones of my retina. This same apple is without taste or flavour until it enters my mouth and its pungency activates taste buds and olfactory cells. These sensory experiences are complex and intensely subjective. The redness of the apple I perceive is not the redness you perceive. To some extent we all live in our own worlds. To some extent we all make up our own worlds, anyway. That is not madness. Either we need to come to terms with a possibility that we are all in some ways a little bit mad, which is a cliché, or we need to consider a much more inclusive, less discriminating attitude towards experiences we do not share and that we do not understand.

In the early part of the eighteenth century the Irish priest and philosopher George Berkeley posed the enigmatic question: "If a tree falls in the forest, and nobody is there, does it make a sound?". Three hundred years later there seems to be a degree of convergence between philosophers and neuroscientists as how to answer this question, which is "no". There is no sound because it is not perceived. Perceiving brings the world into being, and it appears that this is a general principle and not confined to the mad.

William was brought to the unit in an agitated state. He was accompanied by the police to whom he had fled in terror. He was from upcountry and had come to the city in the hope of finding inspiration. He was an artist, a poet, and had been struggling to develop a creative focus. He had found the city distracting and so he had hired an isolated cottage on the coast, about an hour way from the hospital. There, on his own he sought in a state of increasing anxiety to retrieve his creativity which he told us gave meaning to his life. Towards evening the wind had risen. I am familiar with the area. The wind comes roaring and howling down the mountain in fitful bursts of a quite extraordinary force and intensity. In the growing darkness against the slope of the mountain this wind created in the cottage intermittent moaning, keening sounds that as night fell filled him with an increasing sense of dread. It was a sound that was completely unfamiliar to him. It could not possibly be simply the wind. Something else was happening, something much more sinister and foreboding. There was no electricity in the cottage and the only illumination was created by a flickering candle. In this subdued light he perceived what he initially thought were shifting shadows on the wall. Becoming increasingly fearful and disoriented by the wind and the darkness he formed a ghastly apprehension that these shapes were not shadows but stains, and the stains were of blood. He realized with horror then that the mournful sounds that had been tormenting him were not due to the wind but were the pitiful cries of infants in great distress. These laments seemed to emanate from above him, in the loft area below the roof of the cottage. His senses increasing deranged, but in a desperate attempt to find the source of his distress he found a ladder and climbed into the loft. Here in the virtual darkness he gazed in horror on a mass of bleeding, mutilated children, some dead, some crying out to him, their blood copiously flowing and seeping down the walls of the god-forsaken cottage. He fled, found his car somehow in the darkness and raced to the police where he gave a frenzied and incoherent account of what he had encountered.

It was almost immediately assumed that he had lost his mind and so he was brought in the middle of the night to the hospital. When seen by the doctor on duty it was apparent that his great distress was intensified by the realization that the police were not going to act on the information that he had given them and that they were not going to rescue the children. To add to his horror he understood that they had dismissed him and that they thought he was mad. Later in conversation with William it was evident that he was an extremely intelligent and imaginative man who used his talents creatively in the composition of poetry. A number of issues had started to trouble him including conflict with a girlfriend and financial difficulties among much else. He sought to escape, to clear his mind he said. On that terrible night he acknowledged that he was not himself. He could not make sense of the bewildering sounds, yet, partly because of his vivid imagination he felt compelled to investigate. Not knowing what was happening, in the storm of the outside world or within himself was a cause of anguish. He had to have an answer, however dreadful it might be.

There was another memorable encounter with William after he had recovered. I was involved in making a documentary about schizophrenia and I asked him whether he was prepared to talk on film about what had happened to him. He agreed enthusiastically. He wanted us to know what it was like. We took him to a sound studio and the engineer created a range of sounds for him to identify which most closely matched the quality of his hallucinations. I have an abiding memory of him dancing about the studio, delighted that the particular sound had been created and that we now knew what he had experienced, that he was no longer isolated by it and that it was shared.

It had been a madness but it was also in some way understandable. Part of the problem contributing to the burden of stigma is the notion of madness or psychosis being intrinsically ununderstandable, and therefore beyond or outside us and fundamentally other. The question must arise as to whether this is inevitable, that it is part of human nature and that the need for the other in a way represents our own failure of imagination. This tension between a continuum or a spectrum and a dichotomy or polarity is not of course limited to mental illness. In the fields of sexual politics there is a fairly recent shift away from a binary construct of male and female genders, with an understanding of the distress experienced by those who do not fit into these simplistic and inadequate categories. This pertains also to race and class and any other way in which we might identify ourselves or become confined. It is not clear why this does not extend into the domain of madness, and whether or not there is an equivalence, or whether some other, unknown force drives the apparent need to construct madness, with all its then avoidable and lamentable consequences.

2

The need for the other

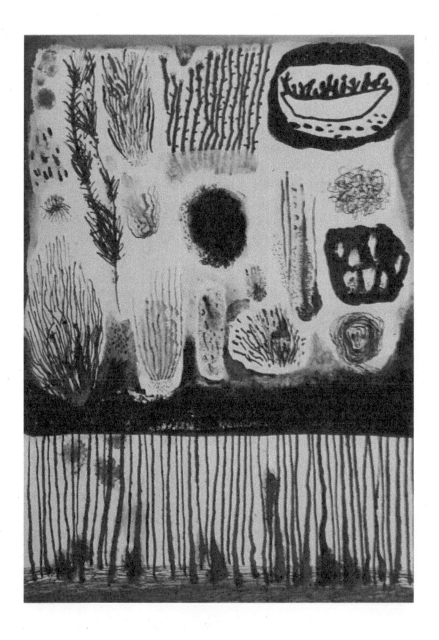

Despite a wide range of determined efforts the problem of stigma persists. We seek strenuously to educate. "Psychoeducation", both of the family and the "client" are considered mandatory in the management of schizophrenia. Students and specialists in training are taught this. Research is presented to dispel the notion that madness is associated with violence. Evidence is shown that a large part of the suffering of those living with schizophrenia is due to stigma, or the exclusion that arises from this.

This phenomenon prevails, possibly to a varying extent across cultural and socio-economic class divisions, and, perhaps with varying degrees of intensity, and with different consequences it persists over time. It is difficult to account for this mystifyingly tenacious and persistent problem. It does not seem to be a matter simply of information. There seems to be a need for the other.

Valkenberg Hospital where I work continues to appear in the imagination of many in the city as a place of fear and dread. "Jy is mal: jy hoort in Valkenberg" ("you are mad: you belong in Valkenberg") persists as a refrain of dismissal and alienation. You don't count. You are not one of us. You don't belong with us. You are too different from us. You threaten us. We do not feel safe with you in our midst. You need to be put away. You need to be in Valkenberg, anywhere, but away from us, outside, beyond the gates of the city, across the river.

Being away, outside, appears to be the priority. What might happen within these zones of exclusion is of lesser consideration. The driving concern is not care but separation, as if madness is contagious or contaminating. This has a particularly harsh and tragic resonance in South Africa. Many factors contributed to the emergence and persistence of the apartheid system, but a central driving force seems to have been fear, and more particularly fear of the unknown, of contamination by the heathen, and of loss of land and privileges, and with regard to madness, the loss of the fragile faculty of reason.

The asylum was not created simply out of fear. A genuine concern for the mentally ill cannot be dismissed as a motivating concern, but the physical exclusion that this entailed was in all probability a powerful perpetuating factor. Causes and

consequences become confused. It would be simplistic to argue that the problem of stigma is a consequence of the exclusion represented by the development of the asylums in Europe in the eighteenth century. The more recent trend towards de-institutionalization, again motivated by a complicated range of factors and not solely by a benevolent concern for the mentally ill, has not I believe significantly reduced the burden of stigma.

Some of the difficulties in making sense of the notion of the "other" might be a consequence of this being regarded as an entity, rather than a complex phenomenon arising from a range of interacting socio-political, cultural, historical but also importantly psychological factors. It is necessary to consider the construct in this multi-dimensional way if anything is to be gained in reducing its apparent intractability.

The notion of the other confers an illusion of safety, of order, of normality. There is a paradox in the need to invoke a threat in order to feel secure. Otherwise what is there? Is all contingent, wide open, endlessly vacant, with no fence to demarcate the boundaries, to define who we might be? In early Cape Town the wild almond fence was an entangled haphazard physical expression of an edge between an enlightened European settlement and a savage darkness. The Liesbeeck river is an edge between the ordered, managed and manageable city, and disorder, the imagined turmoil and the threat of madness.

We take something away from ourselves, we excise something deemed inconsistent with a notion we have of ourselves, and put this something other elsewhere, on the other side of the fence, of the river. We should then be safe, we should feel secure. But the early settlers described the unease of gazing from a precarious fortress upon the campfires of the local herders they gradually began to perceive as hostile. The campfires encroached, became menacing. Lines were drawn. The fortress needs an enemy, an assailant, to justify its being. The wild almond hedge is hopelessly inadequate.

The journals of Jan van Riebeeck describe an ambivalent, uncertain shifting attitude towards the local inhabitants. The relationships are at times cordial, cooperative if not wary, and at other times hostile. Over the years there is a drift towards enmity, growing on one side partly due to the theft of cattle, on the other side, due to the dispossession of grazing lands. There were quite possibly at times some moments of peace, some notion of a co-existence, of mutual benefit and a shared future. At what point, and surely there was no point, but over what period of time did this possibility fade? When, and how quite imperceptibly does it arise that the enemy becomes the enemy, that someone or another becomes the other?

The city gazes across the river towards the hospital with some ambivalence, if not unease.

Why the fences? Is this for the protection of those within or those without? The boundaries are porous and arbitrary. Our patients wander out into the suburb of Observatory and they wander back. The average length of admissions is about three to four weeks. Patients are discharged and often after a while they come back. Families, students, workers and staff come and go. The hospital is not a fortress. Yet the divide persists, and it seems possible that in part this might be because it is intangible.

The fort, the fence, the river, all appear to be frail barriers against the unknown. A fence surrounds the hospital on one side of the river. On the other side of the river fences, high walls, barbed wire, alarms seek to protect the houses of the suburbs. The enemy is not on the other side of the river, he or she is roaming the streets of the suburb. The fences are not working. There is no safety. The enemy is not hemmed in. It is free to roam.

At present the city is preoccupied with a court case that involves a horrifying and bewildering family murder. It bears a disconcerting resemblance to a fairly recent murder case that gained international attention. The current case is unresolved, but the accused is a family member. In the prior event the accused was the partner of the lover he was found guilty of murdering. Both cases involved extreme violence, in one the use of an axe, in the other a shotgun. Repeated blows, repeated shots, as if the sheer frenzy and brutality of the murders signified something beyond the killing, as if the murders were an endpoint of what was described as a mounting rage, and, of course, a madness.

The two murders bear a resemblance in another troubling respect. The attacks were claimed to have come from the outside. In the one circumstance the convicted murderer claimed that he had acted on the conviction that the person he had shot was a potential assailant that had entered the apartment. In this belief, sobbing, he said he had killed his lover. In the other the suspected killer claimed that it was not himself but an intruder that had murdered his family with an axe. A middle class family it is claimed is destroyed behind the high walls, in the illusory safety of their suburban home by an invader. A cruel detail is added, to enhance the thrill of horror: the man is laughing as he hacks the family to death. This is an ancient story, a terror haunting the imagination for over three hundred years. The enemy, the outsider, the barbarians have broken down the fence and are swarming over the walls. The defences are overwhelmed. There is a terrifying sense of inevitability about the attack. It was always going to happen. Now it is upon the cowering lover hiding behind the bathroom door, the innocent, bewildered family in the safe house in the secure estate. But the attack is not from the outside, it is from within, and this poisons our consciousness with a deeper, more insidious fear. The threat, from within rather than from without is intolerable. Let it come from outside if it must be. The danger lurking beyond the fence, on the other side of the river, outside the fortress is at least more understandable, knowable. From within, like a madness emanates another kind of fear.

Currently western Europe is preoccupied with the issue of immigration. This is a major item in national elections, it dominates current affairs. It is a cause of intense debate. Anxious reference is made to a "way of life", "national identity" and "terror". Sometimes made explicit, more often not, is the notion of a threat, of an engulfing wave. This threat is perceived as unstoppable. No international law, no policeman on the shore can stop the tide. The fear is spread wide. Now it comes not across the fence, not across the river, but across the ocean, in broken, leaking boats. The fear provokes reaction. There is a rise in extremist, nationalist politics. The barricades come up. Invocation of the other, a threat to a way of life, now from the outside, streaming across borders, has become a useful tool to gain political support.

A wide range of factors contributed to the formation and the maintenance of the apartheid system for most of my childhood. The monopoly of power and wealth in disregard of justice were powerful perpetuating factors, as was, perhaps less obviously fear. A fear that persisting over the centuries, unabated, gathering force and hammering at the gates of the apartheid edifice developed a relentless momentum. Confused with this fear was an ambivalence, an uncertainty as to who or what constituted the other. A mutual dependency confounded customary notions of difference. Exclusion was ineffective. White babies clung to the backs of their black carers. All over the country townships were situated away from the city, but not too far away. Smoke arising from the wood burning fires of the corrugated iron dwellings of the alien workers would have been visible from the town on the other side of the hill or koppie, exciting ancient fears, as the first settlers gazed in apprehension upon the campfires of the encroaching, belligerent herders. These more contemporary but desperately poor settlements were separate but not too separate to be out of mind. A dependable supply of labour was needed. Racial segregation became inefficient, impractical and impossible, yet continued to hold sway as a hollow or cynical political slogan. There being the other was necessary, politically expedient, but now, confusedly, gradually the other became less than the other and lost definition. What to do? Where to turn? Would it be imaginable to be without the need for the other? How necessary, after all these years of an accustomed way of thinking, a habit of fear, is the other in order to define us?

Mtembe is admitted to the unit in a floridly psychotic state. The family seem curiously unperturbed. He has been bewitched. It is clear. He had had some success in a business venture and this had provoked the envy of others. Arrangements were made. Money was spent and the evil spell was cast. Our task was simply to make Mtembe better. The use of standard anti-psychotic medication to achieve this did not trouble the family. We were not required to provide an explanation. That had been sorted out in a way that was satisfactory to the family and the community. The explanation was consistent with cultural beliefs. Any talk of a biological contribution and certainly a genetic disposition was both meaningless and alien. His madness did not pose any threat. The attribution to witchcraft resolved that potential difficulty. Witchcraft as a way of making sense of something that might have caused terror was therapeutic, if not for Mtembe, but clearly for his community. The other was named, became known, and so lost its dreaded force. The serpent lost its fangs. Mtembe was not excluded because he appeared to be mad. The provision of a culturally meaningful explanation rendered the invocation of the other unnecessary.

Those on the other side of the river were perhaps not dangerous. Perhaps with some bartering, some friendly cooperation, some sort of dialogue, possible difficulties might be resolved. Differences might not be insurmountable. Perhaps the enemy is not the enemy.

An attempt to explain the persistence of stigma, the apparent need of the other through recourse to historical events might seem extravagant or rather absurd. It might be argued that the notion of the other is simply part of human nature, but what is possibly more mysterious is the persistence of the need for the other. It has been suggested that stigma arises to some extent from fear, and that this fear in turn concerns the apprehension of the other that becomes all the more menacing as it is unknown and unfathomable. Defining the other, labelling it in whatever way that might be convenient and meaningful both to the patient and the community at least mitigates the unease. It is also probable that the stigma attached to mental illness has less to do with the nature of mental illness itself, or madness, than this perplexing need for the other.

Why the other anyway should necessarily be a source of fear and apprehension is in itself curious. God is unknown and worshipped. The ineffable, the transcendent, the hidden order of things are endowed with a positive, enhancing spiritual quality that have been a source of yearning throughout history. Is it impossible that madness, rather than a source of fear and hence exclusion, could rather require the need or wish to learn, to understand, to extend our notion of who we might be and how we might be in the world? This is less an issue of knowledge than the need for a fundamental change in attitude. An assumption cannot be made that the acquisition of knowledge in some automatic way changes attitudes or enlightens. How do we allow it in ourselves to perpetuate the burden of stigma? Are our notions of our own sanity so tenuous, our beliefs in the order of our world so precarious that we regard the need for the other as inevitable.

3

The frontier: a historical context

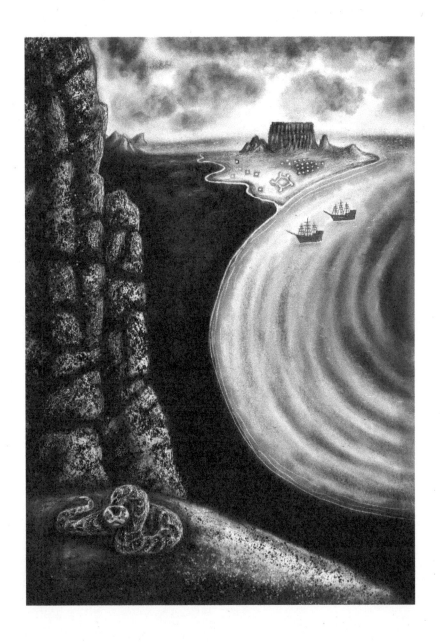

The Liesbeeck river begins on the eastern slopes of Table Mountain above the Kirstenbosch Botanical Gardens. It flows through the suburbs of Bishopscourt and Rondebosch to Observatory where it joins the Black River and ends in Paarden Eiland, absorbed into the Atlantic Ocean of Table Bay. This is the Cape of Storms, or otherwise the Cape of Good Hope. It is in the area of Observatory that the river drifts past the hospital, and divides the hospital from the city.

It is not a long river, the course being approximately nine kilometres. It is for the most part shallow and clogged with the reeds that give it its name. It is not grand. It is an improbable frontier, this thin, inauspicious stretch of water that marks the start of the colonial project in southern Africa, that heralds the dispossession and the conflict that have endured from the middle of the seventeenth century to the present day.

If dispossession is central to the way in which the conflict is understood the year 1657 might be considered as the beginning of this long history of strife. In October of that year Jan van Riebeeck, directed by the VOC (United Dutch East India Company) governors in the Netherlands granted freehold lands along the Liesbeeck to a number of the company's employees. This was in part motivated by the need to control costs in the savings gained by not paying wages, but also by the need for fresh food both for the garrison and the passing ships in Table Bay, and in the belief that this might be more efficiently produced by private enterprise.

A number of violent confrontations between the local indigenous groups and the European adventurers preceded this date. In 1510 Francisco de Almeida , the first viceroy of the Portuguese Indies, following what seemed to have been a botched kidnapping was murdered with fifty of his men by the Khoisan. De Almeida had ostensibly approached the Khoikhoi pastoralists somewhere in the Liesbeeck valley to barter for sheep and cattle. It is not clear what ensued or why the Portuguese attempted to kidnap the two Khoikhoi. There was an altercation. It escalated. The Europeans were violently assaulted, and apparently in seeking revenge were murdered. What had gone so tragically wrong remains unknown. It is not apparent whether an initially potentially cooperative encounter could have been resolved peacefully, or whether this violent outcome reflects an inevitability in the clash of European settlers and agriculturists and the local pastoralists, a conflict that in its various permutations persists to the present. Nor is it clear to what degree arrogance, fear, greed and stupidity, and in the prevailing thinking of the times, a careless dogma of divinely ordained superiority contributed to this harbinger of future turmoil.

Thereafter the local inhabitants were portrayed by the Europeans as barbarians, as dangerous and heathen savages, the embodiment of the terrifying "other".

"Of all people they are the most bestial...they are the reverse of human kind...so that if there is any medium between a rational animal and a beast, the Hottentot lays the fairest claim to that species... they are as squalid in their bodies as they are mean and degenerate in their understandings...their native inclinations to idleness and a careless life, will scarcely admit to either force or rewards... their common answer to all motives of this kind, is that the fields and woods afford plenty of necessaries for their support, and nature has amply provided for their subsistence...so there is no need for work...and thus many of them idly spend the years of a useless restive life" (1)

This contempt conflicted with need. The Dutch were sick and starving, gazing with hope and envy and fear upon the herds of the Khoikhoi, moving into the fertile valley of the Liesbeeck for pasture as part of a transient nomadic rhythm. Hope would have arisen from an expectation that they would be able to barter for sheep and cattle, the wealth of these "bestial vermin", and fear from the notion of the "other" the encroaching hordes on the banks of the river, the campfires at night, and what must have seemed the vulnerability of the fort on the edge of an unknown continent. Fear then, on both sides of the river, on the west side, of death by starvation or violent attack, of annihilation, and also, perhaps the anxiety of being alien, of being too far away, of dislocation, and on the east side, on the side of a vast continent, the dread of dispossession, of the beginning of an end.

The problem of stigma is an enduring theme in these essays. It is a complex phenomenon, and a wide range of factors contribute to its mystifying endurance, given the amount of information available to support its damaging effects. It would of course be simplistic and inappropriate to consider the events described as in some way causative, but it can be argued that ignorance, and arising from ignorance, distrust and thence exclusion are significant historical and cultural factors that shape the local expression of this iniquity that contributes greatly to the suffering of those deemed mentally ill.

An instance of this ignorance and its calamitous consequences emerges from the beginnings of this engagement on either side of the river. Van Riebeeck is confounded. His men are quite desperate. They see the ample herds of sheep and cattle across the river and cannot understand why the pastoralists are unwilling to barter.

Van Riebeeck in frustration and disdain records in his journal: "Would it matter so much if one deprived them of some six or eight thousand cattle? For this there would be ample opportunity, as we have observed they are not very strong". (2) Almost from the beginning of the arrival of the Europeans on the southern edge of the continent, a delineation of power on either side of this slack, inconsequential river is established, a notion of harmonious co-existence is set aside and the resort to force is proposed as a solution, as if this is reasonable and just. For the time being, van Riebeeck is constrained by the company, and urged to barter rather than seek war.

There is from the start a failure to understand that for the Khoi livestock, not land represent wealth. There is a further and dangerous misapprehension regarding the occupation of land in the failure to recognize that the land occupied by the company employees formed an integral part of the pasturage routes of the Goringhaiqua and the Gorachoqua. The marine shoreline also provided subsistence for the Goringhaicona, and the Cochoqua moved their grazing routes south from the Swartland during the summer grazing pastures in the Liesbeeck valley. (3) The VOC settlements lay in the path of these routes. The Khoikhoi pastoralists could not fathom why a vastly wealthy company, recently arrived from a distant country should assume any right to impede their movement, and the settlers, with a different notion of land ownership combined with a belief of racial superiority were affronted by the failure of the Khoi to acquiesce. They were also in all likelihood in fear of their lives.

In 1657 with these increasing pressures on land and with tensions rising van Riebeeck persuades the VOC to allow a number of its servants to be released from the company and establish themselves along the banks of the Liesbeeck as "free burghers". This is the moment at which Cape Town becomes no longer a mere "refreshment station" but a settlement. The lands on the west side of the river are occupied, owned. A frontier is established: an edge is defined.

The Khoikhoi pastoralists demand to know where they are to graze their cattle. Van Riebeeck suggests they move inland, to the north and west, putting them at risk of conflict with the Cochoqua or "Saldanhars". This proposal is rejected. A leader of the Goringhaiqua or "Kaapmans", Chief Autshumato is lured to the fort on the shores of Table Bay and a hundred of his cattle are captured by the Dutch. One Kaapmans is shot dead and another wounded. Autshumato is dispatched to Robben Island from where he escapes eighteen months later. The Kaapmans respond by stealing cattle and burning the homesteads of the "free burghers". The two sides are effectively at war.

On the 19th May 1659 the council of which van Riebeeck is head meets at the fort and issues a declaration that will set the country on a path of conflict and acrimony and mistrust for the centuries that are to follow:

"Since we see no other means of securing peace and tranquillity with these cape people, we shall take the first opportunity practicable to attack them with a large force, and if possible, take them by surprise…we shall capture as many cattle and men as we can…the prisoners we shall keep as hostages, so that we may restrain and bring to submission those who may evade us…the council prays that it may please the Lord God to attend us with His Blessing and His Help. Amen" (4)

In his journal van Riebeeck reports on and dismisses the grievances of the Khoikhoi. He writes: "They strongly insisted that we had been appropriating more and more of their land, which had been theirs all these centuries, and on which they had been accustomed to let their cattle graze. They asked if they would be allowed to do such a thing supposing they went to Holland...", and "as for your claim that the land is not big enough for us both, who should in justice rather give way, the rightful owner or the foreign intruder?..." Eventually they had to be told...that their land had fallen to us in a defensive war, won by the sword, as it were, and we intended to keep it." (5)

This was the justification, of dispossession and ruin by force. There is no attempt to provide a moral argument, perhaps there is no sense of a need as God was considered to be on the side of the Europeans, as it was assumed there was divine support for the fateful election of the Nationalist government almost three hundred years later. So there was no further need to accommodate, no need for compromise, no need for sharing, no more need for caution: to the victor went the spoils of war.

The "other" having been defined and conquered, exclusion of course had to be established and maintained and defended. A series of palisades and watchtowers were erected along the banks of the river, with a system of flag signalling to the fort to warn of danger. In addition the planting was ordered of a bitter almond hedge and other fast growing brambles and thorn bushes to prevent intrusion and to protect the land and cattle of the settlers. These were the precursors of the high walls and the barbed wire that have become a feature of present day predominantly white south african suburbs.

Flags, bitter almonds, barbed wire: it seems impossible to imagine that these frail measures would provide an adequate degree of security, or peace of mind, as if the exclusion of the mentally ill could bring under control the fear of madness, as if being safe and normal were possible. Yet, at the time of writing and for the foreseeable future the sluggish Liesbeeck river divides the hospital from the city, and in this division perpetuates the fear of the unknown and the stigma of mental illness.

The unknown does not necessarily generate fear. Wonder at the unknown seems entirely possible, and maybe one way of coping with the uncertainties of life and the mysteries of the universe. If Valkenberg Hospital represents an edge, of sanity and order, and a space for the examination and treatment of the turbulent inner workings of the mind and brain, another adjacent institution separated from the hospital by a narrow gravel path turns outward to examine the edges of time and space.

The first permanent observatory was developed on the Observatory site adjacent to the hospital in October 1820. From this point on the edge of the river, at the time menaced by poisonous snakes, (the rocky mound on which the observatory was erected was initially named "Slangkop"), and surrounded by leopards and hippopotami, the shape and edge of the southern hemisphere was determined and the mass of the moon and Jupiter were measured. The distance of the sun from the earth was estimated and this remained the standard for nearly half a century. In the later part of the nineteenth century the observatory was involved in a major international effort to produce a detailed photographic "Map of the Heavens".

Order, precise measurement, and in this scientific ambition the control of chaos is brought to the edge of the river and of the city and the continent. On either side of this narrow gravel path, but on the same side of the slow drift of the river two city institutions co-exist, the one turned inward to the turmoil of the mind, seeking illumination to aid recovery, and the other turned outward, searching through measurement to find order in the chaos of the universe.

Visitors to the city are surprised at 12 o'clock each day except Sundays by a loud explosive retort that reverberates across the city bowl, a booming echo of assault. In a flash and a puff of smoke there occurs momentarily a memory of danger. The pigeons in the company gardens rise from the oak trees in an agitated flock, having no such memory, confused by the signal of apparent threat. There seems to be nothing to confirm this, no sustained clamour of violence, and the birds return to the trees and the city resumes its customary rhythms.

This reed clogged river emerging from the southern slopes of Table Mountain and flowing slowly through the southern suburbs of the city, past the hospital and the observatory to join the Black River and enter the sea in Table Bay is a centuries old frontier. It represents a margin, historically of a European settlement, of a claim of ownership and dispossession, and the beginning of enduring conflict and mistrust. It persists as an edge, on one side of the gravel path, of measuring time and space, and on the other side, of precarious notions sanity and madness.

References

1. John Ovington, Master of the East Indiaman Benjamin, quoted in Raven-Hart, R. (1970). Cape of Good Hope 1652 to 1702: The First Fifty Years of Dutch Colonisation as Seen by Callers. Cape Town: A. A. Balkema, cited in Mostert, N. (1992). Frontiers: The Epic of South Africa's Creation and the Tragedy of the Xhosa People. London: Jonathan Cape, p.107.

2. Thom, H.B. (ed.). (1952). Journal of Jan Van Riebeeck, Volume 1, 1651-1662. Cape Town: A. A. Balkema, p.16.

3. Worden, N., Van Heyningen, E. & Bickford-Smith, V. (1998). Cape Town: The Making of a City. Cape Town: David Philip.

4. Resolution of the Council of Policy of the Cape of Good Hope, 19 May 1659.

5. Thom, H.B. (ed.). (1952). Journal of Jan Van Riebeeck, Vol 1, 1651-1662. CapeTown: A. A. Balkema, pp.195-106.

4

Living with uncertainty

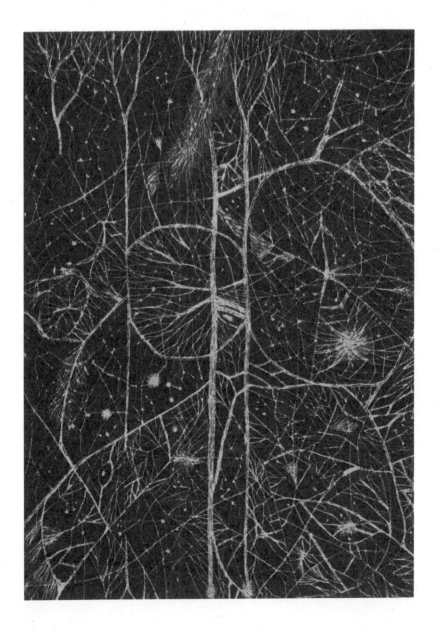

A frequently encountered criticism of psychiatry, and implicitly a way of differentiating psychiatry from general medicine is its incertitude. With this comes a range of assumptions, that psychiatry is vague and therefore unscientific, that in comparison to general medicine its basic tenets are ill-understood, and possibly as a consequence of this, that its treatments are ineffective. According to this scenario general medicine progresses triumphantly and seamlessly. If there are uncertainties these are expected to soon be dispelled by the inexorable forward march of biomedical science. This dichotomous way of thinking is entrenched in medical school training and in the institutions of medicine, in the separation of psychiatry from other specialties, and in modern, materialist cultural ways of thinking.

Psychiatry is about the mind, and since there is no clear understanding about what might constitute the mind psychiatry is uncertain. It does not fit with general medicine; it is a "Cinderella" discipline. In the popular imagination it quite possibly belongs more to early twentieth middle Europe than the twenty first century. For many the ridiculous image still prevails of the psychiatrist as a middle aged man with a beard, sitting at the head of a couch taking notes, while a younger middle class woman lies turned away from him, rambling on interminably about her dreams and her sexual fantasies.

This dualist way of thinking, this separation of mind and body, of the psychological and the physical, formalized in the separation of psychiatry from general medicine is not helpful, has no basis in contemporary neuroscience and is more probably harmful. Defining a problem as psychiatric leads to the neglect of physical aspects of the presenting problem and is all too often perceived as dismissive. "It's all in the mind" is interpreted as "it's not real". Conversely, defining a problem as physical leads to the neglect of important psychological factors that require attention. Depression might be a manifestation of a neuroendocrine problem. Being unaware of the likelihood of a person living with a terminal cancer being depressed seems cruelly reductive, unimaginative and unhelpful. The status of the dementias is unclear. The symptoms, certainly in the early stages are psychological and the biological basis of the process are fairly well elucidated. This group of disorders seem to be both psychiatric and medical. With the rapidly developing understanding of the biological basis of the schizophrenia spectrum disorders this group is increasingly being described as "neuropsychiatric" in nature. The duality does not seem to hold.

While I was working in a community clinic a young woman was referred to me by the medical officer working in an adjacent office. The referral note was absurdly brief. It read: "Known psychiatric patient. Now complains of headache. Please take over management".

I asked this young woman to clarify what the problem was. She looked at me vaguely and then her head sank to the desk where we were both was sitting. She was fortunately accompanied by her mother who told me that her daughter had been perfectly well until three days ago. She had then suffered the sudden onset of a severe headache. It was described as a blow to the back of the head. She had later become drowsy during the day, was agitated at night, and more recently had begun to vomit. The headache had got steadily worse. This was not a psychiatric problem. This was a medical emergency. She was showing features of a raised intracranial pressure, in this context most likely to be due to an intracerebral bleed. She needed an urgent CT scan, not the attention of a psychiatrist.

This encounter raises many issues, one being the discrimination so often observed against patients with psychiatric disorders. Having a mental illness somehow disembodies one. Symptoms are without justification attributed to the psychiatric problem. A proper history is not taken. The necessary examination is not performed. The problem is not taken seriously. This has dangerous, possibly life-threatening consequences.

The medical officer appeared to have been certain that the symptoms were not due to a medical condition, but to the unspecified psychiatric disorder of which a cursory mention had been made. This is inferred because the necessary history and examination had not been undertaken to justify the diagnosis which was not a diagnosis but a careless assumption. In clinical medicine certitude requires great caution. Making such assumptions is rarely feasible and it is hazardous.

The discipline of psychiatry is uncertain, but so is general medicine and so is science. I had studied for a bachelor of arts degree before I started medicine. In our seminars in the arts faculty we were encouraged to question, to reflect and analyse. There were few facts and even this was open to debate. Is James Joyce's Ulysses a good book? Why is it important? Why do we study one text and not another? We learned some rudimentary tools to think critically, or at least that was the aim of our teachers. For these reasons and many others starting medicine was a struggle for me. I perhaps naively transferred this critical way of thinking to the basic sciences. How do we know? How can we be sure? How can we be certain of this when we know that what in the past was considered certain was subsequently proven to be false. I must have been a very irritating and exasperating student, and I was not helping myself, but I did develop the rather vague notion that medicine represented another culture, and that it required a different way of thinking. I coped somehow, but the feeling of not being sure about being sure persisted.

As junior doctors a most difficult and miserable task was to impart bad news to patients and their families. I cannot remember ever having been told how to do this. "It is cancer. It is advanced. It is inoperable. There is nothing more that can be done". Inevitably the question follows as to how much time is left. I of course had no idea and I did not know how to answer the question. Nor it transpired did many of my seniors at the time, or not with any degree of certainty. We did not have an opportunity to discuss these important issues at any meaningful level but I did form the impression then that a confident authoritative posture was to be recommended. A professional certitude was for some unknown reason assumed to be more reassuring and consoling than an admission of incertitude. Not being certain became elided with not knowing, or not knowing for sure, and this seemed to be considered unprofessional or merely incompetent.

I have been prescribed statins by my general practitioner because of high cholesterol and a family history of cardiovascular disease. A study was recently published concerning the benefits of statins in preventing cardiac events, or deaths due to heart attacks. Two respected daily newspapers reported the findings. One declared that millions were taking statins unnecessarily, the other that every male over the age of sixty should be taking statins. Two very different conclusions were drawn from the same study. Despite the most strenuous and skilled endeavours the benefits remain unclear. Furthermore there are drawbacks to taking this preventative medication, including not only the side-effects. The act of taking the statin is a constant reminder of one's vulnerability. With the swallowing of each wretched tablet the bell tolls of an assured mortality.

Obesity in prosperous and lower and middle income countries is a cause for concern, yet the factors that contribute to this and what to do about it remain uncertain. Smoking causes cancer but it is not that straightforward. Person A smokes forty cigarettes a day for most of his adult life and dies in his eighties of unrelated causes. Person B who smokes the same amount is dead as a result of a bronchogenic carcinoma at the age of fifty. How to treat a relatively benign prostatic cancer in an otherwise healthy seventy year old man is uncertain. The benefits of surgery for lower back pain are uncertain. Clinical medicine if fraught with uncertainties. The more we seem to know the more we do not know, or the uncertainties move to another level. An ischaemic event or a heart attack owing to a thrombosis in a coronary artery appears to be fairly straightforward, the many interacting genetic and environmental factors that contribute to the formation of the thrombosis are much less clear.

For many years I was required to present an update of research in the field of schizophrenia to the department's weekly journal club. This became challenging. Every year in the literature there was a familiar refrain. These were exciting times. We were on the verge of discovering the causes of schizophrenia. Ten, forty then over a hundred genes were identified as being contributory. The expectation was that with the elucidation of the causes more effective treatments would become possible. This has not happened, or whether it has happened or not is open to debate. It is by no means certain. After so many years, after so many endeavours and so many millions of dollars spent on research the causes of schizophrenia and its effective remedy remains elusive.

Some time ago I probably annoyed my colleagues by presenting an image of a half-filled glass, and saying that with regard to schizophrenia research I was not sure whether the glass was half full of half empty. I don't think this has changed significantly but that does not mean the research is going nowhere or that the pursuit of the causes of schizophrenia has been futile. It is just more complex than had perhaps been thought, and with complexity comes uncertainty.

The history of science is replete with ideas and beliefs that at the time were held to be certain and in retrospect have been proved false and absurd and even embarrassing. On a visit with colleagues to see a new hospital in Kimberley in the northern Cape we were given a tour of the big hole, a massive excavation pit. A brochure informed us that the most eminent geologist of the time had been tasked by the colonial government to survey the area for possible diamond deposits. After doubtlessly extremely thorough investigations he declared with great certainty that no diamonds were to be found in the area. Within five years the most extensive diamond deposits in the world were discovered at the site. Incidentally, thereafter the geologist, apparently undeterred, formulated an ostrich hypothesis. He had in fact not been mistaken. Ostriches in a distant diamond rich area had swallowed the diamonds and moving to Kimberley had chosen to defecate the precious stones there, on a massive and very generous scale.

Uncertainty is not confined to clinical medicine or psychiatry but appears to be an integral aspect of basic science. The very fabric of reality is uncertain. Uncertainty is intrinsic to quantum physics. The nature and extent of dark matter and dark energy is not known, nor is it clear why matter should be, rather than there being nothing. It does not seem to be known whether we inhabit a universe or a multiverse. Why time should have a direction, and the origins and the ultimate fate of the universe or multiverse are profound mysteries. The world is made up of matter and force particles comprising, we are informed, a deeply mysterious web of fermions, up and down quarks and bosons. That is where things are for the time being it seems, but in a discussion with a young physicist recently he told me that there was uncertainty in his circles about what might actually constitute a particle, or whether a particle might perhaps be a length of string, or a wave.

Uncertainty does not have to be a problem. It can be a source of wonder. It is a driving force to answer important questions, to solve mysteries. Certainties can be oppressive. There is no further to go. Doors close. The problem perhaps has more to do with how we live with uncertainty, as if in some way in order to survive we need to believe in some things being certain, however illusory that might be.

A vastly complex array of factors contribute to acts of terror, but one possibly neglected factor might be the yearning, independent of religion, for certitude. The modern world is too complex and too various. It is not possible to reconcile this alien world with the teachings of the ancient texts. Values are no longer absolute but bewilderingly and contradictorily relative. A fundamentalist position represents more solid ground. The notion of fundamentalism itself is fraught with uncertainty but one aspect would seem to be an inclination to interpret the texts in a more concrete way, a disinclination to tolerance and as a consequence a higher risk of seeking transcendence in the rapture of oblivion and martyrdom.

Perhaps the most personal and existential uncertainty of our lives is when and how we will die. Most of us live with this uncertainty, but that we get older rather than younger is certain as is the fact of our mortality. Even this is however disputed by some of our more technologically inclined fellow beings who imagine and plan to defeat death by having themselves, whatever those selves might be, frozen or uploaded into the cloud. Yet there is no escaping incertitude, as it unknown whether this disembodied software might or might not be a desirable state of being.

Given the positive nature of incertitude, of not knowing propelling us forward to knowing, or seeking, it seems that we nevertheless have to come to terms with the very human unease of having to live with inevitable uncertainty. Certainties are consoling. We comfort children, we seek to persuade ourselves that the world is a secure place, that there are landmarks and signposts and beacons that will reliably guide us on our way. We are not inclined to contemplate the chaos of the universe.

We seek patterns or shapes of meaning in order to make predictions so that we can plan and hopefully gain some degree of control over our lives. It is a tentative process. Living with uncertainty is discomforting but being in a world that is entirely certain is unimaginable. It is also hazardous, inducing an inertia that may undermine the seeking necessary for survival. A total certainty or predictability would make our lives empty and devoid of any need to make choices or take action. A paralysis of boredom induced by the illusion of certitude seems an undesirable state of mind or being, or certainly lacking in the joy of surprise.

It is a matter of finding some balance between a degree of predictability in order to cope as best we can, and accepting but not being overwhelmed by uncertainty. This all goes to pieces in psychotic states. There is no balance.

The parents of Rudewaan listen to me anxiously. He has been recently admitted to our unit and I don't think that there can be any doubt that the diagnosis is that of schizophrenia. "But doctor how can you be sure?" "How long will it take for him to get better?" "Will he get better?" "Will he be able to work?" "Will he be himself again?" "Will he be able to lead a normal life, study, work, marry, have children, look after us when we get old?" These questions get asked again and again, and I wish that I could answer them with a certainty that I know would be unjustified. I am the consultant. I am the senior doctor in the unit. There is nowhere else for the family to turn, to get the answers they so understandably need. It is difficult to accept the diagnosis of schizophrenia, and all the more difficult to come to terms with the many uncertainties that such a diagnosis entails.

I try to explain the problem to the students. We attempt a discussion as to what constitutes a diagnosis. The diagnosis of tuberculosis is not the same as a diagnosis of schizophrenia. I talk of a "tentative, provisional hypothesis" and it is clear that they are dissatisfied. They are not impressed. Science is to do with facts, with certitudes. Therein lies its great successes and that is unquestionable. Without the solid basis of empirical, objective verifiable factual information the status of biomedical science becomes tenuous. The inclination to certitude is understandable and leads to a growing confidence and the proud claim of being a professional. Doubt is difficult. It gets in the way. It is messy but it is necessary.

Finding the balance is the goal but that is often difficult and the goalposts shift. It is not helpful to anybody, not to patients nor families nor practitioners to wallow in a sea of uncertainty and doubt and confusion. It is also not helpful to adopt a position of confident certainty when the circumstances do not allow it. Some things are inevitably uncertain, some things less so, and sometimes it is appropriate to be certain and sometimes it is not. Attitudes and styles of performing also change with time, and the practice of medicine is subject to cultural shifts. Generalizations are to be avoided, and I am not sure if this might have been due to my lowly position as a medical student, but I do have the impression that the consultants when I was a student were more arrogant. They seemed to be more unquestionably certain of their superior knowledge and their unfailing capacity to solve whatever challenging problems they encountered. They were often referred to ironically as gods and often they behaved like gods, being literally minded. I don't think it is like that any longer, or certainly not to such an extent. Why this should be so is yet another uncertainty. There are surely many factors involved but it does seem plausible that the sheer accumulation of information has had a paradoxically humbling effect, that such hubris is inappropriate and certainly that knowing everything is impossible.

5

Being a doctor

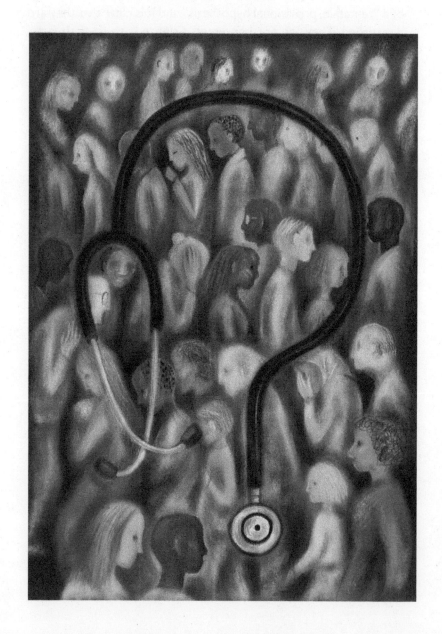

The daughter of a colleague has just graduated in medicine. She excelled, gaining the degree with distinction and it seemed to us all that she had a bright future ahead of her. But she is not sure. She is not sure at all. She is not happy in her chosen career. She is not confident that she made the right choice. She dreams, she possibly yearns for an alternative. She is young. She says it is too much for her at this stage of her life. The pain, the suffering, the sheer burden of being responsible, of making decisions that will affect other peoples' lives is too much. She wants to be light. She wants to be frivolous, carefree. This makes her feel old, she says. Clinical medicine makes her feel trapped. It is too grim.

It is not so much the work itself she says. There is some gratification in making a difference, in being helpful and seeing her patients get better because of what she has done. It is perhaps what is happening around her that she finds the most difficult. It is the cynicism, the disappointment, the joyless grind of the work that both perplexes her and burdens her. Her young colleagues are not sympathetic. They say she is indulging in a naïve and romantic notion of medicine. They tell her she should simply get on with it, with the expectation that at some stage things would be different, and that her choice of career would prove worthwhile.

Nor are her seniors, an assortment of registrars, consultants and lecturers particularly helpful. When she expresses her concerns they do not respond. They shrug, they nod their heads, they turn away. Nor, she complains can they be regarded in any way as role models. They do not seem in any way to enjoy what they are doing. They seem tired and resigned. They seem older than their years. They are grey. The women doctors especially seem to have made sacrifices that in retrospect they tell her they doubt were justified. One young consultant has urged her to leave medicine before it is too late, before she said she would become absorbed in the system, the long and relentless career path, and lose any belief that she had any choice in determining her future.

The work itself can too often seem relentlessly harsh and oppressive. This young woman had just finished a three month duty in a local day hospital. One component was working an eight hour shift in the trauma unit. Friday nights were the most dreaded. Young men would come in with stab wounds and occasionally gunshot wounds. These injuries were mostly incurred in gang related feuds. The victims were often intoxicated. They were uncooperative and abusive. She described a routine of cleaning and suturing and inserting chest drains and waiting for the shift to end. She said she became dulled. A point was rapidly reached when she felt that she was learning nothing new. She was developing no new skills. It was just a bloody and joyless routine. There was no reward. She did not feel she was making any useful contribution. Anybody with the most basic skills could be doing the same thing, and anyway the same young men would be back the next weekend, with a new injury, sullen and resigned, so that she began to think that both she and her patients were trapped in something beyond their control. She was too tired to think she said. She did not know what to do, other than to persist and endure what she felt was an ordeal until this period of her internship ended.

She had been dragged down. She hoped it would be different in another area of work, but it was not, and the same weight and a sense of futility pursued her. She began another duty in the outpatient clinic of the hospital. On her arrival at the beginning of the shift the queue of patients waiting to see her stretched down the passage. It seemed endless. She did not know how she could possibly cope. Most often the complaints were minor, aches and pains and anxieties and the need for some sort of explanation and reassurance, but each required an adequate assessment and this took time. Outside the queue got longer. Patients became restless and complained. She felt she was being held to blame. This seemed unfair to her, but again she did not know where to turn and what to do.

The growing, gnawing sense of the pointlessness of her endeavours was aggravated by the belief that what she was doing was not medicine, or certainly not the sort of medicine that she imagined she would be practicing when she embarked on her training. It was a sort of patching up. The cleaning and the suturing became a metaphor for medicine. It was not what she envisaged, and she became disheartened and demoralized. This was compounded by an impression that the majority of the complaints were not of a medical nature, and not amenable to any sort of medical solution. The aches and pains and the tiredness and the anxieties seemed more to do with the hardship of her patients' lives. Her despondency deepened with a sense of her involvement being not only futile but in a way fraudulent. There could be no medical answer to social and economic woes, and it seemed wrong to her to perpetuate this false or unexamined assumption, but again she felt too overwhelmed and too weary to stand back and think clearly and make appropriate decisions. The certainties that she assumed to underpin the clinical sciences appeared to be ephemeral.

She felt guilty in describing her struggle with these issues to her colleagues. They did not seem to share her experience, or were unwilling to talk about their own difficulties. It was not clear to her whether or not they were unhappy, or whether admitting it would only make things more difficult, or whether their unwillingness to divulge any concern was due to an unarticulated notion that any complaint was a form of weakness.

Amongst more senior colleagues the problem was perhaps less fatigue than disillusion and disenchantment. She was told that things would get better, that once she found her direction the work would become more gratifying, and that somehow they had all got through it, and no damage was done. It was a rite of passage, and again there was this ill-defined assumption that because of these ordeals they had become who they were. What that might be was unclear, but there was a pride in the achievement. If not inspiring role-models they were at least stalwarts. This understandably did not impress or reassure the young doctor.

My own colleagues were beset by another range of problems. They felt beleaguered by administrative and bureaucratic tasks. Every quarter of the year we were required to undergo a staff performance management system assessment. This was in theory a self-evaluation of one's performance in association with a senior colleague. It was supposed to be a collaborative, collegial exercise, but of course it was difficult not to feel you were being judged. There was no escape from this. Whatever senior position you might hold there was always someone ahead of you or above you to mark you, to estimate your performance and your value. It seemed to me that an inordinate amount of time was spent on identifying goals, targets, objectives, action plans, developmental and training needs, key performance indicators and a whole panoply of other apparently important aspects of my work that were mysterious and foreign to me. It seemed that a whole language had been imported from a different, managerial culture, and whether or not it was appropriate to clinical medicine had not been sufficiently considered. It had certainly not been discussed with ourselves, the victims. Increased productivity was given as one of the more important goals of this exasperating exercise. The criteria to define what might constitute increased productivity for me as a senior clinician were obscure. Should it be more admissions, more discharges, more publications, more courses attended, more audits of this or that, more and more of something or another to qualify for a higher notch, a possible monetary reward?

Responding to this time consuming and to me wasteful task by stating that one was simply trying to do one's best in difficult circumstances, and with limited resources was dismissed as being ridiculously inadequate. We had to work through the various items and eventually agree upon a score. Within the limits of the department's budget this in turn might qualify the aspirant for a bonus. Like our more junior colleagues we wearily submitted to this charade. It was too much of an effort to oppose it, and to what end? Perhaps some of us were more enthusiastic, and assiduously collected the points necessary for a reward, but for many it was an insidiously degrading and demoralizing process.

I am not sure to this day whether the devisors and practitioners of this management system are sufficiently aware of its subtle and pernicious effects. It was less evaluative than devaluing. A system was supposedly being managed but it seemed to many of us it was ourselves who were being managed. We had become items or units of labour and our worth or value to the system was to be measured in terms of a notion of productivity that was wholly inappropriate to our field of endeavour. I don't think this was much spoken about in an explicit way, but I do believe that it was a contributing factor to the cynicism and despondency that grew slowly amongst too many of us.

Many of my colleagues considered moving into the private sector with the expectation that they might then be more free to practice the medicine they wanted. This proved to be illusory. Doctors in private practice complained bitterly about their seemingly endless battles with the medical aid schemes. It was not a dissimilar situation. What was considered to be a clinical decision was evaluated and authorized or overruled by a manager, or perhaps more specifically a decision was made less according to clinical need than economic viability or profitability. They also complained about how hard they had to work to make their practice financially worthwhile, the difficulty for the same reason in taking holidays, and the isolation of their work. They did not seem to be a particularly joyful, liberated group, and some also expressed a disquiet in attending to a relatively small and privileged sector of the community. It was not what had been intended. I think very few of us embarked on a career in medicine with a notion of enriching ourselves. If we had it was surely in any case a dim-witted choice, and computer or actuarial science, or business studies would have been more lucrative career options.

Being a doctor carries other burdens which to an extent are self-imposed. Modern medicine has created expectations of cure which are too often ill-founded or inappropriate. The notion of cure applies to a very limited number of medical conditions if it is considered in a strict fairly reductionist sense. In this respect the cause of the presenting problem has been identified and eliminated, and there are no further symptoms nor any probability of a recurrence. Yet there is no cure for cancer, for diabetes, for many respiratory and cardiovascular problems, for dementia, nor for schizophrenia and many more of the afflictions of the modern world.

Nevertheless a fairly tentative triumphalism pervades the culture of medicine. It is believed that there is a steady but sure progress towards the cure, towards the elimination of pain and suffering, as if death itself could be treated. Many of our patients seem to believe this in various ways and to various degrees, but so too does the medical profession. The result is that when confronted with a problem that is not amenable to a cure, let alone the likelihood of successful treatment, we are confounded and at a loss as to how to respond or cope. We can very easily feel inadequate.

This burdens both patients and their doctors. It is reflected in the language often used with regard to cancer. X or Y is "bravely fighting" this feared disease. Z has "lost the battle". Failure is implicit and inevitable. Compounding the suffering of loss is the cruel message that Z was weak, he or she did not try hard enough, that somehow there will always be a way to defeat cancer. This has no scientific basis, and it is nonsense, but it persists and extends beyond the diagnosis of cancer. There is a problem. There is no problem. The doctor will fix it and if he or she does not they are not good enough doctors and you go elsewhere.

The news has recently been dominated by a particularly tragic case. A young couple have been unable to accept that their infant son is suffering from a progressive and incurable disease and is going to die. They are frantically and desperately seeking a cure, and false expectations have been created, only to prolong the anguish. Crowd funding has been sought internationally for a cure that has no hope of success. Politicians and religious leaders have become involved, as if money and support and the authority of leadership could help when medicine fails. In this case medicine at the most sophisticated level, and conducted by the most skilled and dedicated practitioners was very loudly and publicly judged to have most miserably failed.

This happens on a more mundane level in every clinic on every day. A patient drags him or herself through the door, slumps in the seat and delivers a long list of complaints including a range of vague physical symptoms combined with an account of insurmountable personal and social and economic hardships. This baggage is dumped on the desk of the usually young doctor who feels overwhelmed by just listening to this litany of woes. The patient reclines in the chair, as if unburdened, and an unspoken message floats in the oppressive air of the clinic: "You are the doctor. You sort this out. It is your duty now to solve my problems".

"What am I doing here? Why did I become a doctor?" I distinctly remember thinking, and I do not doubt that these same concerns continue to trouble my colleagues to various degrees and in a wide range of settings, and to which of course there is no simple answer.

Some answers are that being a doctor is thrilling and intense and privileged and engaging and intellectually profoundly stimulating. It is thrilling and intense because you are inevitably engaged in situations that are dramatic, not necessarily because they involve life or death issues ,but because they affect people's lives and you are not an observer but a participant. You can make a difference. It is privileged because a doctor is drawn into a situation of trust. The principle of confidentiality, however complicated it can be at times is the bedrock of clinical practice. A very particular intimacy is circumscribed by professional boundaries. By entering what often seemed to be another world we made close contact with our patients, sometimes simply by laying a hand on another's, or at other times bearing witness to intense suffering. In this way it seemed our lives were extended, deepened and made more various. This was not simply vicarious. It was required and expected of us that we should be engaged. Nor was it relentlessly grim. There were times of comedy and absurdity and also joy.

The intellectual stimulation is varied, but one element is that although medicine is based on scientific principles, a strictly scientific model in clinical practice is insufficient. In the process of evaluating a clinical problem and making an adequate decision the particular context needs evaluation, and psychological and social and cultural factors need to be taken into account. There are no given answers. Despite what our managers might think there are no formulae, no standard operating procedures. Every situation must be regarded as unique and this requires the imaginative use of both a scientific and a creative approach. Facts but also values are necessarily considered and weighed in the attempt to do the right thing at the right time in the particular context. This might seem aspirational or even romantic, but if this position could be gained, that beyond the drudgery and the oppression there are rewards that are profound, the struggle is worthwhile. I cannot imagine having done anything else in my professional life. I regard myself as most fortunate. I hope the daughter of my colleague will find her path.

6

The boundaries of mental illness and the problems of living

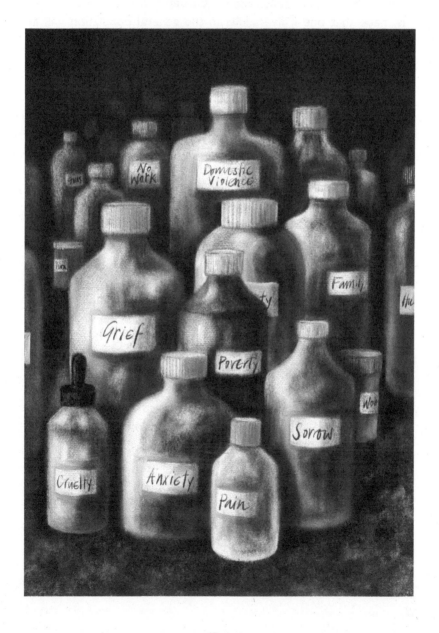

The boundaries of mental illness are over extended. A number of factors contribute to this fairly recent phenomenon. One driving force is a reaction to the relative neglect of mental illness in the past and a concomitant lack of funding for research into the causes and the effective treatment of these disorders. In order to emphasize the prevalence and the burden of mental illness a claim is made that one if five adults in the general population will at some stage in their lives suffer from some form of mental disorder. It is not clear whether such a claim furthers understanding and reduces stigma or is unhelpful and potentially harmful.

One aspect of possible harm is that given such a broad definition of what might constitute illness the claim will be dismissed as a misrepresentation of the problems of living as symptoms of a mental disorder. The Diagnostic and Statistical Manual of Mental Disorders (DSM5) published by the American Psychiatric Association has been dramatically expanded. Problems such as "bereavement disorder" and "opposition defiant disorder" are included, raising concerns as to whether these are new, meaningful categories, and whether or not invoking the notion of a disorder in this respect is helpful or might instead undermine coping strategies. Diagnosed as suffering from a mental illness a bereaved person might understandably be more inclined to resort to medication than seek the support of family and friends.

The great majority of mental disorders making up this twenty percent of the general adult population constitute anxiety and depressive disorders. The problem arises as to what might be considered a valid, reliable threshold for making such diagnoses. Anxiety and depression are problems of living. These difficult, at times deeply unpleasant and agonizing emotional states prompt responses that can be, and probably are for the most part beneficial. Understanding and support are enlisted. The intensity and the incapacity also tend to pass with time. A diagnosis of mental illness is more likely to slow the process and confound strategies for recovery. How one copes with suffering is a question of values, and there should be great caution in prescribing how one should cope with adversity. Problems arise when scientific attitudes intrude with claims of objectivity and a panoply of operationally defined diagnostic guidelines.

The difficulties posed by boundaries or thresholds also pertain to the rather arbitrary distinction between serious and other mental illnesses. Schizophrenia, bipolar disorders and the most severe depressive disorders generally fall into the serious category. The majority of anxiety and depressive disorders do not, and it is this group that account for the escalating, worldwide diagnoses of mental illness. How "other" in distinction of "serious" is defined is not made explicit, but "unserious" or "not so serious" is surely implicit, and it is difficult to imagine someone in the throes of an anxiety attack or in the anguish of a depression not being enraged by such an apparent disregard.

The notion of a not serious or not severe illness is ridiculous, and raises the question why this should be considered an illness at all, and what purpose there might be in invoking illness or a pathological process, other than to profit the pharmaceutical industry.

Further problems arise with regard to the allocation of limited resources and with regard to appropriate management. An argument is made that the expansion of the diagnoses of anxiety and depression diverts attention and resources away from schizophrenia and bipolar disorders, representing greater burdens in terms of disability and suffering. This is disputed and depression is estimated to be one of the major causes of disability in the near future. A diagnosis implies the need for treatment and this raises further difficulties in that it is not clear what are the most appropriate and effective treatments for anxiety and depression. Controversies abound as to whether medication or various forms of psychotherapy, or a combination thereof are more appropriate, and the matter is further confounded by some evidence that treatment of whatever nature is less effective for these disorders than for the more serious forms of mental illness, given the inadequacy of this term. It stands to some reason that grief will not be diminished by either a diagnosis or an anti-depressant.

There are lethal consequences to this possibly rather abstract notion of definitions and boundaries and thresholds. At the time of writing concern is rising in the USA of an epidemic of opioid addiction. Deaths from overdose are similar to those caused by motor vehicle accidents and among the most common causes of mortality in those under fifty. It is also big business. Opioid painkillers amount to billions of dollars in sales, as do treatment programs for addiction and overdoses. It seems doubtful that the escalation in the prescription of opioids corresponds directly to a recent rise in the phenomenon of pain. It is more probable that the escalation is in the diagnosis of a pain disorder, considered to warrant this potentially lethal treatment. The problem is of course compounded by misuse, abuse and addiction, but the opioids are prescribed initially for what are judged appropriate and effective treatments for pain.

Opioids are effective treatments for acute pain, much less so for chronic pain which far outweighs acute pain as an indication for treatment. Opioids for the treatment of chronic pain are of doubtful efficacy and are clearly dangerous. It follows that the diagnosis of a chronic pain syndrome has potentially hazardous consequences, and that for this reason the validity and the utility of the diagnosis must be carefully scrutinized. For the most part a diagnosis is probably not made, and the presentation of the symptoms of pain is considered sufficient justification for the prescription of an opioid.

Pain is a universal phenomenon and it has value in protecting the body from actual or potential harm. In its chronic form it without value. It is an expression of suffering, and in this respect may be considered to be a problem of living. The translation of chronic pain into a medical problem with a medical solution is too often not helpful and too often harmful.

I met Magda only on one occasion, in a busy community clinic on the outskirts of the city. She had been referred to us by the medical officer. The complaint had been of widespread pain. This had become steadily worse over the past six months and was becoming intolerable. She had been examined by the medical officer who could find nothing to account for her symptoms. The referral note was brief, and indicated that in the absence of any physical findings the problem must be of a psychiatric nature. No mention was made of an even cursory mental state examination to support this conclusion.

She recounted a story of many misfortunes and seemingly insoluble problems. After years of abuse she had eventually been deserted by her drunken husband. She had no work and she was in dire financial straits. Her teenage daughter was pregnant and she was sure that her son was abusing drugs. He had dropped out of school. She felt desperate and she did not know where to turn. She was exhausted all the time and her body ached. I told her I thought she was suffering. Her body was feeling it. It was all too much. She seemed relieved by this. "Yes. Yes." She said. "Dit is my senuwees dokter ". (it is my nerves) She sought an explanation not a diagnosis. There was no evidence of a medical problem, nor of a psychiatric disorder. She did not need to be told that there was anything wrong with her. This was more likely to make her feel worse and further undermine her very limited resources. She was struggling, certainly. The situation was painful. Her pain was understandable. Her suffering needed to be acknowledged. She was not depressed and not unduly anxious. There was no need for medication nor any particular form of counselling other than for me to register and acknowledge her predicament.

Clinicians often describe being under pressure to make a diagnosis and to prescribe medication, and often admit to an unease about this, recognizing that they do not believe it will do anything good but feeling a need to do something. With regard to Magda this seemed more likely to be interpreted as a paternalistic dismissal of the extent and gravity of her problems. These actions are not neutral and not without consequences. Problems of living are transformed into medical or psychiatric problems and are then treated in a way that is not helpful and all the more likely to lead to a perception of not being in control, and thence a downward spiral to helplessness. This woman was proud. She was dignified. Her circumstances were dire and unjust but she was not in any way broken. She needed to be respected. Being a doctor it seemed important to me then not to be a doctor.

In circumstances such as these the diagnoses of fibromyalgia or chronic fatigue syndrome or myalgic encephalomyelitis are often invoked. This is the language of medicine, of pathology, and the terms are probably most commonly used in the specialist domains of neurology and rheumatology. In psychiatry the categories of somatoform disorders, or somatic symptom disorders, or medically unexplained symptoms are more likely to be used, and all are unsatisfactory. Somatoform disorders or somatic symptom disorders are unhelpful because the terms indicate a psychiatric disorder which many presenting with such symptoms would understandably find offensive, interpreting this as dismissive, and medically unexplained symptoms is an unsatisfactory term because it is unexplained. These terms are also problematic in that there is no evidence to support a diagnosis of encephalomyelitis nor the rather arbitrarily defined fibromyalgia, if objectively verifiable biological pathologies are considered necessary for such alarming sounding diagnoses to be made, rather than the symptoms of pain and fatigue.

Sebastian described a range of shifting emotions and thoughts and behaviours after his father to whom he was very close had died suddenly and unexpectedly.

"From the start I cannot remember the feelings, specifically of grief. I was more confused or disorientated. It seemed to be a different world. Things that were meaningful or important changed. Light and colour drained away. I don't think I cared very much about anything any longer. I did not think about the future. I didn't think I would be part of it. I didn't care very much about myself. I don't think I was self-destructive, but certainly, looking back I took stupid risks. Life was empty. It seemed to be a charade. I did not care very much if I was alive or dead. Then, very slowly, colour and texture in the smallest detail began to emerge in my world. Cautiously I retrieved meaning and purpose in life. I became engaged in work, marriage and children. I have not forgotten the loss, of course. It will always be part of my life, and I suppose I would not be whoever I am without what has happened to me. That goes for all of us surely. Somehow we find a way of going on. I can't compare my experience with others but things are possibly now more intense, or precious and vivid".

He did not seek a diagnosis. He did not think that there was anything wrong with him. He did not consider that a diagnosis would in some way affirm his struggle to cope with the death of his father. He regarded the struggle as something inevitable and believed that the symptoms he interpreted in the context of mourning would pass with time. A diagnosis of a bereavement disorder in this circumstance seems wrong and unhelpful and invalidating and an insult to one's efforts to cope with adversity.

Intrinsic to the notion of a diagnosis or the construct of some form of disorder, whether psychiatric or not is the expectation of a cure or a solution. A clinician might seek to qualify this and claim that for many disorders the belief in a cure is inappropriate, and that effective management might be the best that can be hoped for. This might be so but in the lay imagination the provision of some form of cure is what follows from a provision of a diagnosis. The symptom is identified and treated with the assumption that it is then eliminated. The problem is solved and the person who is no longer a patient gets on with his or her life. But loss is not something that can be solved. The hardship and social and economic adversity contributing to the symptoms of pain and fatigue are not going to go away, and to allow that this might not be so with the provision of what is called treatment is simplistic and patronizing and mendacious.

The pharmaceutical industry might profit but amongst members of the general more critically minded population the response to this process of pathologizing problems of living is likely to be scepticism and cynicism and an increasing disenchantment with modern medicine. This phenomenon is evident in general medicine as it is in psychiatry and is reflected in a trend towards alternative or complementary forms of medicine. This is no answer but psychiatry is not furthering its cause by reaching beyond its limits.

7

The confounding limits of science

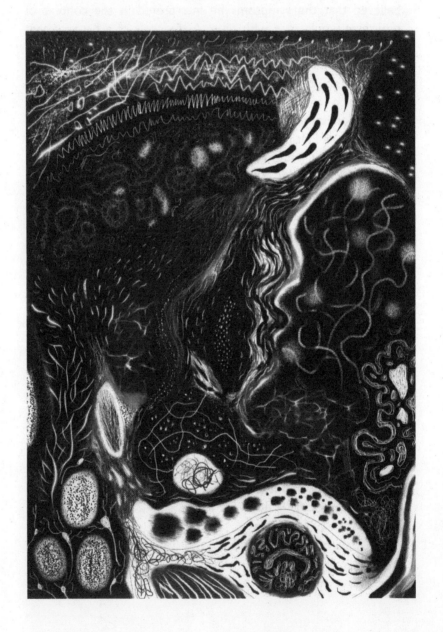

"I feel they want to know about me...they want to influence me detrimentally...they want to know what I am doing in the breathing world...I go under attack from the outside world...people affect me...my pulse... my heart beating...my breathing..."

"I cannot take it any more...he was making me crazy...I had to throttle him...the voices were telling me to shut him up...he is the king of calamity...I am the king of peace..."

"I am Jeremiah...I am Allah...I am responsible for the downfall of mankind...I am deaf...I am blind... I am being punished for the Fall...but I said Eve don't do it...Eve! Don't eat the banana! But she ate the banana, and now I am punished...and we are all doomed..."

What these idiosyncratic utterances have to do with the neurobiological basis of schizophrenia is a mystery. Dopamine dysregulation, or a fault in the expression of an array of interacting genetic variants or a dysconnectivity of neuronal networks in the higher centres of the brain cannot explain the strangeness and the anguish implicit in these accounts. Nor is any common denominator evident, which might be expected if there is a shared pathophysiology, other than distress and a sense of threat and injustice. This disjunction reflects a deep and ancient philosophical problem and so should not surprise us. How mind arises from the matter of the brain is an enduring and enigmatic problem.

Psychiatry concerns itself with disorders of the mind and claims to be a scientific discipline. Definitions of what constitutes mind are various, but include notions of subjectivity, intentionality, agency and autonomy. Subjectivity is integral to the concept of mind and the feeling of who we are and what we are not. A problem then arises as to how to provide a scientific account of the mind and its maladies, if central to the scientific method is a requirement of objectivity.

An indication of the scientific aspiration is the development of operationally defined diagnostic systems in psychiatry. Schizophrenia is defined by a set of rules. For example delusions and hallucinations and some degree of functional impairment must be evident, and the symptoms should not be accounted for by a general medical condition or substance abuse. These rules are explicit and objectively verifiable. The diagnostic process therefore in terms of a degree of reliability meets basic scientific criteria. This does represent progress in that the diagnosis of schizophrenia with all its potentially damaging implications is not left to mere intuition, or as I was taught in my undergraduate years, "a feeling".

I remember the professor imparting this to us by waving his fingers in the air in a vague fluttering motion, as if to communicate the inadequacy of words. I recall being frustrated at the time. This did not conform to my youthful notions of scientific rigour, but in retrospect he was perhaps saying or suggesting something important that has become lost in a triumphalist belief in scientific progress. Then we believed in some vague way that it was just a matter of time, and that soon the cause of schizophrenia would be discovered, and with the known cause would come the cure. The reliability of the diagnosis was at least the first step.

A number of problems have arisen in this regard that have placed limitations on such optimism. Schizophrenia has come to be regarded less as a provisional, hypothetical construct than a thing out there, on object of scientific enquiry. The subjective dimension which is central to any study of the mind and its disorders is marginalized or neglected.

Related to this is an uncertainty regarding the diagnostic validity of such a reified construct. Schizophrenia is not a thing that can be measured or verified by some validating objective marker. To this day, and confounding the expectations of the past there is no genetic test or neuroimaging study that can confirm the presence or not of schizophrenia. In another language, whether or not a person is suffering from schizophrenia is, at least at present beyond the realms of science. Suffering is not amenable to measurement. It would be absurd to seek to estimate the quantum of suffering appropriate for a broken leg or a broken heart.

The question also arises as to whether the term schizophrenia can provide an adequate or meaningful account of the protean expressions of the disorder, and whether such an abstract formulation problematically neglects schizophrenia's phenomenology, or the lived experience of schizophrenia. There is a tension between objective verifiable third person accounts of mental states and subjective deeply personal first person accounts. In order to develop an adequate and useful understanding and explanation of the problem of schizophrenia neither perspective can be put aside. The objective and subjective positions are not binary opposites but complementary. Coming to some basic and useful understanding of psychotic phenomena must incorporate first person accounts however difficult, incoherent and obscure these might be. Dismissing these phenomena simply because personal perspectives fail to meet the conventional criteria for scientific objectivity limits understanding and lack the rigour and comprehensiveness which is surely an important part of the scientific method.

In current standard practice there is a gulf between diagnostic explanation and a sufficient understanding of the predicament of an individual in a specific personal, social and cultural context. This reaches beyond the confines pf psychiatry. It is a frequently heard complaint in general medicine that one is treated merely as an object by a harried clinician, a mere assembly of symptoms. It is difficult to imagine how the fear of an early death can be separated from a diagnosis of cancer, or how an abusive partner or socio-economic deprivation or grave personal losses might be considered irrelevant to a complaint of chronic pain and fatigue.

An adequate understanding for example of the phenomena of schizophrenia is lacking. It would require at least some degree of integration of three levels: the neurobiological deficits or derangements, the cognitive and emotional correlates and the subjective experience of these aberrant processes. It would not be helpful, and it would have grave implications for the pharmacological treatment of schizophrenia if for example we chose to associate delusions with diminished rather than increased dopamine transmission, or vice versa with regard to problems of executive function. We would be aggravating not alleviating the problem. Psychotic symptoms are not simply eliminated by anti-psychotic medications. A more nuanced and precise definition of the nature of the psychotic symptoms is required.

Diagnostic explanation and meaningful understanding cannot be regarded as dichotomous and need to be integrated in clinical practice and in research programmes. This is required both to foster an improved therapeutic alliance and to clarify the neurobiological basis for specific symptoms rather than overarching disease categories. It is not being merely nice and polite or culturally sensitive to ask what meanings might be attached to symptoms such as hearing voices. It might amongst many other things guide us as to whether any form of intervention is warranted in the first place. Focusing on specific symptoms rather than broader diagnostic constructs might also guide us towards more precise and valid neurobiological correlates.

Related to the uncertainties regarding the validity of psychiatric diagnoses are the arbitrariness of many operationally defined criteria, the considerable overlap between diagnostic categories and the very indistinct boundaries between mental illness and what might be considered to be within the bounds of non-pathological human experience. This applies most obviously to problems such as anxiety and depression but extends also to psychotic phenomena. There is a debate as to whether psychosis should be most appropriately regarded as a category or a dimension and this again seems to be caught up in the tensions between the requirements of validity and reliability. Reliability favours a categorical formulation: understanding psychosis in dimensional terms might be a more valid approach but eludes reliable determination.

The trend towards understanding psychotic phenomena on a spectrum has been given impetus in recent years by attention being paid to the prevalence of psychotic experiences in the general relatively healthy population. Many people simply find ways of coping with psychotic symptoms. Various strategies might be adopted but very probably include granting meaning to these idiosyncratic experiences and embedding the phenomena in personal and cultural contexts. These can be effective ways of alleviating the distress associated with an experience that might otherwise be further complicated and aggravated by being perceived as pathological. It is bad enough believing that others want to do you harm. It is made worse by being told you are sick or mad.

Possibly enabled by Facebook a young man in the out-patient clinic told me of hearing voices asking him if they could be his "friend". These voices were not perceived as malicious or pathological. They were consoling to him. There was no reason to take them away. In another context a young man appeared to be reassured that the voices he heard were communications from his ancestors.

Merely defining these experiences as auditory hallucinations seems restricted. The meanings attached to the experience are more likely to be more important to the person than the definition of psychopathology. This is of concern because it determines what form of intervention should be made, if any, and this has ethical ramifications. There is an important difference between paternalism and a more respectful collaborative way of trying to help people living with psychotic experiences. It is less the symptom itself than the distress and the impairments it might engender that is of concern. In an ideal world, and if a degree of insight is retained it is then for the person who is experiencing psychotic symptoms to decide if help is needed and what form that help should take. The assumption that psychotic phenomena are inherently pathological and should therefore be suppressed needs to be reconsidered.

Another assumption underlying the way in which psychosis is understood and consequently treated is the notion that there is a fault in the way a person with psychosis perceives the external world in contrast to the more accurate appraisal of the world by those not affected by psychosis. This rather simplistic distinction is called into question by current neurocognitive formulations of how the world is perceived and enters into our consciousness. It is evident that sensory signals are relatively crude or elemental and that a time lag exists between the activation of receptors and the entry of these signals into our consciousness. Perceptions in this regard are conceptualized as inferences or beliefs about the world. I see what I believe rather than I believe what I see.

These rather abstract considerations do have implications with regard to how we imagine and treat severe mental illnesses. Symptoms of psychosis are constructions not dissimilar to the way in which we all try to make sense of the world, and in the context of psychosis may be understood as attempts to give some form to what might otherwise be experienced as intolerable noise. These endeavours then need in some way to be acknowledged rather than eliminated or merely neglected. Modulation of salience, limiting distress, and enhancing the capacity to cope might be more helpful and appropriate goals of treatment than the suppression of experiences that are desperately real for those who suffer.

The fundamental pathophysiological deficits and the ultimate causes of the syndrome of schizophrenia remain unknown. Looking beyond the signs and the symptoms and attending to the experience of psychosis, and linking this to observable phenomena and known neurobiological shifts may yield more meaningful results and more valid diagnostic constructs. First and third person perspectives need to be integrated if advances are to be made in the elucidation of these enigmatic phenomena. The rigid implementation of reductive scientific models has generated a bland and bleak depiction of psychosis that does not accord with the strange and extraordinary stories we encounter in our wards.

The limits are especially confounding because in contrast to other fields of scientific endeavour little progress seems to have been made in the field of mental illness and in particular schizophrenia. This might be disputed, but in my experience the expectations at the time when I was beginning my career in psychiatry have not been realized. There are many possible reasons for this, one being that as the human brain is the most complicated thing in the known universe this observation should not be surprising. Related to this is the notion that the human brain does not have the capacity to understand itself or the nature of consciousness. An argument could then be made that it is merely a matter of time, and that with the rapid development of artificial intelligence that obstacle will be overcome. A smart machine will solve the problem.

A further conundrum then arises in that if we do not have the intellectual capacity as humans to know the nature of ourselves it is unclear how we will be able to know that our brains have been superseded. We will not have the intelligence to grasp that there is an intelligence superior to our own. If that might be so it is uncertain as to how we might be able to use the information derived from this superior intelligence in an intelligent and useful way. Another difficulty lies in the order of investigation. It is curious that we should imagine that we can begin to understand how things go wrong when we do not understand how they work in the first place.

8

The biology of madness

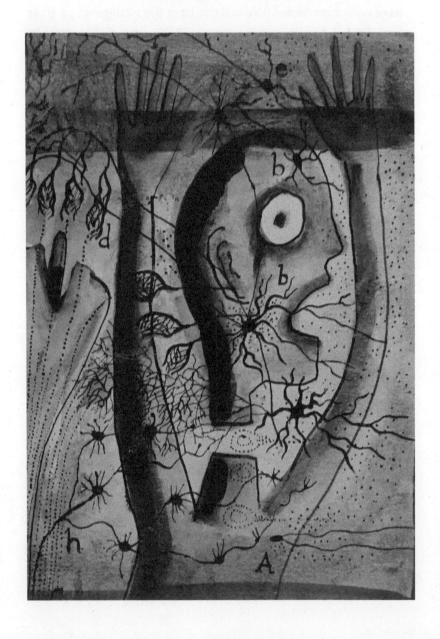

There are two universities with medical faculties in the western cape. They are approximately fifty kilometres apart but traditionally are culturally, historically and politically distinct. Both faculties have departments of psychiatry and for much of the time while I was a student, and until quite recently, these departments held different and at times opposing positions with regard to the nature and causes of mental illness.

The one department was considered to be "biological" in orientation. Mental illness was caused by an array of biological factors and in this respect a "biomedical model" was considered most appropriate. This required the identification of a number of specified signs and symptoms for a diagnosis to be made. The predominant form of treatment was medication, intended to treat the biological factors that were presumed to be the causes of the illness characterized by the specific diagnosis. This was more or less in line with a European way of thinking about psychiatry. Psychiatry was a medical speciality. The as yet undetermined causes of mental illness were presumed to be biological and therefore the treatment was essentially physical.

At the adjacent institution, on the other side of the river, an alternative way of thinking prevailed. Mental illnesses were of a fundamentally psychological nature. The causes were due to psychological conflict, often arising from childhood experiences. These conflicts were for the most part of an unconscious nature, and treatment involved bringing these repressed events to the surface, with the assumption that in this clear light of consciousness the symptoms would resolve. Not much attention was paid to making diagnoses. Of greater interest were the psychological processes giving rise to the presenting problems. This position was more aligned to a predominantly American psychoanalytical tradition. Treatment was therefore more of a psychotherapeutic nature and there was much less emphasis and interest in physical treatments. Psychiatry was not really a science. It occupied an uncertain space between medicine and the humanities.

Partly as a consequence of these divergent positions the one department had a much stronger tradition of research than the other. Viewing the phenomena of mental illness objectively enables scientific enquiry. Identifying symptoms according to operationally defined criteria, using rating scales to measure changes, for example in the mental state in response to one or other medication, employing randomized controlled clinical trials to investigate the effectiveness or not of various treatments brought psychiatry into alignment with general medicine. Psychiatry should no longer be regarded as a marginal discipline, rather embarrassingly lagging behind the other disciplines in its lack of scientific rigour and compromised by its uncertainties.

These differences have over the past few years diminished, and possibly withered away altogether. The psychoanalytical tradition has waned in influence, particularly with regard to serious mental illness or the psychoses. This is in all likelihood due to a number of reasons including rapid advances in the neurosciences, but also perhaps in an increasingly scientific world, an embarrassing lack of evidence to support often extravagant claims, and an equally awkward absence of evidence that psychoanalytical treatments are at all effective.

At the time I remember these two different ways of thinking giving rise to a quite teasing, mostly healthy rivalry. The one "biological" position was dismissed as crude and reductionist, the other as non-scientific and vague and this led to discussions and debates that were for the most part friendly and possibly creative. I do not remember any real antagonism and perhaps this reflected an awareness that this dichotomous way of thinking was false and far too simplistic a conceptual framework for the understanding of a fundamental problem implicit in the tension between the two positions. This arises from the persisting and profoundly mysterious relationship between the mind and the brain.

Regardless of current neuroscientific and philosophical thinking it seems very probable that for many if not for most of us there is an unwillingness or a refusal to consider that who we are might arise from mere matter. It is intolerable, it is an affront to believe that our most intimate thoughts, our deepest feelings, our very souls might be mere ephemera, or the epiphenomena of central nervous system electrochemical signalling bound within the absurdly confined limits of the skull. This disquiet is reflected in debates about what might constitute the nature of mental illness and how it should best be managed. Sometimes this is explicit: more often the assumptions that inform our thinking are implicit. We are uncertain, at some level, as to whether madness is an affliction of the brain or the soul, and then as to whether it should be treated by a doctor or a priest or a shaman.

We might feel squeamish or we might regard it as abhorrent that a psychotropic medication, a tablet that blocks dopamine transmission in certain parts of the brain should be used to treat the profound perturbations of our souls or our psyches.

The difficulty seems to arise again from a dichotomous way of thinking, an unexamined belief that it is one thing or the other, that it is either biological or psychological, reflecting a seventeenth century dualism that persists to the present day. It is very probable that these fundamental philosophical issues underpin many of the debates and controversies in contemporary psychiatry. Yet many of those advocating one position or another would quite probably doubt the relevance of philosophy to the question as to how mental illness should be conceptualized. It seems also less of a scientific issue than a problem of belief or dogma. Over the many years that I have worked as a psychiatrist it has been disappointing that these polarities seem to have persisted. This is despite remarkable advances in the understanding of how the brain works, and what happens when it does not work, and in the philosophical domain despite advances way beyond the dualism of Descartes, however vexed the question might still be regarding the nature of consciousness.

The difficulties might arise to some extent from the limitations of science, or a scientific way of thinking. Who we are, the way we think and feel and behave, and consequently the nature of the aberrations of these very human faculties are not a matter for scientific investigation. These are issues of belief or of faith. This transcendent and consoling edifice of our notion of ourselves, our humanity, can surely not be reduced to mere matter, the stuff of the brain. It cannot be that this cathedral we imagine of ourselves might just be a precarious construction of bricks and mortar and broken glass. This is a refusal of the evolution of our species, but also of contemporary thinking in the neurosciences about the complex relationships between mind, brain and the environment. Binary thinking might appear to make things simple, but in all likelihood the issues become more muddled and distorted. Related to the problematic mind-brain dualism is another prevalent question, usually also framed in a dichotomous way, as to whether the causes of mental illness are either biological or environmental. The question poses its own problems. A more appropriate enquiry might be to consider the nature of the interaction between biological and environmental factors that give rise to mental illness. The way we think about these matters is further confused by assumptions made about causation being both linear and uni-directional.

David is drinking too much, his wife complains because he is depressed. He is depressed because he has been fired from his job. He got fired because he was drinking too much. Perhaps he was drinking too much because he was depressed at work. Perhaps the depression was caused by his drinking getting out of control. Perhaps we complicate things for ourselves by trying to see things in linear terms when a rather more messy complex of interacting factors might be more valid interpretation.

Nemba was admitted to our unit after what appeared to be a long history of gradual deterioration in health culminating in a dramatic escalation of overtly psychotic symptoms. He had been cared for by his grandmother. The father had reportedly suffered from some form of mental illness. He had abused alcohol and died in a violent altercation when Nemba was aged six. The father had abused the mother and possibly as a consequence the mother had herself resorted to a dependency on alcohol. This eventually led to her death in her early forties. Nemba struggled from the beginning of his life and this was perhaps understandable in the circumstances. He began to fail at school and was admonished by his teachers for being stupid and mocked by the other children for his odd appearance. He was eventually sent for an assessment and a diagnosis was made of a mild to moderate intellectual impairment associated with the features of a foetal alcohol syndrome caused by his mother's alcohol use in pregnancy. With little or no family or professional support and with no confidence in himself Nemba started to avoid classes and then drifted away from schooling altogether. The grandmother applied for a disability grant on the basis of his intellectual impairment and this was granted.

In these circumstances it was almost inevitable that Nemba should become involved in the gangsterism that was rife in the townships. He was extremely vulnerable and the small income he gained from the disability grant was very attractive to the gangsters who soon exploited his desperate wish to belong by selling him drugs and enlisting him in criminal activities. Things took a miserably predictable course. He drifted downwards, his behaviour became increasingly erratic and disorganized and eventually the police were called when he threatened his grandmother with violence. He said he would kill her if she did not give him money for drugs. When the police arrived he was raving in an incoherent manner and it was apparent to them that he was ill. After three days in the psychiatric unit of the local day hospital there was no change in his behaviour and he was transferred to our hospital.

It is clear that no single cause can be identified to account for this lamentable trajectory, and that many factors interact in a circular manner to contribute to his decline. It would be utterly inadequate for example to conclude that the drugs were the cause of his psychosis. His use of drugs was made all the more likely by his lack of any form of social support and his membership of a gang that itself was made all the more predictable both by the lack of any stability in his life and his inability to assert himself due to his intellectual disability. The lack of support and the intellectual disability was a consequence of his mothers' alcohol abuse and this in turn was very probably a result of the fathers abuse of her. The fathers' violent behaviour might have been due to alcohol but it might also have been part of his unspecified psychiatric illness. As it would be oversimplifying matters to attribute Nemba's illness to drugs so would it be to attribute what emerged to be a schizophrenia to his father's mental disorder. It was a tangled web of potentially harmful factors, perhaps none of which alone might have caused his illness, but acting in concert that culminated in the psychotic disarray that led him to our unit.

Isolating one or another factor is arbitrary and not helpful. It might be more useful in terms of guiding management to divide the wide range of potentially causative events into predisposing, precipitating, perpetuating and protective risk factors.

With regard to Nemba, for example, his father's mental illness and his intellectual disability may be considered predisposing factors. The drugs and the violence associated with his gang membership were precipitating factors and his lack of any social support and the stress of increasing contact with the police owing to his criminal activities would be likely perpetuating factors. Sadly it is difficult to identify any protective factors in this unhappy story, and so it was difficult for us to feel in any way optimistic about his future.

It is extremely rare, and I struggle to recall any psychotic episode in my clinical career that might have been solely attributable to one or another biological cause. Invariably there is a complex interplay of biological, psychological, socio-economic, cultural and other factors that interact and entangle, leading to the endpoint of a set of unique and specific symptoms, subsumed under the rather inadequate term of a schizophrenia spectrum disorder.

In this respect it is also inadequate to consider a dichotomous gene versus environment theory as the causation of schizophrenia. The futile debate persists, yet it is crude and takes no account of current scientific knowledge particularly in the field of genetics.

Currently over one hundred gene variants for example, have been associated with schizophrenia, and are considered to exert relatively small, non-specific effects. It is therefore highly likely that not one gene variant but a number acting together in various combinations contribute to the eventual expression of schizophrenia. Furthermore it is not either one gene or another, or a particular environmental circumstance that leads to schizophrenia, but a complex interaction of genetic and environmental factors. For example a specific gene variant on exposure to cannabis significantly increases the risk of developing schizophrenia. In theory one could perform the necessary testing and in the absence of this variant puff away quite happily without the risk of going mad. Perhaps this being in theory should be emphasized. There is a persisting two to threefold risk in developing schizophrenia on exposure to cannabis, and it would seem reckless, certainly with a family history of mental illness to take this risk, regardless of one's genetic constitution.

The relatively new field of epigenetics demonstrates the inadequacies and distortions implicit in the enquiry as to whether, for example schizophrenia is caused by one's genes or the environment. Epigenetics concerns the study of the ways in which environmental and other factors modulate genetic expression. We are not determined by our genes. An array of biological, including genetic factors interact with internal and external environmental conditions in a much more fluid and dynamic way than had perhaps been previously imagined. Disposition is probably a more appropriate term than determination. The core element or DNA is composed of a fixed genetic sequence that is read and translated by RNA according to need and circumstance. In another language environmental factors modulate the way in which the genotype or genetic code is expressed as the observable phenotype.

The unease about thinking about the most intimate aspects of our inner worlds in a biological way arises from a vague and erroneous notion that something being biological is in some way fixed and determined. It would be absurd to think that how we think and feel and act is separate from our physical selves. It is another question as to whether these physical processes can entirely account for who we are. Whether the biological basis of our consciousness, of how the feeling of who we are is ever to be illuminated remains for the time being and for many quite happily a profound and beguiling mystery.

9

Medication and madness

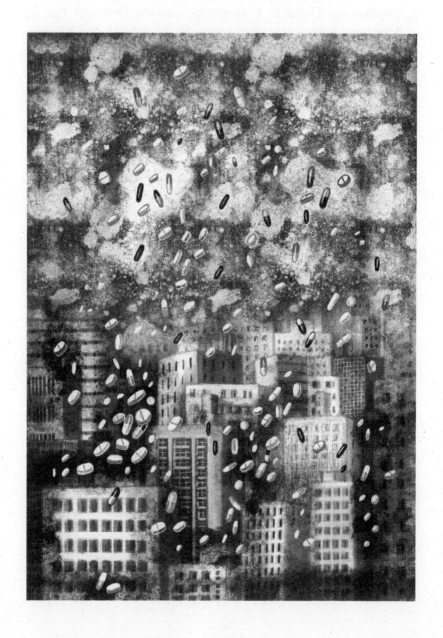

The mere idea of taking medication or using any form of physical intervention to treat mental illness is for many deeply unsettling if not abhorrent. This is meddling with the soul. It is resorting to some crude biological instrument to change something that is infinitely complex and private. In religious terms it is challenging fate, or god. It represents one of the more disturbing and wilder ambitions or expectations of modern medicine: a refusal of the acceptance of suffering, a narcissistic demand for happiness and control of the chaotic contingencies of our lives. It is the manipulation of the psyche for self-advancement or for advantage over others. It is the hubris of biomedical science and it is without boundaries.

One contributing factor to this antagonism is the history of cruel and harmful attempts to bring madness under control. Inducing high fevers and diabetic comas, electroconvulsive therapy without anaesthesia and a wide range of psychosurgical techniques represent some of the more extreme and appalling strategies. One interpretation of this is a cruel demonstration of the power and savagery of the medical profession over the most weak and vulnerable, and a cynical experimentation without heed of the consequences. Hope had been lost and many of the patients or victims had been abandoned in the large asylums with no one to protect and defend them from these zealots or mad doctors.

Another interpretation was that these interventions were attempts by the state to exert control and punish deviancy. Under the guise of medical benevolence the capitalist order sought to maintain a compliant and homogeneous populace as a secure market for the maximization of profit. This was dramatized in the film of the novel "One Flew over the Cuckoo's Nest", a fiction that to this day shapes attitudes about psychiatry and its treatments with damaging effect. That the story might represent a metaphor of how the modern state subtly exerts and maintains control over its citizens rather than an honest and accurate account of the practice of modern psychiatry is of little relevance. Psychiatry is perceived as sinister and its treatments aimed to maintain social and political order rather than to benefit those suffering from mental illness.

Another way of trying to make sense of this grim past is to understand these interventions as arising from desperation. The expressions of madness were profoundly distressing and confounding and often dangerous, and the fear of madness was compounded by its origins being unknown and by the absence of effective remedies. At a time of medicine developing an increasingly scientific basis, psychiatry was separate. It was fundamentally mysterious. It lacked a biological basis. It failed to conform to the principles of the biomedical edifice. A gastroscope could reveal a bleeding ulcer to be the cause of abdominal pain. An electrocardiogram could demonstrate the reason for somebody suddenly putting a flat hand to their chest and gasping for breath. No scope or x-ray could demonstrate the underlying cause for a psychosis, for something that was so obviously and so pervasively and distressingly wrong. Nor with increasing technological sophistication could CT scans, functional MRIs, SPECT or PET scans or any other instrument yield the neurological basis or the biochemical or any other correlate of mental disorders.

This is yet another cause for the disquiet and the inhibitions regarding medication and madness. It arises from an anxiety about a fundamental lack of understanding about the nature of the mind and its disorders, and about the relation of mind to its physical substrate the brain. These concerns arise in turn partly from dualist assumptions. The mind is separate from the brain. Medication can quite conceivably alter the functions of the brain, but if a fundamental substance dualism is accepted it is less clear, or it is inconceivable as to how medication can affect the mind, or effectively treat mental illness. The problem is not a problem if a more materialist conceptualization of mind and brain is accepted, but these are discussions that do not take place in the turmoil of the admission unit nor in the relative calm of the out-patient department. For the most part these discussions do not take place at all, but are implicit in many of the qualms that abound regarding pharmacotherapy.

The distinction between general medicine and psychiatry is not distinct and nor are the methods of treatment. The precise ways in which an anti-hypertensive agent or a statin might exert their effects are not entirely clear, nor certainly in primary prevention are the benefits of these agents self-evident. Why some malignancies respond to certain cytotoxic agents and others do not is uncertain. The pharmacological treatment of a problem as common and costly as chronic pain remains controversial. There are currently no effective treatments for the dementias, or certainly no agents that significantly reverse the degenerative process. Many drugs work to a certain extent in a certain number of cases without there being a clear understanding of how and why this should be so, and this is also true of psychotropic medications.

How electroconvulsive therapy exerts its dramatic effects is unknown but that it can be an extremely beneficial treatment in specific circumstances is not in doubt. That I have not ever prescribed this form of treatment has nothing to do with any misgivings about its effectiveness despite the side-effects. Misconceptions about electroconvulsive therapy nevertheless persist and do harm. The image of men in white coats holding down some writhing patient, usually an attractive but wild young woman, while some harridan applies the electrodes to her cruelly shaved head continues to thrill and horrify gullible theatre and film audiences. It needs to be borne in mind that the vast majority of patients choose this form of treatment because they believe in its benefits and they are willing to tolerate the side-effects. I have not worked in any hospital anywhere where ECT was administered involuntarily. I accept that this only my own experience, and that practice is different elsewhere, but it would constitute abuse and a grave injustice.

A commonly used group of anti-depressant agents, the selective serotonin reuptake inhibitors presumably exert their benefit through an action on the serotonin neurotransmitter system. At a physiological level this is fairly immediate and why a therapeutic response can only be expected after two to three weeks is unknown. Nor is it known with any degree of certainty how anti-psychotic agents work, what complex array of inhibiting and stimulating neurotransmitters are activated, what receptor sites and secondary and tertiary messenger systems upstream and downstream are engaged, and what endophenotype changes may be required for a therapeutic response to be achieved. Not knowing how something works might be awkward or frustrating, but it does not have anything to do with whether or not it works. A pragmatic attitude is required.

There are over fifty patients on the waiting list. I have to do whatever I can to make the patients currently in the ward better enough to be discharged in order to begin admitting those on the waiting list. Without effective treatments, without medication the system would grind to a halt within weeks. We would be neither able to admit nor discharge. When my time comes and I do not have the capacity to make informed decisions about how I should be treated ,I hope I will be given whatever it takes to get me out of a situation that I have come to understand is intolerable.

A friend sent me a disturbing e-mail yesterday. A friend of hers and a patient of mine had committed suicide by jumping from a building in the city centre. The mail was of sadness and loss but was also tinged with anger and exasperation. The medication I had prescribed she wrote had made him normal. "Normal" was written in capitals and followed by an exclamation mark. He had nevertheless chosen to stop the treatment. She considered his tragic and unnecessary death a consequence of this act. What madness, what other kind of madness she wondered had driven him to take this disastrous decision.

This is a familiar lament. "He was doing so well doctor. He was back to his old self. He even said that the medication was helping him". Then things fall apart. The vast majority of readmissions to our unit are as a result of stopping medication, often in association with substance abuse and of course the two are related. The term non-compliance is discouraged in favour of non-adherence. Non-compliance suggests a passive acquiescence to treatment rather than an active participation in decision making with regard to treatment options. It is surely obvious that somebody will be more willing to take the prescribed treatment if they themselves have been involved in the choice of whatever treatment might be most appropriate.

The causes of non-adherence are various and complex and interacting. It is pointless and unhelpful to blame somebody for stopping treatment although this happens all the time. Those prescribing the treatment also bear some responsibility. It is rare that despite the clear benefits of adherence one would wilfully and for no good reason stop whatever has been prescribed. A common cause for non-adherence are side-effects and these can be severe and from a patients' perspective outweigh the benefits of treatment. With regard to the newer "second-generation" anti-psychotic agents weight gain, blood lipid changes, cardiac arrhythmias and somnolence are major problems. People living with severe psychiatric disorders have a reduced life-expectancy of ten to twenty years. Many factors contribute to this disgraceful estimate. Those suffering from schizophrenia for example are very likely to smoke, not to exercise and not to take sufficient care of themselves. This in combination with the side-effects of the anti-psychotic medications put them at high risk of cardiovascular problems or heart attacks. Common side-effects of the widely used serotonin reuptake inhibitors for depression include a range of sexual problems. It seems very possible that a person would be unlikely to raise this issue with the prescribing doctor, either out of embarrassment or on the assumption that the sexual difficulty is a consequence of the depression. It is also very likely that as a result that person would choose to stop the treatment.

There is also a rather bizarre assumption among many doctors that it is ill-advised to inform patients of the side-effects that can be expected on taking medication. This is confused. It is not as if by not informing of side-effects they are less likely to occur. The reasoning seems to be that the patient will be deterred from taking the medication. On the contrary, somebody is much more likely to adhere to the prescribed treatment if they are informed of the reason why the medication is being prescribed and what side-effects can be expected. They might then hopefully be in a better position to make an informed decision, weighing possible benefits against the predictable side-effects, and therefore much more likely to adhere. Not providing adequate information is patronizing and unhelpful. Such information is not limited to possible side-effects but should also include among many items the indications for the treatment in the first place, a possible delayed onset of action and the necessary duration of treatment. It is difficult to imagine why one should be expected to begin whatever treatment is prescribed without knowing why. The anti-depressant effects of the selective serotonin reuptake inhibitors can only be anticipated after two to four weeks. It is to be expected that not being informed of this delayed onset of action a depressed and angry patient will throw the tablets down the lavatory. It can also be anticipated that somebody would be very likely to stop the treatment once they felt better, certainly if side-effects were experienced. It is not at all self-evident that one should continue the prescribed psychotropic for six to twelve months, as one should, even though there has been a positive response. Blaming a patient for non-adherence in such circumstances is ridiculous. These difficulties are of course not confined to psychiatry. Any doctor prescribing treatment for usually chronic conditions, commonly tuberculosis or HIV in this country will be familiar with these problems that are not insurmountable, however confounding they might at times seem.

There are many other prosaic but important reasons why somebody might not continue a form of treatment that confers a benefit, or at least reduces significantly the likelihood of a readmission to hospital. The cost of transport to the clinic, the habit of gangsters to congregate near the clinic to prey on those collecting disability grants, the stigma associated with attendance at a separate psychiatric clinic are common explanations given by both patients and families. There are other perhaps more subtle and difficult factors that are less remediable. On each occasion that a medication is administered an onerous and possibly contradictory message is given, that one is mad, that without the treatment one would be in hospital, that deep down one is sick and it is only this extraneous, banal pharmacological thing that controls or suppresses this miserable truth. In this context a lack of enthusiastic adherence is understandable. There is no escape.

There is another factor contributing not necessarily to a

refusal of treatment but a reluctance or ambivalence. Psychotic symptoms in the form of delusions and hallucinations may be conceptualized as secondary phenomena, or attempts to give meaningful form to biological or neurological events that are experienced as intolerable and menacing. Psychotic phenomena may represent a struggle to recover control, and however incomprehensible it might seem from the outside, to restore meaning and coherence in a terrifying and formless world. The phasic nature of symptoms is perhaps not sufficiently registered. Psychotic symptoms come and go. Patients say: "Somebody is trying to kill me. I know you think I'm mad but it's true", and then, "I felt as if somebody was trying to kill me" and then, "I was crazy. It's gone". It does not seem inconceivable that at least in some instances symptoms represent strategies to lever oneself out of the abyss.

For as long as I have known him Manuel is cheerful and enthusiastic. When I see him in the out-patient clinic he greets me warmly. He is dishevelled. His hair is long and unkempt and his clothes are unclean. Although it is summer he is wearing a thick jersey. He is a graduate of the university I attended. He won the class medal in the physics department and was embarking on a doctorate before this wretched illness turned his life upside down. He appears unphased. He tells me he is delighted with his medication. It is "perfect" he says in wonder. He sternly insists that I am under no circumstances allowed to alter it. He is floridly psychotic. The reasons for his apparent excitement, and his expressed gratitude for this supposedly successful treatment are mysterious to me. I have not taken the symptoms away. He has not recovered yet he appears to be content. This it seems is what he wants, or this is sufficient. His ailment is acknowledged. He is receiving treatment and that appears to be more important to him than any benefit that might be gained.

This calls into question the goals of treatment, or more specifically anti-psychotic medication. In my practice I wanted to change the term to neuro-modulation, which might be rather abstruse. My ambitions met with no success. If symptoms do possibly represent tentative steps to recovery the elimination of these symptoms would not necessarily be helpful and leave merely a void. The distress and disability associated with psychotic symptoms are the more appropriate focus of therapeutic attention. To acknowledge and affirm a person's vivid experience and the struggle towards recovery and simultaneously seek to modulate or attenuate the intense distress and confusion that is part of the process requires a difficult and at times elusive balance.

10

Traditional healers, Freud Jung and other interpreters

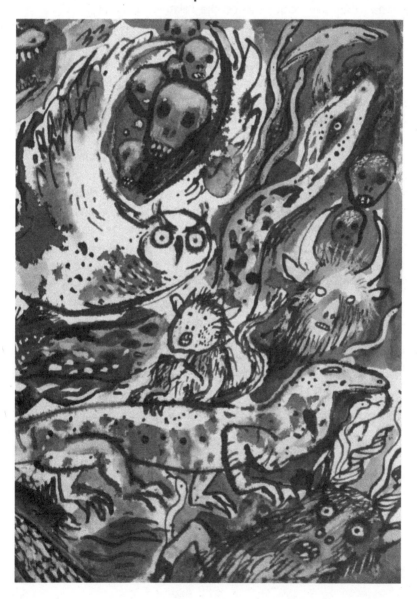

"She comes to fetch me… she comes to fetch my heart…she comes to fetch my breathing…"

Michel is a 21 year old single unemployed man originally from Burundi. He made his way slowly through Tanzania to Mozambique, and thence to Kwazulu-Natal and finally to the Western Cape. He was initially accompanied by his father but when they had both reached the relative safety of Tanzania the father had returned to Burundi to collect his wife and a younger son. The father and son were killed in Burundi and the mother disappeared and was presumed to have also been killed. As Michel moved southwards, without family or any other form of support he gradually developed the belief that his body and his life had been overtaken by a woman he named Maji Khali. In desperation while in Kwazulu-Natal he had sought help from a traditional healer. He had been advised to perform certain rituals and was given a red rope to tie around his waist. This was to no avail, and having moved to Cape Town he tried to hang himself because he found the presence of this woman intolerable. He was admitted to hospital where he again requested the help of a sangoma. He said. "You can't do magic, I can't do magic…only magic can help me…"

He said that he was not angry or afraid but he acknowledged that he was profoundly depressed. A large part of the depression was his helplessness. He was in the wrong place. There was no possibility that we could help him by keeping him in the hospital. The only solution appeared to be magical, and that could only be provided by a traditional healer. We did not do magic and so we were also helpless. It seemed that the desperate nature of his situation called for the certainty of a solution of magic, however impossible that might be. He sought a cure for his intractable problems. He was not interested in how this belief might have arisen, or how Maji Kali might have emerged in his world. He held Maji Kali to account for his predicament. She was to blame, and so of course he had to get rid of her. He needed a remedy that would guarantee her expulsion from his world. An interpretation had been made and now it was for the sangoma to do whatever was necessary to solve the problem, to undo the tragedies of his life, to do the magic, to make things whole again. We were keeping him in hospital against his will.

On a psychological level clearly Michel felt that he had lost control over the circumstances of his life. This control had then been granted to Maji Kali, who provided in some sort of concrete way an explanation to account for the losses he had suffered. She was the explanation and her eradication was the solution. How to manage this posed a certain difficulty in that the delusion provided him with a meaningful account of what had happened to him. With successful treatment in terms of the elimination of Maji Kali what should then be made of his predicament? We would be taking away a solution, albeit magical. We would be taking away a hope of restoration, however illusory.

Michel was treated with conventional anti-psychotic medication and arrangements were made to bring a traditional healer to the hospital to advise on traditionally meaningful ways of dealing with Maji Kali. After approximately two weeks Michel was discharged from the hospital to a refugee centre. Maji Kali had disappeared. It is unclear as to what extent the belief in her, and the rituals of her expulsion contributed to his recovery. What was more sadly clear to us in this context were the limitations of what might constitute recovery. He was a young man in a foreign country with no family and no support and with no better prospect of a future than before he had come to our hospital. The sangoma was not able to undo his terrible misfortunes and nor were we.

Mandla was a law student at the university to which the hospital was affiliated. He was in the third year of his course and he was flourishing academically. He was the pride and hope of his family who lived in the eastern Cape. His colleagues and teachers had become increasingly concerned about his erratic and uncharacteristic behaviour. The alarm increased when he stopped attending lectures. Eventually he was admitted to our unit in an overtly psychotic state. He was not in any way distressed but rather elated or illuminated. He had received the calling to be a traditional healer he told us. This was ukuthwasa, and it could not be resisted. Refusal to answer the calling would cause displeasure to the ancestors and would result in prolonged personal suffering. There was no choice other than to abandon his career as a lawyer and to embark on his training to become a healer.

This caused consternation and dismay among his family. Informed by the university of his admission to our hospital they immediately made their long way from the rural eastern cape to the city. They dismissed his claim of having been called. That was the past. That was traditionalist and had no part in the future they envisioned for him as a bright young professional in a western world. He could not be allowed to drag them backwards after all the sacrifices that had been made to get him as far as he had come. They were angry and anxious and pleaded with us to ignore his talk of ukuthwasa and treat him conventionally so that he could be discharged as soon as possible to resume his studies.

In accordance with the family's wishes and as he did not refuse treatment the conventional anti-psychotic medications were prescribed and the symptoms resolved. At the time of his discharge Mandla seemed mystified by what had happened. He did not want to become a healer. He was determined to become a lawyer and a source of pride to his family and to his community. He was to be part of the vanguard of the new South Africa.

He was readmitted within the next six months. He was not so sure now about what might be happening to him, and nor was his family. Perhaps this ukuthwasa was true although they did not want it to be true. Perhaps it was just too powerful to be refused. Perhaps they would have to put aside their dreams of a different future. Another course of anti-psychotic medication was not going to resolve these issues.

Enquiries were made and we managed to find a healer that was prepared to come to the hospital and meet with us to decide on how we should proceed. I think we were a little disappointed when he arrived. Perhaps we were hoping for something more exotic, for him to be covered in animal skins and some sort of headdress with feathers to terrify and cast down the evil spirits. Mr. Malosi was dressed in a suit and tie with only a simple string of beads and a staff to signify his calling. He was pleasant and mild mannered but curiously insistent that I should address him as

"Professor" while he called me "darling". It was not to be a conventional clinical meeting. Everybody involved was in attendance, including Mandla and his family, Mr. or Professor Malosi, our clinical team of doctors psychologists social workers and occupational therapists and a number of bemused nurses and students. I said that I did not think that Mandla was going to be able to manage without the medication. Mr. Malosi proposed a collaboration. We should continue with our treatment and inform him when we planned to discharge Mandla. Following discharge Mr. Malosi insisted that he would ensure that Mandla continued his medication while at the same time undergo the necessary rituals to become a healer. Nor did he think that being a traditional healer was incompatible with being a lawyer. He advised that Mandla continue with his studies and again he promised to provide support and to supervise. I think we were all relieved and also reassured by this flexible and imaginative course of action. I don't know if it worked but we all fervently hoped it would when we wished him well on his discharge a week later.

This encounter raised the hope of a more constructive relationship between ourselves and the traditional healers who are for the most part consulted by our patients before they get to us. Given the far greater numbers of healers in the communities of southern Africa, and a shared culture and a meaningful idiom of misfortune and disease there seemed to be an important opportunity to work together, a possibility of integrating understanding and explanation in the provision of a more effective service to our patients. Another encounter cautioned us against any naïve assumptions, although I continue to believe that finding imaginative ways of collaborating between traditional healers and more western evidence based approaches is necessary and important and a possibly innovative and creative way of dealing with otherwise intractable problems.

Xolani had been discharged from our unit six months earlier. The diagnosis had been made of a schizophrenic illness and he had responded well to the prescribed anti-psychotic medication. The details of what happened subsequently are not clear. He had returned to be with his family in a rural area of the province. It seems very possible that he had stopped his medication at some stage. He had become ill and his family had taken him to consult a group of traditional healers. The diagnosis on this occasion was possession by an evil spirit. The remedy was to place stones over an open fire, and then to throw water on the stones with the expectation that the scalding heat would drive out the evil spirits. When Xolani struggled against the terrible pain of his burning skin this was interpreted as evidence of the evil spirit fighting against the treatment and he was held down over the stones with greater force.

On his return to our unit Xolani had been mutilated. He had lost most of his nose to burn injuries, he was blind in one eye and he was missing fingers on both left and right hands. Whatever evil spirits there might have been were dismissed within a few days of anti-psychotic medication. His family were grief-stricken and enraged.

One of the many issues raised in this story is the problem of interpretation. Seeking evidence is not the sole province of a western oriented scientific approach to medicine. In this account of what had happened to Xolani psychotic symptoms were interpreted as evidence of being possessed by evil spirits. In a further cruel elaboration his understandable struggle to escape was interpreted as further confirmatory evidence of possession. The unbearable suffering inflicted by the treatment was then rationalized as a necessarily extreme measure to heal this most unfortunate man. In some grotesque way, and most likely to the perpetrators of this abuse it might have all made sense and been justified.

It is perhaps needlessly provocative and ridiculous to associate Freud and Jung and others with these practices. The argument is against interpretation. It concerns the possible harm done in not attending to what is presented, but rather in interpreting the problem that presents itself in terms of something else. That something else might be the belief in evil spirits or some other less malign school of thought or doctrine or ideology.

In my training to become a doctor and then a specialist psychiatrist psychoanalysis had very little influence. I am therefore in no position to make any critical comment about the theory and practice of the various schools of psychoanalysis other than to recount my own troubled experience. For a few months I was required to attend a specialist and renowned psychoanalytic unit in London. It was at the time of great concern about the sexual abuse of children and how this should be managed. As students we watched through a one-way mirror as a family was interviewed. It was suspected that the father had abused his daughter. Much is made in modern medicine and in psychiatry about the need for evidence but this raises again the question of what constitutes evidence. In this miserable circumstance it seemed that the father's silence or his failure to divulge was considered evidence of his complicity. The long awkward pauses, the confusion and the excruciating tensions were interpreted, or at least it seemed to me as confirmation of repression and denial. The family was trapped. The truth would be revealed and if not that was indicative of the power of defensive strategies. In all my years of training I struggle to recall a time when I have felt more ill at ease, as if I should not have been there.

At the same institution my senior colleagues talked enthusiastically of the "material" that was brought to therapy sessions. This again caused us disquiet, as if the deeply personal and complex stories of distress and pain were being used to confirm and bolster an abstract edifice that could not have made any sense to those bewildered participants in the therapy sessions. To have your private anguish interpreted by a remote and dispassionate therapist as a repressed desire to have sex with your mother and kill your father or any other myth seems more likely to offend and alienate than to be helpful. It also seemed at the time to us as students absurd.

The causes of schizophrenia and of autism remain unknown. In the psychoanalytical culture of the middle part of the 20th century this did not deter proponents from declaring that the causes if not blame for these immensely complex disorders lay with the mothers. Without any evidence, but in accordance with psychoanalytic doctrine the cold disengaged mother was held to account and in this way heedlessly and unnecessarily compounded the distress of affected families.

Jung and others within the psychoanalytic tradition have had even less impact on standard psychiatric thinking and practice at the beginning of the 21st century, certainly with regard to serious mental illnesses, given the problems that that terminology entails. More specifically the interpretation of dreams in regard of schizophrenia is irrelevant although Jung did not seem to hesitate to make a diagnosis of schizophrenia on the basis of his interpretation of dreams. This seemed to take precedence over a patient's personal history and social context. The interpretations anyway very often seem idiosyncratic if not bizarre and had more to do with Jung's spiritual, mystical and neo-pagan preoccupations than anything to do with his patient's predicament. I should admit to being discouraged by his own account of what he seemed to regard as a "blissful" revelation involving God defecating on a cathedral with such explosive force that it was destroyed. The young Carl Jung describes weeping with joy and gratitude at his interpretation of this lurid image as an indication that "one should be utterly abandoned to God". On rereading this account in Memories, Dreams and Reflections it is opaque to me as to how he came to draw this enraptured conclusion from the divine detonation.

The issue is less with the details of these various and fragmented and at times mutually hostile explanatory models. The concern is with an inappropriate foreclosure, an explaining away, whether that might be as evil spirits or an oedipal complex or some arcane governing archetype of a collective unconscious. This does not indicate a presumptuous rejection of these schools of thinking, and it is possible that the experiences described merely reflect a crude and reductionist application of sophisticated psychoanalytical principles, and that these ways of thinking might have greater meaning in other domains of psychiatry. It does suggest that with regard to the understanding and treatment of schizophrenia and other serious psychiatric disorders psychoanalysis has a minimal and waning relevance.

11

Coercion

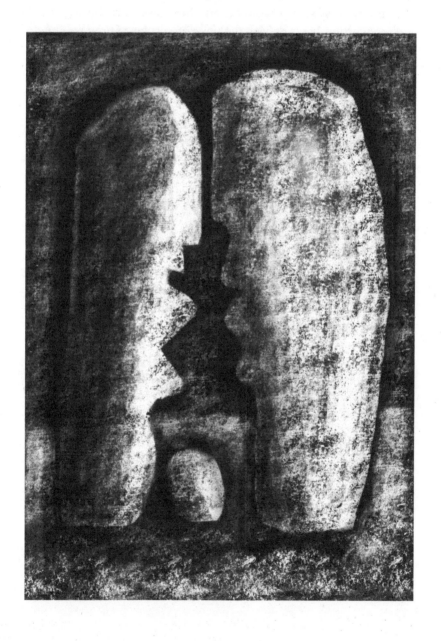

This is a fiction that might be familiar to many of us, in various permutations.

Someone has gone crazy. He has run amok. He is charging around shouting and screaming. He is not dangerous but he is disturbing the peace. He is rattling the order of things. Perhaps he is embarrassing. Perhaps at another level his behaviour is disconcerting. He is defying the unwritten rules of how we should be together. In this respect he is threatening. He does not belong. Perhaps he is mad in that it is madness not to conform, to know how to behave in order to serve one's own needs and the needs of society. He is out of control and that cannot be allowed. Anything can happen. Who knows how it will end? He is unpredictable. Perhaps he could become dangerous. Something must be done. He needs to be removed.

The police are summoned. There is no evidence of criminal behaviour so an ambulance is called. It does not matter too much how he is removed as long as peace and order are restored. Men in long white coats bundle him into the back of the ambulance and perhaps a siren is sounded as he is rushed away to some dark and foreboding asylum beyond the outskirts of the city. There he is injected with powerful sedating substances. He is not assessed in any way. There is no examination. There are no formal admitting procedures. He is put into a uniform and dragged semi-comatose into a single room that looks like a prison cell. When he regains consciousness he is frightened and angry. He protests loudly and three burly and menacing male nurses restrain him and sedate him again.

When he again recovers he decides to adopt a different strategy. He tries to reason with the nurses. He says he is well now and he does not belong in hospital. Something happened that he does not fully understand but it is over now and he needs to go. This to the staff is a clear indication that he has no insight and that he should remain in hospital and receive further medication. The patient becomes increasingly distressed. He demands to see a doctor.

Eventually a psychiatrist is summoned. This is a sinister, rather dishevelled middle aged man in a grubby long white coat.

Perhaps he sneers. Perhaps he has a tremor. He is drunk. No, better, he is a drunken psychopath! The doctor is wrestling with his own demons! He does not ask any questions but he peers at the patient as if he is a specimen. He confers with the nurses. Not understanding the need for further treatment the patient is deemed uncooperative and more medication is prescribed. Perhaps the race angle needs to be addressed: the doctor is white and the patient is black. Violence is perpetrated on the black body. There is no good reason to stop at race. The doctor is privileged, middle class, a beneficiary of an unequal socio-economic and educational system. The patient is disempowered. The violence of structural and historical injustices is enacted and perpetuated.

The patient perceives his situation as hopeless. He has no voice or his voice is disallowed. He becomes apathetic. He refuses to eat and drink in some confused way as an act of self-assertion. This is interpreted as indicative of a depressive disorder. Electroconvulsive therapy is prescribed. No permission is sought as he is considered to lack the capacity for informed consent. This could go on and on. Maybe it could be taken to a further extreme. A lobotomy is proposed, either due to his perceived failure to respond to treatment or as punishment for his intransigence.

This ludicrous scenario may be regarded as a harmless fiction. It is not. It is odious and deeply offensive and it causes harm. Our ways of thinking are shaped insidiously by such ghastly and sensational depictions. Reality is too grim, or too prosaic or too boring.

I am not sure to what extent this lurid depiction of cruel and coercive activity informs thinking about current psychiatric practice. It certainly reflects, to a greater or lesser extent portrayals in popular film and theatre. The problem then arises that it is too easy to dismiss these absurd and melodramas as mere fiction, or the shrill and hostile distortions of one or another anti-psychiatry or propagandist position. Insufficient heed is then paid to the very real and complex problems of relations of power, and the associated quandaries of coercion in the practice of psychiatry, however well intended and formalized in law these practices might be.

An alternative scenario might be described, based on a composite of a number of clinical encounters in which I have been involved in the admission unit of the hospital where I have worked for many years.

Nxaba has begun to act strangely over the past few days. He has become withdrawn and hostile towards his friends and family. He starts to mutter to himself and refuses or is unable to say what might be troubling him. The family of six live in a two roomed shack in an informal settlement. The mother begins to worry about the safety of the younger siblings who share a room with Nxaba. A crisis develops in the early hours of the morning when the mother wakens to the smell of burning and the terrifying crackling sound of flames. Nxaba has set fire to his bed and he has locked the door of the room, trapping his younger siblings. The father calls for help and with the help of neighbours manages to break down the door and rescue the children. They also manage to douse the flames and prevent a conflagration engulfing the adjacent dwellings. Nxaba is unable to explain his actions. He appears to be confused. He tells his father in a disjointed jumble of words that he felt compelled to burn down the house, that the voices were telling him that this is what he had to do. He shows no sign of remorse and no awareness of the grave dangerousness of his actions. The father stays with his son in the one room for the night. Nobody can sleep. Everybody is afraid.

The next morning the father tells Nxaba he is taking him to the local clinic. He says he thinks the son is not well, that he is sick and that the situation is dangerous. The whole neighbourhood could have gone up in flames. Nxaba refuses to accompany his father. He says there is nothing wrong with him. With the help of the angry and frightened neighbours Nxaba is forced into a taxi and taken to the clinic. There he is assessed by a nursing sister and he is examined by a doctor. There appears to be no evidence of a medical condition to account for his strange behaviour. A number of investigations are performed and exclude any likelihood that drugs might have been the cause. Nxaba continues to behave in a hostile and disorganized way. He insists that he has to leave the clinic and in a rather menacing way says there are things has to complete, that there is unfinished business. Although he does not say anything in an explicit way it becomes clear to the clinic staff that he is responding to voices over which he appears to have no control.

The staff form the opinion that he is probably suffering from some form of mental illness, that he is refusing or unable to accept that he is ill and needs treatment, and that as a consequence he poses a danger to himself and to others. The father signs a form and both the nursing sister and the doctor sign the necessary forms for involuntary care. Nxaba continues to insist that he must go. For his own safety and the safety of others a decision is made that he should be kept in a closed ward. He is assessed again the following day and the day after by two medical practitioners who agree that he is ill and needs treatment. After three days there is no sign of improvement and therefore the legal forms are completed for Nxaba to be transferred to a specialist unit. These forms are sent to an independent review board whose task it is to ensure that the rights of a patients in predicaments such as Nxaba's are respected. The forms are also sent to a judge in chambers in order to ensure the process is in accordance with the letter and spirit of the mental health care act.

However well intended to protect against the possible abuses described in the first scenario, these processes are fraught with complications. One right may conflict with another. One ethical principle may be inconsistent with another. Nxaba has a right to receive treatment. He also has the right to refuse treatment. The principle of beneficence requires that he be treated for what quite obviously is a serious illness that is causing him and his family great distress. This conflicts with the principle of autonomy, in this circumstance the need to respect his refusal of treatment. The difficulties arise to some extent from the problematic notion of insight. An argument could be made that due to his impaired insight the right to refuse treatment is ceded, and for the same reason beneficence should take precedence over autonomy. This might be dismissed as being paternalistic.

Another difficulty is that insight is a rather abstract concept and it is not an all or nothing phenomenon. There are degrees of insight and the degree of insight might shift over time. Nxaba for example might have some insight that he is unwell but no insight into the need for treatment. Differences in cultural attitudes can compound these difficulties. Nxaba may accept that he is ill but attribute this to bewitchment. On these grounds he might insist that he be seen by a traditional healer rather than be treated in a western oriented evidence based context perceived by him to be alien. In this regard it seems very likely that he would regard decisions made about his care according to the principle of beneficence as being coercive.

These cultural differences arise not infrequently and need to be addressed with great care. It is not at all helpful to have one's belief in, for example amafufunyane dismissed as having no scientific foundation. Regardless of the science it does provide at least some form of an explanation. It grants meaning. An explanation of synaptic dysconnectivity in the central nervous system is not going to be meaningful to Nxaba and his family, nor does any kind of scientific explanation answer the urgent question as to why the problem might have arisen in the first place. Disregard of the cultural context, and the meanings and explanations families and patients attach to the symptoms of mental illness can constitute another less concrete form of coercion.

A scientific evidence based approach does not need to be antagonistic to a more traditionalist culture specific position. There is no good reason to believe it is one thing or another, and a more creative complementariness needs to be adopted. Understanding and explanation should not be considered to be in binary opposition and there might be many levels of explanation, some more speculative, others based on sound evidence.

Some degree of coercion might be inevitable in the management of extreme psychotic states, given that a defining feature of the psychoses is a lack of insight. That lack of insight might be into the dangerousness of psychotic phenomena such as command hallucinations or persecutory delusions. This can of course only be ethically justifiable on the basis of an assumption that the treatment given involuntarily can reasonably be expected to be effective in relieving the symptoms and hence reducing the risk of dangerousness.

Maluti says: "I don't want to die but the voices are telling me to kill myself. If I don't obey my whole family will be killed. My village will be burned to the ground. There is absolutely nothing I can do about it. You cannot and you must not stop me. You do not understand. I am not ill. I do not need any treatment. I just need to do what the voices are telling me to do. Leave me alone. I have to die. The voices are telling me this".

Quama has savagely attacked his mother and nearly killed her. He insists that it is not his mother but an evil spirit who has taken the form of his mother and bewitched him. He had to destroy this evil spirit to protect both himself and his mother.

Wishing to avoid coercion I have made errors of clinical judgement that have had tragic consequences. A young student was admitted to our unit following a suicide attempt. After about five days in the high care unit he pleaded with us to be allowed out for a day. He did not ask to be discharged. He said that he was feeling restless and confined. The noise on the ward was distressing him and he was having difficulty in regaining the strength of mind and the determination necessary to resolve the problems that had led to what seemed a precipitous attempt to end his life. He was not psychotic. He spoke with insight and reasonably. His concerns were understandable. A turbulent admission unit accommodating for the most part behaviourally disturbed psychotic young men, many from very different backgrounds to his, and possibly perceived by this young student to be threatening was clearly not an environment conducive to his recovery.

"You have to let me out for a few hours. I promise you I will come back. I won't be on my own. I have got friends who will look after me. I don't know why I did that. It was something impulsive and I do not feel that way now. I don't want to end my life. I want to live. But being here is not helping me. Please. You cannot understand what it is like being locked up here. How can I possibly get better? It is safer for me to be out of here. I am not going to do anything silly. I will be alright. Please. Let me go, just for the night. I will come back. I promise. I know I need help. I want to get better. You must trust me. Please."

His friends confirmed that they would look after him. They would be vigilant. They would take turns to watch over him and they would return him to the unit the following afternoon. If all went well I made an assurance on my own part that we would plan to discharge him within the week.

Early the next morning I was informed that he had been found hanging in the bedroom of the friends' home.

To this day I am not sure that in retrospect I would have made a different decision. It was nevertheless a terribly bad decision, and I regretted it profoundly. I needed to show trust in him. I wanted to act in good faith. I wanted there to be hope but I was wrong and a bright healthy young man died. It could and should have been prevented and it was not possible for me to think that I was not responsible.

Acting under pressure from colleagues, from families, from managers and in this last awful incident from patients themselves escalates the likelihood of things going wrong, but I struggle to imagine how things might be otherwise. There is no escaping risk. There is no escaping uncertainty and there are no guarantees that the decision made is the right decision.

In these deeply distressing circumstances it is difficult for me to imagine how a degree of coercion might not be avoidable, as a temporary measure, with the intention of acting in the best interest of our patients, and given their lack of capacity owing to illness.

It is nevertheless one of the most difficult things I have had to cope with in clinical practice. It was always regrettable and seemed to represent a compromise and a failure of the health care system to prevent the dangerousness of these situations from arising in the first place. Having arisen it seemed too often that there was no other safe option, and yet it was always distressing to all those involved.

12

Violence

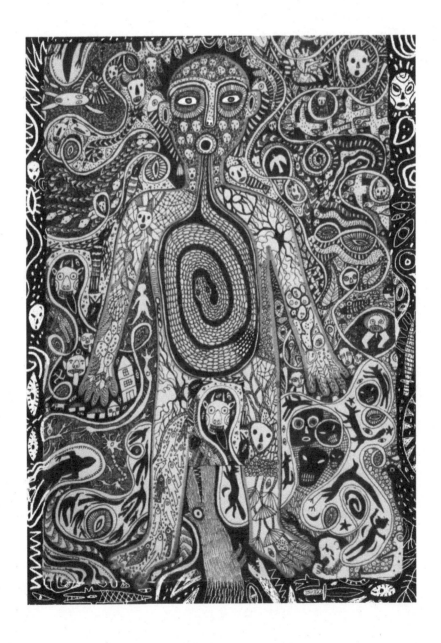

"I am an assassin".

"An assassin?"

"Yes. I am the assassin".

"Who do you plan to assassinate?"

"The president. Of course".

"Oh, the president. Of which country?"

"This country. Of course".

"When do you plan to undertake this assassination?"

"When the time is ready".

"Why do you want to assassinate the president?"

"I don't want to assassinate him. It is just something that I have to do".

"What do you mean, it is just something you have to do".

"There are forces, very powerful forces or spirits that are compelling me to do this. It is outside my control".

"Don't you think it is wrong, to kill anybody, whether or not it is the president".

Unathi is vague.

"Yes, I think it is probably wrong, but it is not up to me. It is not for me to decide whether or not it is the right or wrong thing to do. It will just happen. When the time comes".

"How do you know when that will be?"

"When the forces of energy reach my penis".

"What do you mean?"

"The forces are moving slowly through my body. I can feel them moving from my head into my chest. They are moving very slowly. When they get into my penis I will know the time has come".

"How will you know that the forces have reached your penis?"

"When it gets long".

"How long?"

"Nine inches".

"When your penis reaches nine inches in length you will know it is time to kill the president of the country".

"Yes. That is right".

He speaks without emotion, but patiently, as if explaining something that is self-evident, as if I should know these things. He is untroubled.

"You do understand I have responsibilities?"

"What do you mean, responsibilities?"

"If I have reason to believe that the life of the president of the country, or anybody else for that matter, is in danger I have a duty to inform that person".

"No. That is ridiculous"

"What do you mean it is ridiculous".

"His life is not in danger".

"Why not?"

'Because my penis is not long enough".

"And when it is?"

Unathi hesitates.

"Then I will be the assassin".

"How will I know that your penis has become long enough for you to be an assassin?"

"I will tell you".

"You will come and tell me when your penis is nine inches long so that I can inform the president that his life is in danger? How can I rely on you? You understand that I must inform the security services of this plan to assassinate the president. There is a risk".

"Yes". He seems nonchalant.

"And what if you are then arrested, and charged with a very grave offence?"

He shrugs. This appears to be of no concern to him.

"I don't know. Things will just happen. I can't stop anything. It is not for me to decide what to do".

I am in a dilemma. I do not doubt that Unathi will act when the time comes. I do not doubt that he poses a danger, but the danger is not imminent.

It is also difficult for me to imagine contacting the president's security office to inform them that my patient intends to murder him when his penis has reached a length of nine inches. It seems quite possible that they will become suspicious of me. "Do I think this is amusing? Am I trying to make a joke of the threatened assassination of the president? Are psychiatrists all mad?"

I make an appointment to see Unathi in a months' time. On this occasion he is quite cheerful. He seems to want to reassure me. The forces are still in his chest. They have barely moved. They are nowhere near his penis. I must not worry. There is no immediate danger to the president.

"I am fine. You must not worry. Everything is okay", he tells me. He is not yet an assassin.

We wait.

The association of violence with mental illness is a significant contributing factor to the burden of stigma. The crazed killer is a familiar figure in the popular imagination, fuelled by fictional accounts in film, theatre and other media that feed on our apparent need to be titillated by violence. Psychopathy is elided with psychosis. He was attacked in a psychotic frenzy. A psychopathic killer is on the loose. He, and invariably it is a he, has to be a psychopath because of the evil brutality of his actions. The terminology of mental illness is used without seriously implying that these acts were committed owing to mental illness. It is merely a matter of degree. The acts were beyond the pale, inhuman. This evil could not possibly have been committed by a sane person, by one of us. Madness is carelessly invoked.

At the time of writing two mass killings have occurred in the United States over one weekend. The president has attributed the murders to mental illness. There can be no other, more complicated explanation. It is simple. Violence, in the absence of any other indicators, in the opinion of this most powerful figurehead becomes a defining feature of mental illness.

Mental health care workers, a term used to indicate the very wide range of professionals engaged in the field strive to correct this misapprehension. Most of us consider it our duty to do everything we possibly can to reduce the alienating and harmful effects of stigma. To this end we make the claim repeatedly that persons with mental illnesses are no more violent than those without a diagnosis of mental illness. This applies particularly to the spectrum of serious mental illnesses or psychoses, accepting the problematic nature of this terminology. It is not in any way suggested that anxiety and depression are not serious mental health problems, but these conditions are not associated with violence.

The claim of a lack of association with psychosis and violence needs to be qualified. A person living with schizophrenia, with adequate social support, who does not use drugs and who is adherent to treatment is no more likely to be violent than a member of the general population. This does not apply to a young man with a long history of a severe psychotic illness with frequent relapses owing to non-adherence to treatment and substance abuse problems and who has no social support. The risk of dangerousness increases when such a person is responding to command hallucinations, telling him or her to do things over which they feel they have no control. "Kill her, she is a witch!" "You are a worthless person. You do not deserve to be alive. Why don't you just end it? Do it! Now!"

In this respect Unathi has to be considered as potentially dangerous. He feels he has no agency, he has no option. He has been compelled by external forces to become an assassin. There is no assumption of a freedom of choice, of ourselves as autonomous or of the will being free. He is fated to be the assassin.

Yet I do not believe that Unathi in his present state poses a danger to the president of the country. This is a clinical judgement and I might be gravely wrong in which case there will be severe repercussions with regard not just to the life of the president but also to my career. There are a number of reasons to consider this not to be a matter of urgency, one being the banal observation that the president is inclined to surround himself with a phalanx of bodyguards, and to travel around the country in a cavalcade of security vehicles with flashing blue lights and menacing outriders. Another reason is the very nature of his psychotic illness.

Although he is highly intelligent Unathi's resources for planning and problem solving have become severely impaired, this being associated with his diminished insight and judgement. It is highly improbable that Unathi has the capacity for the very complicated processes that would be required to successfully take out the president. A more likely scenario would be that when the time came he would make his way to the Houses of Parliament. When asked by the security staff what his business was he might quite possibly say politely and with due deference to authority that he has come to assassinate the president. He might even be asked why he should want to do such a terrible thing and when he answers that his penis is now long enough things would take a predictable course. This seems more probable but it is not certain. Violence is unpredictable.

It is also complex. A wide range of differentially weighted factors contribute to the emergence of violence. Because somebody has a diagnosis of a mental illness it cannot be assumed if that person commits an act of violence it should be attributed to the mental illness. More specifically if a person suffers from schizophrenia or any other psychotic illness there is no reason to believe that an act of violence committed by that person may be directly due to the psychosis. Other problems, most obviously substance abuse may provide a more plausible explanation. Probably more common are social and economic factors. A person with a diagnosis of schizophrenia is very likely to experience exclusion, and as a result of the illness and the incapacity to work to drift down the social scale. A predictable recourse to drug use and the absence of any meaningful social support will put that person at high risk of violence, either as a victim or as a perpetrator. In this scenario mental illness is certainly a contributory factor but the absence of social cohesion as a protective influence and the substance abuse as a precipitating element might have a more significant bearing on the commission of violence.

Command hallucinations, or a voice or voices experienced in external space instructing somebody to do something, usually in the context of schizophrenia poses a particular threat of violence. This again needs qualification. There are degrees of agency. A person might hear a voice telling him to kill his mother but have a sufficient sense of self or autonomy to refuse this action. He might have a degree of insight leading him to recognize the commanding voice as a symptom of his illness. He might on the other hand believe he has no power at all to resist the voices, commit an act of violence and thereafter deny any responsibility, insisting: "It was the voices that made me do it. I had no control.

How could I do such a terrible thing. It was not me".

It is the early afternoon of the 6th September 1966 in the House of Assembly in Cape Town. The Prime Minister Dr. Hendrik Verwoerd has just entered the House for the afternoon session. He makes his way to the front bench and exchanges greetings with his parliamentary colleagues. Just as he takes his seat a uniformed parliamentary messenger bustles across the floor from the lobby entrance. The name of this messenger is Dmitri Tsafendas. Without warning Tsafendas draws a sheathed knife from his clothing. He bends over the Prime Minister and withdraws the knife from the sheath. He stabs Dr. Verwoerd in the neck and the chest four times. Members of Parliament rush forward to subdue Tsafendas. Others, among them four medical doctors go to the aid of the Prime Minister. Frantic attempts at resuscitation are made. Dr. Verwoerd is rushed to Groote Schuur Hospital where he is pronounced dead on arrival.

Dmitri Tsafendas was born in Lourenco Marques to a Greek seaman and a Mozambican woman of mixed race. He was sent to live with a grandmother in Egypt in the first year of his life. He returned to Mozambique five years later and then at the age of ten he moved to South Africa. He attended a primary school for two years and then returned to Mozambique where he enrolled at a church school for two years. From the age of sixteen he worked in various places in various capacities. In the 1930's he joined the South African Communist Party. He became a seaman in the Merchant Navy in 1941 and he served on a convoy ship during the war. He travelled, or wandered thereafter for twenty years. During this period it appeared that he began to experience symptoms of psychosis and was hospitalized for short periods in various countries. During a detention on Ellis Island in New York a diagnosis of schizophrenia was eventually made.

In South Africa Tsafendas was classified as white in terms of the country's apartheid system at the time, but was shunned by the white community as being of a darker hue and an outsider. Shortly before the assassination he applied for reclassification from white to coloured in order to legally live with his mixed race girlfriend. This was refused.

After the assassination the anti-apartheid movement distanced themselves from any association with Tsafendas. Although he is reported to have told the police shortly after the murder that he killed Verwoerd because of his disgust for his racial policies, any political significance that might have been attached to his act of violence was denied to him. At the trial Judge Andries Beyers declared Tsafendas not guilty of murder by reason of insanity. He had been diagnosed with schizophrenia and it was claimed by police and his defence that he was inhabited by a giant tape worm that spoke to him.

Following the trial he was initially accommodated in a cell on death row in Pretoria Central Prison where he spent the most part of the remainder of his life. When asked in an official enquiry how he was being treated Tsafendas made no complaint and told the inquiry that he was particularly pleased with the carrots that formed part of the meals that he was given. The carrots were good for the tape worm he said. He seemed to care for this tapeworm. It was not his enemy.

He was a calm placid person. There was no prior history of violence and no violent behaviour after the assassination. It appears to have been an isolated and extreme act. Dmitri Tsafendas was eventually transferred to Sterkfontein Psychiatric Hospital where he died in 1999 at the age of 81. He was buried in an unmarked grave outside the hospital grounds. Fewer than ten people attended the Greek Orthodox service.

To this day it remains unclear what prompted Tsafendas to murder Hendrik Verwoerd. It is uncertain in what ways a lack of any secure attachment in his early years, his restless wanderings around the world and his lack of identity with any community contributed to this one act of appalling violence. It is not known whether the madness of Tsafendas, or the tapeworm, or his alienation from the world or a sense of political injustice led finally to the assassination of Verwoerd.

Yusuf sits quietly in the ward round. He answers my questions in a polite and respectful way. No he does not understand why he attacked his father. Yes he understands that it was a terrible thing to have done. No it will never happen again.

Yes he will take his medication. I am sitting close to him. Under the placid surface he seethes with a violent rage. He is not open to me. I have no understanding what fuels this. I do not know whether it is his illness, or some dark secret in the family or his rage at the circumstances of his world that make him as dangerous as I think he is.

On the ward he is withdrawn. There is no indication of aggression and there is no violence. He is passively cooperative with the staff and in his relations with the other patients. Soon I will have to discharge him. He will return home and after a while he will stop taking his medication and it is highly predictable that he will then again ferociously attack his father. The father refuses to lay charges against his son which would enable us to transfer him into the forensic sector. He says his son is sick. He is not a criminal. The father knows the risk. I fear for his life.

There is nothing inherently violent in the nature of mental illness and more specifically in the nature of the psychoses. This misapprehension probably extends to psychiatric hospitals, where violent behaviour might be expected amongst young men confined involuntarily, but violence is much more likely to occur in emergency units and in the context of intoxication. In the many years I have spent in acute units with predominantly psychotic patients I have never been the victim of a violent assault, nor do I remember fear of any such incident. The widely held assumption that there is an association between mental illness and violence does harm and contributes to the alienation and suffering of those living with mental illnesses. Even in the specific circumstances of command hallucinations in my clinical experience the voices are more likely to instruct a person to do harm to themselves rather than to others. If there is violence associated with mental illness it is more likely to be turned against the self than towards others.

13

Unreason

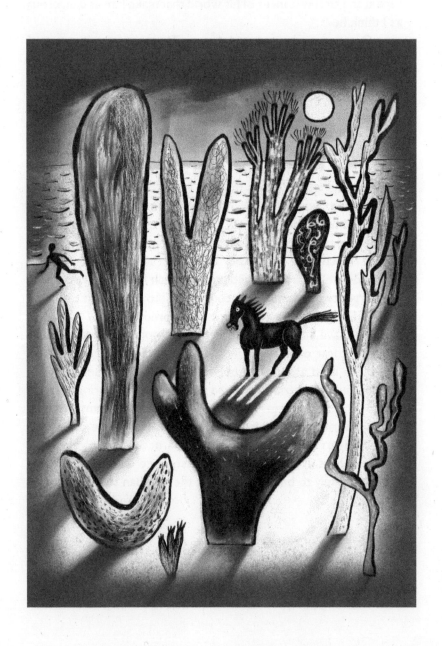

Reason is god. Reason is what defines us as human, or as superior humans. We proudly identify ourselves as homo sapiens. We aspire to reason. We transcend ourselves through reason, becoming god-like in our emancipation from our awkward contingent selves. Reason is imagined as independent of emotion. We attain the status of civilization, or simply of ordered civil society by employing reason to control the disorder and possible chaos of our emotional selves. We are evolved beyond the unreason or the lesser consciousness of the lower orders of being to holding notions of power and control, and a moral authority and entitlement to exert this control. We justly benefit from what is due to us through the exercise of the faculty of reason.

This triumphal edifice is dismantled by unreason. Unreason undoes us and we are rendered mad. We are fearful, and cause fear in others because it is imagined that we are less human, without reason. We become troubled that the power and authority of reason is illusory or more precarious that we would like to imagine. We are ill at ease with the sense that we are vulnerable, that reason might not protect us from madness. We are unable to console ourselves with the fallacious nonsense that serious mental illness only afflicts those who are in some way morally weak, or fail to use reason to protect themselves.

"Sometimes I am so persistently aware of the curiosity with which I must criticize each moment, as the conversation unwinds, that I must criticize myself out of my presence of mind...so that I lose focus in the crisis...a vague epileptic panic rises...on realizing one's own forgetfulness at trying to be lucid...so that I need to keep moving in order to have continuity, as I walk through the silhouetted environment, causing a feeling of calm because of the changing frontiers at the periphery of my vision".

This is one of the many scribbled letters formally addressed to myself and shoved under the door to my office by Govan, a patient I have known for many years and who has remained persistently thought disordered. I struggle to make sense of what he is saying. Sometimes I imagine that I might have some inkling of what he is attempting to articulate and then whatever sense there might be drifts away in a shifting fog of incoherence. Perhaps initially he is describing an excessive form of self-consciousness or self-reflection, to the extent that with some insight he "loses focus". I am not sure what is meant by "forgetfulness at trying to be lucid" but it does suggest a struggle for clarity of thought. If he is seeking continuity it is not clear why he should find some calm in the "changing frontiers", nor why this should be at the periphery of his vision.

Govan is a highly intelligent and very troubled young man. I think he is trying to communicate something very abstract and important to himself but it is not clear. It is not effective. It is convoluted and disorganized, and at some level it seems very possible that he is aware of this, and that must only compound his distress. Perhaps that is why he has to keep moving, as if to be still and be forced to contemplate the disorder of his mind would be intolerable. The calm, he suggests is ephemeral.

In another passage he writes: "Dear Dr. B. the incongruity of my situation here lies in the normalcy of what is denied as impossible and not the possibility of abnormalcy to which intelligence is applied…in terms of what goes on and the mystique around my hundred thousand million dollar acquisition…necessary to provide employment opportunities in terms of landscape gardening the wilderness on Table Mountain so that at least honest labour becomes viable…so that modernists can terrace and lay drainage with a view to social conservation and crop rotation…with a view to decentralization and the restructuring of a global village with parks and orchards in Ruritania…despite this grandiose dream I only wish to pursue my personal talents as best I can enjoy them and to plead for the fate of a disorganized global village under the auspices of the United Nations and the World Bank cannot afford bankruptcy. Sincerely, faithfully yours, Govan."

There is again a glimmering of sense in this and a curious and unexpected insightfulness. He acknowledges the grandiosity of this vaguely articulated scheme, but Table Mountain is oddly relocated in Ruritania, and why the "modernists" should be responsible for the terracing and drainage is deeply mysterious. Words such a "normalcy" are invented, and towards the end of this passage the syntax becomes scrambled. The letter opens and closes with an anomalous formality, and despite or beyond or beneath the disorganization there is a rather whimsical tone of benevolence, of wanting to make the world a better place.

James, an older patient whom I have also known for many years has developed a similar habit of sending me copious amounts of densely scribbled and earnest musings, reflections and complaints. He also stuffs these bewildering missives under my door, and disconcertingly when I see him in the out-patient clinic he demands to know whether I have studied them, and what did I think, and what should he do. I usually prevaricate in some way and he becomes distracted and to my relief does not pursue his interrogation.

Both Govan and James write in a way that is for the most part incomprehensible. There are elements at times of coherence but I am not sure whether whatever sense is discerned might be due more to my reconstruction or imagining than what was intended. Regardless of the uncertainty both these intelligent and literate patients are communicating in a disorganized manner. This should not obscure their fervent need to explain themselves, to be acknowledged and understood. That is understandable. It is not unreason. In both there is a clear sense of frustration, of feeling compelled to tell their stories, yet being painfully aware of their inability to do so in an adequate or lucid way.

Marcus tried to explain what was happening to him in another letter of elusive meanings and pained ambivalence:

"Elements of precognitive thoughts overwhelm me. I think I've been born with a psychic link to mankind...I want to use this to grow but it's vexating being bombarded by too many psychic forces...I thought I was capable of producing earthquakes...it's fantastical, it sounds delusional...that I was capable of exerting an influence on the world...I'm not elated by these powers...I just accept it...they have this surveillance, this inner knowledge of me...eventually I align myself...balance out...get back my privacy...with the medication I get more barriers...without treatment I worry more about myself, my whole being becomes painful...people attack me because of my influence...sometimes they don't intentionally do it...it just comes out of them...it's just got to do with humans...it's just the pain of life...I've come to accept it...I'm trying to raise the consciousness of people on earth...I did the striking of the legs and then there were five earthquakes across the world...at the same time I don't create earthquakes unnecessarily...the funny thing about this is that I take it terribly seriously".

Much of this appears to be without reason. What might constitute a necessary earthquake is unfathomable, as is the belief that one might cause an earthquake by "the striking of the legs". "Precognitive thoughts" makes no sense, and attacking others, whether or not intentionally, being "just human" is difficult to grasp, or needs elaboration to be meaningful.

Much of this is nevertheless clear. Marcus feels that he is under some form of attack, and he is making a strenuous attempt to protect himself. He is both powerful, which he experiences as burdensome, and painfully vulnerable. It is possible but not clear that the one state might compensate for the other. It would be wrong to dismiss these utterances as being entirely without reason, as if reason and unreason are in polar opposition and there are no intermediate spaces. Things surely can be reasonable to a degree, and much might depend on our being willing to understand and to grant meaningfulness.

On a biological level the delusional belief reflects a formulation at the neocortical level, recruiting often peculiar and deeply personal idioms, of what can only be assumed to be a state of unremitting anguish or noise mediated at lower levels. Owing to the impairment of an abstracting capacity, which is a feature both of schizophrenia and damage to the dorsolateral convexity, this construct is made concrete. It is a solution and yet it is not a solution. Being bombarded by psychic forces provides Marcus with an explanation, but the experience of it is "vexating".

The dates are debatable, but evidence from tool making, cave art and rudimentary musical instruments approximately seventy five thousand years ago reflect a capacity to reach beyond the phenomenal world and form alternative representations of reality. This capacity seems to have developed as a function of a critical mass of synaptic or neuronal connectivity in the higher centres of the central nervous system. This seeking of alternative representations does not represent reason. It might be imagined as a yearning beyond reason, beyond the surfaces of our quotidian lives, with a neurological correlate that represents the most developed and sophisticated aspects of our embodied and limited selves. Reason it seems is not enough. We need something more, perhaps something transcendent and unconfined by reason to grant some necessary meaning to our lives. That need seems to be something quite fundamentally human, whether or not we are considered mad.

Some months ago I was gazing in perplexed wonder at a Rothko in the National Gallery in London. The painting was entirely abstract. It was devoid of any representational references and the colours were sombre. I have no understanding what drew me to this painting nor what moved me about it. There is no reason in it at all, but it would be ridiculous to then conclude that this might diminish or undermine the mysterious power the painting held over me.

Regarding reason and unreason in a simplistic binary relationship, that is that something is either reasonable or not reasonable, without any murky intermediate degrees of reasonableness, makes little sense and has damaging consequences with regard to how we understand and treat mental illness.

Madness is in part defined by unreason, its expressions causing fear and exclusion through being ununderstandable and inexplicable. Being more sceptical of the worship of reason, being a little more aware of the tenuous role that reason plays in much of our lives might then incline us less to consider the mad as being other and dispose us more to inclusivity.

We live for the most part probably by unreason. We are sustained by our desires which are without reason and we cope with life by an understandable yet unreasonable refusal of our mortality or a denial of its certainty. It is strange to fear unreason when it seems to govern so much of what we feel and think and do.

14

Wonder

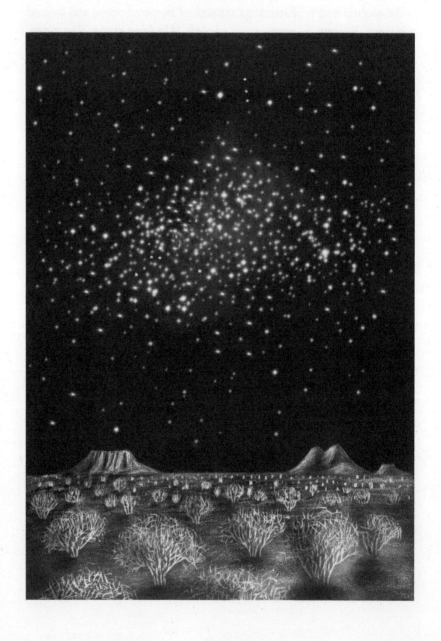

We are sitting in a circle in the ward round room. It is a Wednesday afternoon and we are discussing the new admissions. Renos was brought in during the latter part of the previous week. At the time of his admission his behaviour had been chaotic and aggressive but according to the nursing reports he had settled fairly rapidly. We make an effort to see all the new patients. It is partly to introduce ourselves and to explain the procedures of the ward, but also hopefully an attempt to put them at their ease in very difficult and often bewildering circumstances.

Renos was remarkably relaxed. He seemed quite bizarrely content. I asked him how the weekend had been, a ridiculous question because it could only have been miserable as he had been confined throughout in a closed, very noisy and very probably frightening ward. He beamed, to our great surprise, and declared that he had had a most wonderful weekend. We enquired tentatively as to how this could have been possible in such difficult circumstances. It seemed a remarkable achievement. Again he smiled broadly and with some pride pointed to his fashionable and expensive running shoes. He indicated a coloured disc on the side of the shoe which I think enables one to adjust the pressure in the shoes' heel. "You see Doctor, all I have to do is press this button, which is what I did on Friday night, and whoosh, I am flown to the moon. It was a fantastic flight, and guess what, who should be waiting for me on the moon? It was Beyonce! She was stark naked! She was so excited to see me. We made the most incredible love throughout the night. She wouldn't leave me alone. I was exhausted. Finally, when it had almost become too much for me I said goodbye and thanked her for this most wonderful adventure. I pressed the button again on my shoe and whoosh I was back in the ward. I am not complaining. I need the rest. It was amazing, fantastic!" He leaned back in his chair, it seemed to us in a state of blissful satiation, and yawned. "Wow", he sighed happily, gazing around at his astonished audience, "wow, all you good people, what a fabulous weekend".

A medical student was struggling to suppress her laughter. The rest of us were probably nodding earnestly, trying to decide how to respond appropriately to this strange and rather wonderful story. A caution is necessary in merely considering the notion of wonder in regard to madness. It might be considered false or romantic and in this way undermine the gravity of mental illness. It might lure us into complacency in that if there is some wonder things cannot be too bad, or that treatment is then either misguided or unnecessary. Yet it seems sad and rather impoverished not to acknowledge the strange wonder of these stories. This becomes even more of an issue if these idiosyncratic narratives, confabulations or delusions, or however they might be labelled, are construed as a struggle on the part of our patients to give some form and meaning to what might otherwise be experienced as intolerable noise. Renos is admitted against his will to a chaotic ward. He is frightened. He has to get away. He flies to the moon where he has a prolonged erotic encounter with a world renowned pop star. He flies back willingly to the hospital. It's very curious but it is one way of coping. Certainly it has done nobody any harm. On the contrary it seems to have given him a great deal of pleasure.

I was attending a meeting in the ward when a commotion arose. This meeting was rather oddly called a "climate" meeting, the idea being that myself and the nursing staff would sit in a circle with the patients and listen to whatever issues they wanted to raise. This was a fairly formal, regimented event, the nurse in charge allowing only one patient to speak at a time and limiting their time to a few minutes. On this occasion any semblance of order dramatically broke down. One young man Tswalo began to shriek and howl. He grasped his abdomen as if in severe bouts of pain. I think to everybody's amazement it appeared that this young man was in labour, or that is what he seemed to believe. He fell to the ground and writhed about. The other patients milled about, initially bewildered by what was going on. Then they decided to take action.

They became purposefully engaged, one running to get wet towels, others attempting to soothe and comfort the now terrified Tswalo. The nurses stood back, bemused. This went on for a while. Each patient was occupied with some helpful task. Nobody laughed. Nobody was impatient or angered by this extraordinary performance. The pain increased, the wailing and shrieking reached a crescendo, and then parturition appeared to take place. I had no idea what was going on as the patients were now huddled over Tswalo who was lying on his back weeping. They were stroking and comforting him and two took a dirty bundle of rags away from him. Eventually calm ensued. Everybody seemed to be exhausted by these dramatic events but there was an atmosphere of excitement and celebration. Tswalo had regained his composure and managed to get back on to his feet. I was about to leave the ward when he approached me with the dirty bundle cradled in his arms. He was smiling coyly and seemed proud. The other patients were gathered about him, making cooing noises. It was clearly my duty as the doctor on the ward to admire whatever he had produced. Wrapped in the rags were a pair of dirty shoes. I had no idea how to respond. This is not part of one's training as a medical student nor as a specialist in psychiatry. I hope I made some sort of positive affirmative response, but I certainly could not match the excited enthusiasm of the patients who had attended to him. I left the ward a happy place.

What might have prompted Tswalo to believe that he was in labour was a complete mystery, and I imagine that no amount of psychoanalytical investigation would have made it less so. He was a robust young Xhosa man. He had shown no indication on the ward that he might think that he was a woman, let alone a pregnant woman. The labour, and the birth of the shoes was a surprise to all of us, but what was perhaps more of a surprise to me was the engagement and the kindness of the other patients. It seemed genuine. I did not form the impression that they might possibly have been bored and welcomed the distraction. I did not sense that they were amusing themselves by participating in an absurd charade. They wanted to help the young man. They wanted to comfort him and get him through the crisis, although they must have been as mystified as I was by his behaviour.

It seems important to me to acknowledge this kindness, which seems quite wonderful, beyond the strange and at times frightening behaviours associated with madness. The kindness is not madness. It might be a special kind of kindness, recognizing that somebody is mad, or behaving madly, and yet is in distress and is in need of care and attention. It is all the more remarkable and moving that this kindness came from a group of very troubled and frightened young men who were struggling to cope with their own psychotic demons.

James and Justin are two cousins whom I see every month in the out-patient department. Their stories are sad, even tragic, and yet the dignified way in which they both cope with their illness fills me with wonder. James was working on a doctoral degree in nuclear physics when things started to go awry and then fall apart. It is not clear whether it was perhaps the stress of his academic work or a strong family history of schizophrenia that led to this collapse. In all likelihood it was a combination of factors. An admission to our unit was required and there was a fairly prolonged struggle to gain control of his symptoms. He regained a degree of equanimity but he never fully recovered. His studies were suspended but eventually it became clear that he would never be able to complete the doctorate. He had become disabled to the extent that he would probably never be able to work again, or not in a way that would enable him to live independently. He became dependent on his parents, a father who suffered from a severe degenerative neuromuscular disorder and a mother living with schizophrenia, both of whom had held high hopes for their brilliant son.

When I saw James in the out-patient clinic he was dishevelled and although it was a hot summers day he was wearing a woollen cap and a thick jersey. His hair was uncombed and lanky, his teeth were black and his clothes were untidy and unwashed. I was with a group of undergraduate students. He greeted us enthusiastically and insisted on learning each of their names. I asked him whether he was comfortable with them being with us for the meeting. He responded that he loved being with the students.

From a duffel bag he brought out a number of pamphlets which he proudly distributed. He explained this was an explanation of his philosophy which sought to integrate physics with religion. He told us that he had sent these documents to his former professor at the university, and also to the pope, the then queen of England and the president of the United States of America. He was delighted to have received a card from the pope. It was a photograph of his excellency and a short homily, something that was presumably dispatched to all those who presumed to communicate with the holy man. From his professor he had received a rather curt and dismissive letter, and from the queen and the American president he had received nothing.

He was undaunted. He was joyfully unphased by these negative responses to what he regarded as his life's work. Their affirmation was not that important to him. He would not be deterred from his mission. The students were most welcome to study his pamphlets but he quite understood if they did not. He knew they were much occupied with their studies, that they might feel overwhelmed, and he acknowledged that his grand ideas might not be considered relevant to their medical curriculum. He was considerate and animated and elated. When the meeting ended he thanked us all profusely for the attention we had shown him. He said he looked forward to the next meeting in a months' time.

The students had just started their four week block in psychiatry. I don't know what they were expecting but they seemed surprised and charmed. They wondered how they would have coped in his circumstances, and thought that in all probability they would feel profoundly disappointed and angry and resentful and probably depressed and hopeless. They wondered at his exuberant resilience. He was obviously damaged and he had suffered severe losses but he seemed to us quite heroically undefeated.

His cousin Justin came in after him. He was much more kempt than his cousin and his demeanour was courteous and rather formal. He lacked the excited intensity of his cousin and he seemed more cautious and reserved. He had also had his first psychotic breakdown while studying philosophy at the university, but had quite remarkably recovered to the extent that he was able to resume his studies and eventually gain a bachelors' degree. He also politely asked the students their names and enquired about their backgrounds. He even managed a few words in Xhosa, clearly in an attempt to put them at ease. He was gentle and kind. It was not how the students were used to being treated by patients outside the field of psychiatry. They were more accustomed to being regarded with disdain and impatience, and their presence in clinical encounters was often resented.

Justin enquired earnestly about my well-being and that of my young daughters, as he always does. I am not sure why I answered him on this occasion in the way I did, perhaps it was to indicate to him that I registered his concern and did not dismiss it merely as being polite. Ridiculously I told him that one of my daughters had been in a state of some distress that morning because her cat had eaten her pet mouse. He appeared to ponder on this and then said: "The cat will now become all the more loved because the mouse is inside her".

He was proposing a strange but also creative strategy to console my daughter. Rather than considering this unfortunate event as an act of gratuitous violence on the part of the cat he was suggesting to us a sort of two for the price of one deal in that the mouse was not gone but incorporated into the cat. The mouse had not been subtracted but had been added to the cat. In his kind, albeit rather peculiar way he was trying to help. Another patient might quite understandably have said: "What on earth has your daughters' pet saga got to do with my predicament?". Justin was reaching out.

This is not the more characteristic behaviour associated with schizophrenia, often described as autistic, whereby patients turn inward and become remote and inaccessible. Perhaps it is inevitable that generalizations are made, that we think in terms of stereotypes, but it does harm. Persons are not schizophrenic. That is offensive and stigmatizing. People might live with, or suffer from schizophrenia. We would surely be outraged if somebody was described as cancerous, or tuberculous. Suffering is personal and subjective. Making a strenuous effort not to treat any patients as being the same might go some way at least in mitigating the alienation and exclusion that is so much part of the suffering of the mentally ill. In the same way regarding schizophrenia or psychosis or madness in an irredeemably bleak light is not helpful. There must be some hope and wonder to sustain us all.

There is another element of wonder in this domain that is seldom acknowledged. On many occasions I have thought recovery unimaginable. These young men seemed so immersed in their madness, the symptoms so pervasive and intractable that any way of retrieving them seemed impossible. Witnessing even after a few days, the faltering steps out of madness, the smile, the restoration of spontaneity and of the self was profoundly moving and on many occasions inspiring. The perception that mental illness cannot be treated effectively is wrong and harmful on many counts. Many factors contribute to this misperception. Principally perhaps is the notion of treatment as curative. The great majority of illnesses, particularly of a chronic nature such as diabetes or cardiovascular disease or cancer are not amenable to cure, but can certainly be successfully treated or managed and that also applies to the majority of mental illnesses. Hopelessness and resignation are not appropriate and can only compound suffering. Wonder is defiant and restorative.

Our team was gathered again in a ward round room, on this occasion in the pre-discharge ward. Mashile was ushered in by a nurse. He had a formal, rather dignified authoritative demeanour. I introduced myself and the members of the team and asked him how he was coping. He said he was doing very well thank you and enquired about my own well-being. I in turn thanked him for his concern and then asked him about the circumstances leading to his admission to the hospital. He seemed to be surprised and then said: "But I am the doctor in charge here. I am the consultant". We were all taken aback. I then asked rather hesitantly where that might put me, having been under the impression that I was the doctor in charge. He seemed to think carefully about this and then answered solemnly: "You Dr. B-, you are the Master of the Universe".

This indicated to us that although in a rather grand way he had some sense of a hierarchy operating in the unit, but more importantly it reflected a dissatisfaction with the passive role of a patient as a recipient of care and the wish to fulfil a role that he imagined was more helpful. It also made my day.

A sense of wonder is not indulgently romantic or sentimental but necessary. It does not diminish the tragedy of severe mental illness. We need to attend to the stories our patients tell us. We need to acknowledge at times the strange wonderfulness of these accounts, and the wonder of resilience in circumstances of extreme adversity, and the wonder, sometimes, of recovery.

15

Shame

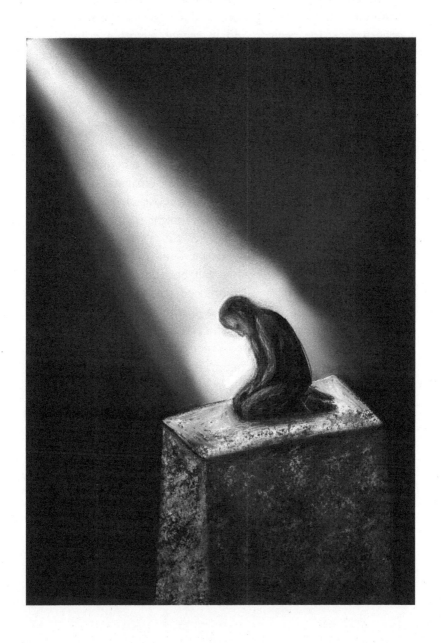

Mental illness is shameful. Suicide and attempted suicide are shameful acts. It is dismaying and perplexing why extremes of human suffering should be considered shameful.

The shame might be personal. It might be felt by the family of somebody afflicted with mental illness. It might the shame of a community for not doing more, and it might be the shame upon government, for neglect, and in recent events a criminal and callous disregard for the mentally ill. It might be the shame we all feel to some extent, for not understanding, or not being able to understand, and not being able to help.

The personal shame is the saddest. It is profoundly wrong that somebody struggling with thoughts and feelings that are unbidden and tormenting should be further burdened by a sense of shame. This shame has many elements, a number of which hover at the edges of consciousness, or emanate vaguely from cultural beliefs to which one might not subscribe yet which exert a pervasive and subliminal influence. I might call myself an atheist but believe or sense in some way that it is wrong to kill myself. The precept might be more explicit. The Koran is emphatic that suicide is sinful and curiously will be punished by everlasting torment in hell. My aunt committed suicide in a post-partum psychotic depression. She was a Catholic and because of the manner of her shameful death she was buried in non-consecrated ground, beyond the hallowed sanctuary of the church in which she had held faith. In this context mental illness has no meaning. It provides no explanation. It is irrelevant. Suicide is sinful. It is shameful. It is taking away from god what belongs to god.

Mental illness in these realms of dogma is a frail construct. It cannot account for or excuse this terrible sin of theft from the almighty. Part of this must be a fear which is part of the human condition. If there is no god who cares for us, for whom it does not matter whether we kill ourselves or not, what is there? An indifferent god is intolerable, and if he or she does not care what are the grounds for leading a moral life, or what is the purpose for anything at all? If we are so terribly free, we are at liberty to kill ourselves, and for many this is abhorrent, and shameful.

This persists beyond religion, but perhaps in a more

attenuated or insidious way. There is a kind of faith in secular humanism, but it is not overt and the notion of shame is less explicit or it is unacceptable because of religious connotations. The faith or the belief is in our humanity. Associated with this is the belief that we and not god are in control of our destinies. We exert free will. We have the freedom of choice. We hold responsibility for the choices we make in our lives. The self is central. It is holy. We cannot blame god or fate when things go wrong. In this context mental illness, or more specifically psychotic states are confounding. There is a loss of the sense that one is in control of one's thoughts and actions. The notion of self becomes tenuous and disintegrates. In this respect one loses one's humanity. Shame is not invoked but it might be felt. Mental illness is an abstraction. It is too vague and precarious a notion to account for this profoundly altered state of being.

It seems possible that these implicit ways of thinking at least to some extent might account for the bewildering persistence of stigma, or the casting of the mentally ill as other, beyond the fold of humanity.

Allied to this is a faith or an assumption that as we are in control of our lives it is our duty to take responsibility for the way we choose to lead our lives. This is undeniable. It is fundamental to who we are. To think otherwise is to deny our humanity. If it is not shameful it is unimaginable.

Eusebius has been struggling with schizophrenia for years. For the moment it is contained. He attends the out-patient clinic regularly. He takes the prescribed medication. He lives in a group home and sees his family over the weekends. He is coping he says but it is difficult. He is well enough to know that he is not well. He has to live with the past and he is unsure of the future. He is not at all certain that he is strong enough to stay as he is at present. The illness is too unpredictable. It is too much for him. He can't undo it. He cannot undo what has happened. He is ashamed and that further burdens him.

When he was ill he assaulted his mother. He cannot understand how he could have done this. It was as if it was not himself he says but it was himself and he cannot make sense of it.

Can madness undo you in this way? What strange illness is this that makes you not yourself? He was running naked in the streets. He was shrieking at strangers. People try to reassure him. They say it was just the illness. He must not be ashamed. He was not himself. He was not responsible for what he did. He will be alright. He must just be careful.

Eusebius does not really understand what that means. Deep down, somewhere in himself he believes this madness is part of who he is and it will never go away. He is humiliated. He is unworthy of self-respect. He is grateful to those who try to comfort him. He nods politely and he says, "Yes I understand, it is just an illness, like diabetes perhaps, and it can be controlled, and it does not have to ruin my life", but I sense that he does not believe this is true.

He is not like the others. His friends from his school years have moved on. Some have already graduated from university. He has been left behind. A bright future has been taken away from him. He wanted to be an architect. Now that seems impossible. There is little or no prospect of him being able to work in a way that will make him independent of his family. He attends an art class and he does beading but he finds it extremely awkward. He is confronted with his disability. He is shamefully unproductive. He has failed.

When he visits his mother he does not know whether it is in his imagination but he thinks he sees fear in her eyes. She cannot forget what he did to her. He cannot live like this and so he stops his medication and within weeks he is back in our wards, ranting and raving, behaving in a wild and dangerous way that will only cause him further embarrassment when he recovers. He is trapped in his illness. Madness is for him a transient and illusory escape that only causes further hurt and shame.

Johannes has recovered from a manic episode of a bipolar mood disorder. He is ambivalent about these episodes. In some respects he tells me that he thrives on the mania. He says it is the best feeling possible. He would not wish it away. He is filled with energy and everything is possible. He believes he is on top of the world. On this occasion he had visited a night club with a friend.

He became intoxicated. He bought drinks for strangers, groped at the dancers and fought with the bouncers who eventually tried to evict him. He had ended the night in a police cell and his daughter was summoned the next day. It would all have been hilarious he said if not for the reproach and the anger he saw in his daughter's eyes when she came to collect him. She said she was ashamed of him and this had hurt him deeply. For this reason he said he would now act responsibly and he would take his medication diligently. He wife had left him years earlier because of his wayward and reckless behaviour. He could not allow himself to now alienate his daughter. He appears to be contrite. He says childishly, "I am going to be a good boy". I am not at all confident. I am not sure whether the sense of shame is sufficiently strong for him to be able to put aside the raptures of his mania.

Jacobus is profoundly depressed. He says he has recovered to some extent. He no longer feels hopeless. There is some vague glimmer of a future. He is no longer hell bent on ending his life. He says he can see things more clearly now, but that means that he can see that he has failed his family, that he is a worthless husband and father to his long suffering wife and children. In one way these sentiments are part of his depressive illness, but in another way this appraisal is valid and understandable. He had lost his job. His colleagues had said the company could no longer afford the many days he took off work because he said he could no longer cope. He had started to drink heavily. He resisted the increasingly desperate attempts of his friends and family to reach out to him. Then one morning he told his wife that he was taking the car out for a drive, he said to try and sort himself out. She became suspicious and went to look for him. She found him barely conscious in the garage with a pipe leading from the exhaust into the car where he sat slumped in the driver's seat. He was resuscitated and there were no adverse effects other than shame. This was the worst part of it he said and he did not see how it would ever go away.

He also believed, and I think with reason that his family was ashamed by what he had done. His wife was religious, and although she was not devout it seemed very probable that she would have believed that his attempted suicide was a sinful act. She might have sought to lessen the burden by saying to me and to her husband that she accepted that he had been suffering from some sort of malady but I don't think she believed it and I think his desperate act lay heavily on the marriage. She told me that she also felt ashamed that she had not been able to help her husband. Shame confused and complicated his depression and it was not something that a pill would take away.

I find it difficult to say to a family that there is no explanation. I sense that they feel there has to be. Where does this madness come from? There has to be an explanation, an answer. Perhaps if there is a known cause there is a solution. I do not think it is helpful to assert causation when the circumstances are most often fraught with uncertainty. Invoking a genetic contribution for example, or environmental stressors can itself too easily lead to self-recrimination and self - blame and then shame. If schizophrenia is an illness like diabetes or tuberculosis there has to be a cause as there are known causes of these illnesses. If there are no known causes we will invent causes: it will be the bad genes or the bad upbringing, or devil possession or an evil spirit or a bad spell or punishment for some transgression. Even if we are able to come to terms with the uncertainties as to why a psychosis might develop we carry the burden of what we imagine our families and communities are thinking: "they must have done something wrong. These things don't just come from nowhere".

There is another cause for shame with regard to mental illness and this pertains to neglect. This manifests in many ways, including the low priority accorded to psychiatric services despite the great burden represented by mental illness on the community, both in terms of human suffering and economic losses. This neglect recently reached a grotesque nadir in the deaths of over one hundred patients in the Gauteng Province of South Africa. These extremely vulnerable persons were removed from Life Esidimeni to unsupervised care in community establishments where they died from a range of preventable causes. This cynical and criminal disregard for human life is a disgrace to the elected government, but we are all deeply affected by the shame of what has been allowed to happen in our midst. It is difficult not to imagine in this atrocious circumstance that the lives of those living with mental illnesses are considered less worthy, and in this respect we are all diminished.

To believe through fear or ignorance that mental illness is in any way shameful is wrong. It causes further suffering and it is as offensive as it is shameful.

16

The dream of the community

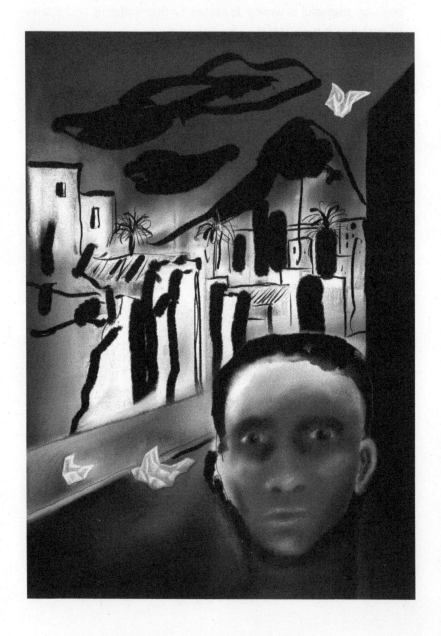

Over a hundred are now dead. There is concern that this number is likely to rise. Many remain missing. For some there are no records. It is not known if they are dead or alive. They have just disappeared. The health ombudsman has found that the most common cause of the deaths was pneumonia, followed by uncontrolled seizures. All but one of these deaths are considered to have been preventable. Extremely vulnerable people have died for lack of care. On average patients died within two months of the transfer from the Life Esidimeni Health Care Group. Esidimeni means "place of dignity". The reasons given for the transfer are given by the responsible health official as "cost-containment".

This is the number of deaths that took place between 23 March and 19 December 2016. Patients were found to be starving and dehydrated. Relatives testify that the patients had been given no extra blankets and warm clothing during the previous year's harsh winter. There are reports of patients being left naked and chained to beds without mattresses and next to dead bodies. There are reports of physical and sexual abuse, of cruel and inhumane treatment. Twenty deaths occurred in an unlicensed care and rehabilitation centre named Precious Angels.

This calamity occurred following a decision on the part of the Department of Health to terminate the contract with Life Esidimeni Health Care Centre in the province of Gauteng, and to transfer patients with mental health care problems to a range of non-licensed non-governmental organizations throughout the province. An estimated 1371 chronically ill patients were transferred from 1 June to 30 June in what was described as a chaotic and shambolic process. The termination of the contract was to save money. State subsidized patients were to be moved from the private hospital group to the care of cheaper community based organizations. The health official responsible for this decision persisted with the plan despite opposition from families, health care experts and activists who warned that these community organizations were not able to provide the high level care that was needed. The aim was to save the province R320 a patient a day. The assumption was that the professional care needed by these patients could be provided by non-governmental organizations for R100 a day.

The report on the "Circumstances surrounding the deaths of mentally ill patients; Gauteng Province" requested by the Health Minister found evidence of human rights violations. There had been a total disregard of the rights of the patients and their families including among many others the rights to human dignity, the rights to life, and the rights to freedom and security of person. Negligent and reckless decisions and actions taken included grossly inadequate preparation for the transfer, the transfer of patients without the knowledge of their families, the transfer of patients to distant locations, overcrowding at community centres that were unlicensed and unregulated, the lack of provision for community health care services, the lack of suitably qualified staff at the centres, and the "precipitous and chaotic" transfer against the advice of experts and mental health care practitioners. The manner, the rate, the scale and the speed of transferring such large numbers of vulnerable patients had been reckless. All these decisions and actions ran contrary to the governmental policies and strategies of deinstitutionalization.

A number of recommendations were made. Disciplinary proceedings should be instituted against the officials responsible for gross misconduct and incompetence. The national minister of health should request the South African Human Rights Commission to undertake a systematic review of human rights compliance and possible violations nationally related to mental health. Appropriate legal proceedings should be taken against non-governmental organizations found to have been operating unlawfully and where patients died. The national Department of Health should review all nongovernmental organizations involved in the project and those that did not meet the necessary health care standards should be deregistered and closed down.

Bewilderment and outrage have ensued. There has been a struggle to find the right words to reach a sufficient pitch of indignation and anger that might possibly be considered an appropriate response to these events. Words such as tragedy and murder have been invoked. Neither seem appropriate. Tragedy suggests a degree of inevitability, a misfortune that befalls us and that is beyond our control. This most emphatically does not apply to those who died following the termination of the Esidimeni contract. These people died because of incompetence and neglect but they were not murdered. I do not think there is any evidence of intent. Murder can only be understood in this context as a criminal disregard for the humanity and the lives of others.

We are confounded. We are horrified. We are ashamed. Amidst this clamour perhaps two points need emphasis. It is difficult not to imagine that such a degree of callous indifference on the part of the officials involved could not have arisen from a certain attitude towards the mentally ill. None of those making these atrocious decisions were health care practitioners. They were bureaucrats and politicians. A terrible confusion of incompetence and avarice and an abysmal failure of imagination seem to have led to a collapse of the most basic humanitarian attitudes. It appears that people with mental illnesses are not quite human. They are not deserving of care and respect. They are mere items of cost. They are a burden to society. They are dispensable. If things go wrong nobody will care too much. We will have achieved the necessary savings. We will have pleased our political masters.

Another profoundly sad and perhaps contentious argument is that although these decisions and actions represent a grotesque extreme they should not be regarded as exceptional. It is not rare nor does it cause an outcry that people with serious mental illnesses are neglected and abandoned in the community. As a result there is further suffering. There is exclusion and ostracization and this might extend in many parts of the world to persecution and demonization. Simple lack of basic care might lead to early death but for the most part this goes unnoticed. We want to believe in the community. We need to believe in care in the community. What has happened here is intolerable. Anger and indignation is of little import if it does not compel us to learn some painful and profoundly disconcerting lessons from these appalling events.

We are about to discharge Mashile and it fills me with foreboding. I don't know how long it will last. His family share these concerns. They also fear for their own safety. When we discharged him previously things fell apart rapidly. Both parents work. There is nobody at home to care for Mashile during the day. There is no day centre in the vicinity. He is vulnerable. Previously gangsters had followed him home from the clinic. They had pretended to befriend him. They had persuaded him to part with a portion of his disability grant in order to procure drugs. When the parents returned home the gangsters were in the home. They threatened the family with violence if any attempt was made to summon the police. It amused them to watch Mashile become intoxicated and then psychotic after using the cannabis. They drifted away after he was again admitted to hospital but the parents knew the gangsters would be waiting. They would find him again at the clinic when he went to collect his medication or at the welfare centre where he needed to collect his grant money. They would follow him home again and they would intimidate the family and use their drugs with impunity. His parents could not protect Mashile and he would get sick again and require readmission.

This is all so predictable: "we are all in danger now so why Doctor don't you keep him? You know he will be back within months, maybe weeks if he manages to stay alive, if the gangsters don't kill him for his grant". The parents know this appeal is hopeless. We have been through this before. I have told them that I cannot keep him in hospital if he has recovered and he is well. We need the bed for those, many like Mashile, who have yet again broken down for lack of care in the community. We cannot use our very limited psychiatric services to treat the historical and socio-economic ills of the city, and besides all this, and perhaps most importantly Mashile wants to go. He says he is better and now he wants his freedom.

The exasperated parents ask what sort of freedom this is, to be abused and exploited by others. When I say we do not have the right to keep him against his will they become angry and say do they not also have rights, the rights to feeling safe in their own home and the rights to the peace of mind that their son is safe and being cared for. They see no end to this. It is a miserable session and it ends with a very clear sense on the part of the parents but also on my own part of dissatisfaction and frustration owing to the limitations of what we can and cannot do. I feel that we are failing this family not because we are refusing to keep their son in hospital but because of the woeful inadequacies of the provision of care in the community.

Political and economic and ideological issues are confounded by confusion about the terms adopted to pursue different agendas. This is apart from ethical concerns and arguments about what might constitute optimal care. Community care is not the opposite of hospital care. Hospitalization is not institutionalization. There is a persisting misapprehension that an admission to a specialist psychiatric hospital means being "put away", and that this is of indefinite duration. This is a reflection of the past, in most countries of the world, and in present times it is indefensible.

A combination of factors, including changes in attitude and psychopharmacological advances render any notion of institutionalization or incarceration redundant and unethical. Yet to this day people possibly squeamish about using the word patient as a demeaning epithet choose the more offensive term inmate, conjuring up however unintentionally the sinister and persisting fear of the asylum.

In the hospital where I work the average length of stay is about four weeks. Some patients do stay longer but the reason for this is most often the absence of a suitable place in the community. Care in the community is a fraught term and is laden with aspirational and ideological freight. Whatever we might wish to believe care in the community too often translates into neglect and abandonment, homelessness and incarceration, now not in hospitals but in prisons. This most emphatically cannot be used as an argument against community care for people with severe mental illnesses. It does require the abandonment of any notion that this might be a cost saving exercise and of an entirely cynical attitude that without the provision of the necessary resources, neglect and a new form of exclusion can be presented as a progressive policy.

In the best of all possible worlds plans are made for Mashile's discharge from hospital. He is referred to a day centre which he will attend immediately following his discharge. There he will be assessed in terms of his needs not his disabilities. He will perhaps join a pottery class and start some basic training in carpentry. He will be part of a group who understand and support each other. He will be introduced to his community nurse who will supervise his care but most importantly provide further support and encouragement. Should he perhaps develop troubling side-effects to his medication the community health care worker will discuss this with the supervising psychiatrist and the necessary changes will be made without Mashile having to wait for hours in a hospital out –patient clinic for a hasty consultation with a psychiatrist to whom he is a stranger. His parents are able to relax knowing that he is safe during the day. He begins to show an aptitude for carpentry and he is invited to join a workshop where he will earn a small income to supplement his disability grant. He takes great pride in his achievements. He is valued by others at the day centre but also by members of the community who see in him no reason to fear those who live with psychotic disorders. His days have purpose and meaning. There is no justification for abandoning what might at present be dismissed as a wishful fantasy.

Beyond the allocation of resources, beyond mere tolerance a fundamental change in thinking is required. It is not simply to be unafraid of otherness, it is to seek it out, to attach value to otherness and in this way to extend ourselves and assert our humanity. It is to refuse the uniformity imposed upon us by the marketplace, the inherited and learned definition of ourselves that shape our attitudes in so many subtle and insidious ways. We need to be willing and accept the need for change in the way we see ourselves and the way we behave towards others. Esidimeni has shamed us all. Perhaps especially in this divided and fractured country we need urgently to extend and complicate our lives by engaging with otherness rather than retreating into familiar territories that can no longer be consoling, the precarious and absurd identities of race and nationality and normality or sanity. It is surely not impossible to imagine that we might be more free if we were to extricate ourselves from the suburbs and fortresses of our fear. We may wish that otherness might not be a source of anxiety and dread but a source of wonder. It is regrettable that so many of us seem resigned to this being merely a dream.

17

The status of disability and its complications

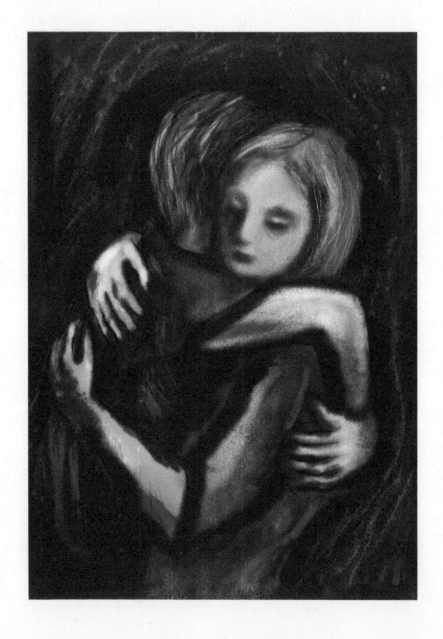

Hannes stares at me vacantly. He is sitting slumped in a chair in the outpatient department. I don't think he wants to be here but on the other hand I don't know where he would rather be. He appears to be disinterested in my questions. He is fine he says. There are no problems. No, there is nothing he wants to raise with me. He has no complaints. He stares through the window at the birds on the river. He sighs and shrugs. He is impatient. He wants to get away. He is ill at ease. The only reason why he is here is for me to sign the application for the renewal of his disability grant. That is all he needs. That is all I have to do. The rest is just noise, a tiresome formality.

I persist and clearly it annoys him. I want to know how he spends his days. I want to know what occupies him. When he wakes in the morning what does he think? What does he hope for? I suppose what I want to know is what gives meaning and value to his life. I suspect the answer to this is that nothing gives meaning and value to his life. These issues are meaningless to him. He drifts along, he gets by, he is alright. I am not to burden him with these irrelevant concerns.

But why not do something, I ask, anything, however small or insignificant it might seem, just to make it worth his while to get up in the morning, just to have something maybe to look forward to? He is impassive. "I am not bored." he says. I tell him, or I try to reassure him that I am not suggesting that he go out and seek some form of formal employment. I know that he is afraid that any kind of work will jeopardize the disability grant. I also know that him finding any kind of paid work is almost impossible. He has no skills, no experience and most importantly no motivation. Yet something, anything, to give him at least some purpose and direction in life I imagine would be helpful. Maybe he could develop some skill, he could learn to cook, he could take drawing classes, maybe he could learn a new language. He looks at me as if I am the patient, as if I am mad. I am unfathomable. I am making no sense. I don't understand. Why don't I just get off his back and sign the wretched form.

I want to say that I acknowledge that he is disabled but not so disabled. It is difficult to find the right language and all the more difficult because he is not interested. It is as if this designation of being disabled has seeped into him and has disabled him at some deeper level.

In another societal domain being identified as disabled can carry with it the added burden of stigmatization. As I am writing this a report emerges in the media concerning difficulties encountered by those trying to provide help for disabled children. A project manager at the Tswaranang District Project Centre in a rural area of the Limpopo province expresses the concern that beliefs linking witchcraft to disabled persons are particularly problematic. One of the major obstacles preventing people from obtaining the limited help that is available is stigmatization. She reports: "there are those who still believe that if you are disabled you are cursed and bewitched. And so we see parents trying to hide their disabled children". Injustice is laid on misfortune: not only are you disabled but you are believed to be cursed, and you are prevented from getting the support and help you desperately need.

The burden of disability in this harsh world is compounded by exclusion. Hannes is extremely vulnerable. One aspect of the schizophrenia he is living with is a loss of drive or volition. This is associated with a very precarious sense of self and agency. There is in this a danger that as in Hannes' predicament one's own perception of disability can compound the disability. A special effort is required to encourage especially somebody struggling with schizophrenia to believe in their self-worth and regain control of their lives. It is not going to be at all possible if the parents of the disabled child believe that he or she is bewitched. This most unfortunate child would be all too likely to believe this.

It is not impossible but it is difficult and unlikely that these issues will be attended to in the turmoil of an admissions ward or in the out-patient department or community clinic, with a restless queue of ten to twenty patients waiting to be seen. It is important, it is necessary, but perhaps most often it seems too much, it is too difficult, too uncertain as to whether the effort expended might result in the elusive reward of somebody regaining a sense of purpose in life and hopefulness. The more likely response, and

I do not think this is confined to the local situation, is a hastily written script and a renewed application for the provision of a disability grant. I think very many of us sadly give up too soon on any expectation that our patients will recover and that their disabilities may be overcome. There is a continuous struggle against a fatalism that affects us all.

This is not in any way an argument against the notion of disability itself and certainly not against the desperate need for the provision of disability grants. It is the expression of concern about some of the ramifications and unintended consequences of invoking disability. Identifying disability, recognizing its extent, and the burden it exerts on individuals and their families and on health services and the economy is of great importance for many reasons. It provides for the allocation of necessary resources and services. It should but does not necessarily stimulate research into the causes and the improved treatment of mental illness. It can and should but does not inevitably lead to a better understanding of mental illness and hence through education and public awareness a reduction in stigmatization and exclusion. Being aware and acknowledging the high prevalence and the great burden of mental illness is the beginning of a long process of dragging madness out of the shadows of ignorance and denial and shame.

A report on the Global Burden of Disease was published in 1990 by the Harvard School of Public on behalf of the World Health Organization and the World Bank. It was subtitled: "A comprehensive assessment of mortality and disability from diseases, injuries and risk factors in 1990 and projected to 2020". In a summary of the findings one observation was made that was described as "startling" by the writers. The burdens of mental illnesses had been seriously underestimated by traditional approaches that take into account mortality but not disability. While psychiatric conditions are responsible for little more than one per cent of deaths, they account for almost eleven per cent of the disease burden worldwide.

Of the ten leading causes of disability five were neuropsychiatric disorders. In the projected estimates of disease burden for 2020 depression was second only to ischaemic heart disease.

There is even greater cause for concern in that indirect psychiatric causes of mortality are not reflected in these figures. People living with serious mental illnesses have a reduced life expectancy of ten to twenty years. There are many reasons for this very disturbing figure but high amongst them are smoking, a lack of exercise and self-care in general that are significant risk factors for premature death due to cerebrovascular and respiratory diseases.

There is no correspondence between these estimates of disease burden and resource allocation or the funding of research. The problems are compounded by a "treatment gap" in that only about twenty five per cent of those living with mental illnesses are estimated to receive the treatment they require. There are again many probable reasons for this, including ignorance and hence stigma and rejection, but it seems that beyond these more readily identifiable factors there is a more mysterious and profound failure or an unwillingness to grasp the grim realities of mental illness.

In many low and middle income countries other factors including poverty, violence and gender inequality constitute risk factors for psychiatric morbidities. Poverty and mental illness interact in a negative cycle of misfortune. For a host of reasons, poverty significantly increases the risk of mental illness and mental illness leads very often to poverty. Certain groups such as children and the elderly are particularly vulnerable. Major social and economic changes and upheavals such as urbanization and migration undermine stable family and community support systems and contribute further to poor outcomes.

The growing awareness reflected in these global epidemiological studies of the global burden of psychiatric disorders, and their enormous social and economic impact is important and potentially valuable in reprioritizing resources and research funding. In most low and middle income countries less than two per cent of the total health budget is currently allocated to mental health services. The figures cannot however indicate the hardships and the inestimable suffering of those struggling with mental illnesses, nor of their families and communities. The plight of the mentally ill, especially in low and middle income countries is lamentable and unjust.

The high prevalence and the burdens owing to disability need to be confronted and acknowledged. This is an important first step in taking the necessary action to prevent and limit disability. The problem needs to be understood as a human rights issue rather than arising inevitably from impairments of psychological and social functioning. Harm arises from the misperceptions of disability as irreversible and therefore as sufficient reason for a fatalistic attitude that there is not much more that can be done other than the provision of a disability grant. Being identified as disabled too often entails the neglect of the necessary effort to foster resilience.

An alternative response would be to identify specific disabilities with the aim of doing whatever might be necessary to prevent a person's life becoming unnecessarily restricted or thwarted. But this is not enough. It might be more helpful to regard disability not as an individual problem but more as a political issue. Social discrimination on the grounds of mental illness is a human rights violation. It also impoverishes us all. Treating this very human and complex problem as a political issue requires us to consider ways of fostering more tolerant and humane attitudes, rather than a more restricted notion of an obligation merely to rehabilitate an afflicted person back into a society that many might regard as itself being sick, fragmented and hostile. The problems are compounded by the changing nature of the world we inhabit. In an increasingly materialistic and technological culture the potential for alienation seems all the more likely to undermine such possibly utopian fantasies. All the more effort is then required to create and maintain attitudes of acceptance and inclusion and compassion.

Perhaps it is wishful thinking but the dream of a community cannot be abandoned to the cynical and banal realities of the marketplace. The disability of an individual should not be allowed to shift attention away from the disabling social attitudes for which we all share a responsibility and which shape our own lives.

A mother wrote to me of her son living with schizophrenia: "While there were times that the situation seemed to be completely hopeless, I gradually became more determined that my son's condition would improve. I refused to accept that he would need to be permanently disabled". She described a number of interventions, including adjusting his medication, his becoming a member of a well supervised group home and her joining a support group. "Our lives are much better now. My son has been stable for years...he is compliant with the medication and even grudgingly accepts that he does have an illness that requires treatment. He has started a small business that gives him the dignity of earning his own spending money and he is learning to drive. These are milestones that I really celebrate. He spends weekends with me and it is a pleasure now to be in his company. But one of the most thrilling events for me is that he has discovered how to laugh again. Not the sort of laughing that he used to do when he was obviously delusional, and which filled me with fear. Now he is able to appreciate humour and he regularly roars with laughter when he recognizes the fun and joy of an experience. I know he will never be the young man that I dreamt he would be, but I have learned to accept that nevertheless he is a sensitive, loving and considerate person and I am very proud of him".

It has been a struggle. She says she has learned to see what has happened to both of them in a different light. In a very imaginative and helpful way she has refused to think of her son as disabled and in this way has retrieved a sense of pride and joy in her relationship with him. Clearly both of them have benefitted. The status conferred of disability should be a means towards helping. It should not be a trap.

18

Pain and suffering

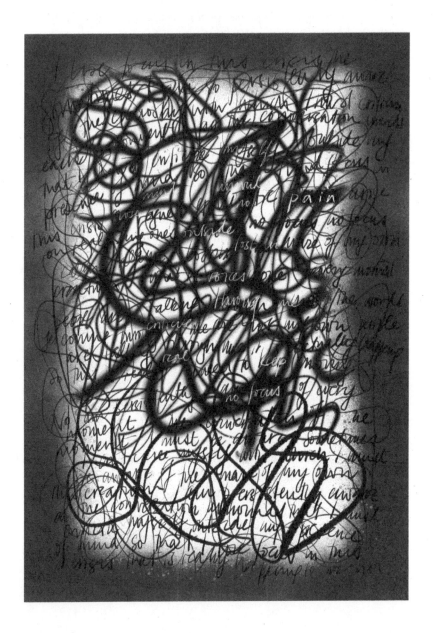

Estelle sits opposite me in the small interview room of the pain clinic where I work once a week. She is a large middle aged woman. She has a downcast but dignified and somehow defiant demeanour. This is the third visit in two months. She is quietly angry but in this there is a curious satisfaction. Nothing has helped. Nothing can help. Her problems are intractable. I and my colleagues who have previously attempted to help her have been defeated. This is too complex, too big for us. The problem gives her stature. She is not in distress. She sits comfortably in her chair and looks at me expectantly. What are you going to do now doctor? She presents the problem as mine, not hers. This has been going on for years. She is used to it. I am not sure that she expects anything to change, but she attends the clinic regularly, insisting that something must be done, that we have failed her.

The problem is pain, and more specifically chronic pain. Of course there is a grey intermediate area but an important distinction needs to be made between acute and chronic forms of pain. Acute pain is by definition of a relatively abrupt onset and for the most part tends to be of a short duration, rather arbitrarily of three to six months. It is usually of biological value, signalling harm or potential harm, and there tends to be a single cause which is more often than not identifiable. In these circumstances a biomedical model is appropriate: a symptom is registered and after examination and the necessary investigations the underlying cause is identified. A diagnosis is made without too much difficulty and the symptom is treated by whatever means considered appropriate and is expected to remit or disappear. The process should be relatively straightforward and treatment is expected to be curative in terms of the elimination of the symptom.

An example may be the symptom of a crushing pain in the centre of the chest. Investigations, such as an ECG or an angiogram might show a constricted coronary artery. A diagnosis is made of cardiac ishaemia. Treatment which might be either medical or surgical, if successful is expected to solve the problem. This is of course simplistic and mechanistic and rarely applicable. The approach is considered to arise probably from an infectious disease model but even in that circumstance it is inadequate. It is not sufficient for example to consider tuberculosis to be caused solely by a mycobactrium. Other factors such as diminished immunity and socioeconomic deprivation might be significant contributory factors that need to be addressed if treatment is to be at all successful.

Chronic pain is a different phenomenon. It is of a more gradual, insidious onset and persists beyond the time expected in terms of current knowledge of basic physiological principles. There is often no single clearly identifiable cause. A wide range of biological, psychological and social and economic and cultural factors act as contributory interacting factors. It is more usefully considered as a problem in itself rather than a symptom of an underlying cause. For these reasons a restrictive biomedical model is woefully inadequate and a broader more systemic biopsychosocial approach needs to be considered. Management is necessarily multidisciplinary and often difficult. Rehabilitation rather than cure is a more appropriate goal of treatment.

Estelle describes being in pain for over ten years. The pain is diffuse. Each enquiry about pain in different parts of her body meets with an affirmative response. The pain is everywhere and it is getting worse. In addition there are other symptoms in other systems. She describes fatigue, a tingling sensation in the extremities, dizziness, the occasional blurring of vision and a debilitating inability to sleep soundly.

She is perhaps more sullen than angry. She has consulted so many doctors, tried so many different kinds of treatment. Nothing has helped. She is resigned. It seems to me now that she does not expect anything to get better. The pain has become part of her world, the way she sees herself.

She lives with an older sister who also suffers from a number of chronic medical conditions. They barely survive on the meagre disability grants they both receive each month. Their many physical symptoms seem to be the main currency of their communication with each other and the outside world.

Estelle describes a deprived childhood. Her father was a drunkard and abusive towards her mother. She is vague and awkward and I do not pursue it but there is a suggestion that she was sexually abused by him in her teenage years. She married young, perhaps to escape from these harrowing circumstances. Her husband repeated the grim story, abusing both herself and her daughter who ran away from the home and whom she now suspects is pregnant at the age of fifteen. Her son is addicted to methamphetamines, is unemployed and steals whatever he can from her pitifully few belongings. It is difficult to listen to this. Misery and helplessness pervade the small room and her life. Pain is not confined to any part of her body. It seeps everywhere. It is the medium of her misfortune.

This is not madness in any conventional sense. Madness more often refers colloquially to the more severe forms of mental illness, and more specifically to the psychoses. This is perhaps stretching the use of the term to its limits, linking madness to an extreme form of suffering, or of a deranged and perturbed way of being in the world. Much uncertainty surrounds the notion of chronic pain, how it may be conceptualized and arising from this how it should best be managed. Part of this uncertainty arises from the limitations of medicine, certainly in the more confined biomedical sense to make sense of the phenomenon. It is more helpful to regard chronic pain less as a medical malady than a form of suffering.

The way we make sense of chronic pain has important and very practical consequences, particularly with regard to how it should be managed. In this regard it is necessary to emphasize that chronic pain in this context is of the vague and diffuse nature described, of unknown or uncertain causes, and frustratingly resistant to treatment. Persisting pain due to cancer, or to the various forms of arthritis do not fit into this broad category and therefore require different treatment approaches. Similarly neuropathic pains or pain due to nerve tissue damage, for example in diabetes or HIV/AIDS or as a consequence of traumatic damage do not meet these criteria. Although the latter neuropathic pains are notoriously difficult to treat these forms of pain tend to be more amenable to medical interventions whereas chronic pain, or what have been described inadequately in the medical literature as medically unexplained symptoms or somatic symptom disorders defy conventional remedies. These might be considered rather abstract issues but the implications of the uncertainties are profound and potentially dangerous. The costs of chronic pain to the economy in terms of lost productivity and the burden on the health services are estimated to run into hundreds of billions of rands or pounds or dollars. The costs in terms of human suffering are inestimable but of great concern particularly in recent years is the escalating death rate due to opioid addiction. This is a consequence of both prescribed and non-prescribed opiates. The great majority are for the treatment of pain. The evidence of benefit of the opiates for the treatment particularly of chronic pain is limited or minimal. Current conventional pharmacological treatments of chronic pain are not effective, are more likely to do harm and are potentially lethal.

Drug overdoses are currently the major cause of death of those under fifty in the United States and are in excess of the number of those who died as a result of HIV/AIDS at the height of the epidemic in 1995. More people are dying as a result of overdoses in the USA than died in the Vietnam and Iraq wars. This is an epidemic that is eminently preventable. The recent surge in these overdoses are due to opioids and the majority of these are prescribed because of a confusion about the nature of chronic pain, and a large part of that confusion arises from the medicalization of suffering that has become a feature of the culture of modern medicine.

I worked in a pain clinic in a teaching hospital for many years. I was asked to join what at that time was an innovative multidisciplinary team and in an early session I encountered Carl. He had been attending the clinic for years and I think he was referred on to me in exasperation, my colleagues feeling there was nothing further they could do to help. He had undergone back surgery many years previously. The operation had failed and he was in persistent pain. He had been prescribed opiates and over the years the dose had increased steadily to a dangerous level. When I first met him he did not appear to be in any distress. His manner was lethargic and nonchalant. He dismissed my concerns about the extremely high doses of morphine he was using. He said he was tolerating it and in a way that was the problem, the need for increasing doses to maintain the same effect.

I think we had become engaged in some form of a bind, in that because the medical profession had failed in regard to the back surgery he believed the opiates were in some way owed to him. I was new to the clinic and perhaps naïve. I felt we had been compromised, and that we were merely maintaining an addiction. I discussed my concerns with my colleagues and I think there was general relief when I discharged him to a chemical dependency unit, although he was resentful. He said pain was the problem, not his addiction to the opiates. How was he to cope without them? I said I did not think we were helping him. The plan was to reduce the opioid dose to a safer level which could then be dispensed by a local clinic but he was not impressed. We parted on unhappy terms. Medicine had failed him yet again.

Some months later I received a message from his mother that he had died. There were no details but the most likely cause of death was respiratory depression due to the opiates. I had no idea what had gone wrong. It was possible that following his discharge from the dependency unit he had managed to obtain the opiates from another source. He was a young man and apart from the pain and the opiates he was relatively healthy. His premature death was all the more tragic because it was preventable.

The first step in prevention would be to not prescribe opioids for chronic pain. With regard to Carl the prescription should have been only for a limited period. Either withdrawing or not initiating treatment with opiates means spending extra time with a patient and a careful explanation of the need to withhold or withdraw what has been conventionally regarded as an effective treatment. This can be difficult and more onerous than simply writing out a script, especially in a busy community clinic with a horde of anxious and impatient patients on the other side of the door. We have all probably done this at some stage in our careers, but we have rarely had to face the longer term consequences of these hasty acts.

The economic burden, the extent of persistent suffering, and the rising death rates as a consequence of treatments that do not work represent a crisis. The concern is that this arises at least in part from a misconceptualization of chronic pain, and that in this respect these grave problems are preventable. The difficulties might arise from the start from what might be considered an abstract or philosophical problem. Dualism is pervasive in medicine and implicit in our ways of thinking. The mind is separate from the body. The mind is intangible. In a materialist culture it is not quite real, or less real than the safe and sound evidence of the physical. In medicine a problem, in this context pain, is conceptualized dichotomously as either physical or psychological. If it is defined as a physical problem it is treated by physical means. If it is defined as psychological things get rather confused. Perhaps it is not really real. Perhaps the problem should be deflected to a psychiatrist. It is one way of at least getting rid of it. This unexamined assumption that a problem is either physical or psychological has serious and potentially dangerous unintended consequences.

Defined as psychological, important physical factors are ignored or neglected. Defined as physical, treatable psychological components, often depression are neglected yet contribute significantly to distress and disability.

Patients were referred to our pain clinic for the most part as a last resort. Within the clinic patients were referred to the psychiatrist as yet a further last resort. It is not difficult to imagine the anger and the exasperation of our patients in this circumstance. They felt both abandoned and disbelieved. "Why am I being asked to see a psychiatrist? Don't they believe me? Do they think I am making this up, that the pain is not real? Do they think I am mad?" were familiar and in many ways understandably indignant complaints. Both at a specialist level and in primary care the results of this practice were predictable. The pain problem became entrenched. The patients were not reassured by any fatuous explanation that there was nothing wrong. They were angered. A further downward step was taken to intractability and a resentful invalidism. In this respect, through misinterpretation and mismanagement chronic pain may be construed as an iatrogenic disorder, or medicine creating its own problems and doing harm.

This problematic dichotomous way of thinking has no basis in neuroscience. There are different pathways in the brain that mediate pain, including very broadly upward stimulating pathways and downward modulating or inhibiting pathways. The upward or ascending pathways activate two fairly distinct centres in the higher centres or the cortex of the brain, one that identifies the location and the intensity of the painful stimulus, the other that mediates the emotional and motivational or behavioural components of the pain. Functional neuroimaging indicates that with chronicity the second pathway becomes more prominent, suggesting that these emotional and behavioural aspects of pain become more powerful perpetuating factors with the passage of time. Appropriate forms of treatment would therefore be to enhance the downward inhibitory systems, usually by pharmacological means, and to address the emotional and behavioural aspects non-pharmacologically, usually with various forms of cognitive behavioural therapy.

Another problem in the way chronic pain is conceptualized and managed is the confusion of causes and correlations. If a mere correlation is misinterpreted as a cause, treating that cause by whatever means is not going to be effective and can do harm. A common example is back pain. An X-ray or an MRI scan might well show abnormalities in the lower spine. It is wrong to assume that these abnormalities are the cause of the pain. Such structural differences are common, are not necessarily associated with symptoms and do not correlate with pain. Surgical treatment will then not alleviate the pain and is more likely to worsen it. This has in recent years become recognized to some extent, and during the years when I worked at the pain clinic there was a significant reduction in surgery for non-specific lower back pain.

Yet another problem is in the direction of causality, or the linear way in which we tend to think of causation. Either A causes B or B causes A. With regard to the common and understandable association of depression and pain the question then arises as to whether the pain is causing depression or whether depression in some way causes pain, or whether chronic pain is a symptom of depression. The relationship is more likely to be circular. Pain and depression interact and lead to a downward spiral. The treatment implication is not to treat either the pain or the depression separately, as a possible cause, but to interrupt the cycle. Trying to identify and treat a single cause for chronic pain in terms of a simplistic biomedical model is doomed to failure. It is more appropriate, and it is not too complicated to address biological and psychosocial factors that might predispose or precipitate or perpetuate chronic pain. Identifying protective factors such as resilience and a sense of self efficacy or being in control is equally important, but in my experience often neglected.

It is probably too late for Estelle. Pain is part of her life now. It is how she sees herself and how she is in the world. It took me some years to question the assumption that our patients attended the clinic for the elimination or the alleviation of their pain symptoms. After so many years there were a significant number who seemed to need, or to hold onto their pain. It had become their way of being, if not coping in the world. Estelle's suffering grants her some form of status and it our duty to register and acknowledge this. I do not think that at this late stage she thinks that we can do anything to significantly reduce the pain yet she attends the clinic regularly. Being a patient, being attended to, waiting for hours for the medications she insists she needs without any evidence of benefit somehow affirms her. She will not allow us to discharge her to the local follow-up clinic. That would be an abandonment, and so we feel trapped in this charade of specialized care. This is probably a familiar experience to many working in pain clinics, a point being reached when you are stuck, when you no longer believe you are doing anything to help and that in reinforcing dependency you might be part of the problem.

It did not, just possibly have to end in this way. If perhaps at the first encounter the harassed junior doctor could have put aside his or her anxieties about the long queue of patients waiting outside and spent a few extra minutes listening to her. A connection could maybe have been made between her symptoms of pain and the many hardships of her life. After the necessary history and examination to exclude a general medical condition the pain might just possibly have been reconfigured as an expression of suffering. In this way no expectations would have been created that the pain could be eliminated, that medicine would solve the intractable problems of her life. It is conceivable that having her hardships acknowledged and the pain given some sort of meaning she might have found some way of coping through the support of her family and friends and her own determination. In this way again it is just possible that by refocusing her attention on the many problems that were causing her distress, rather than the symptoms of this distress, the pain might have withered away or at least not gained control of her life.

Just maybe, imagining pain and madness as forms of suffering rather than mere symptoms or medical problems could lead to more creative and effective ways of understanding and helping.

19

It's all in the mind

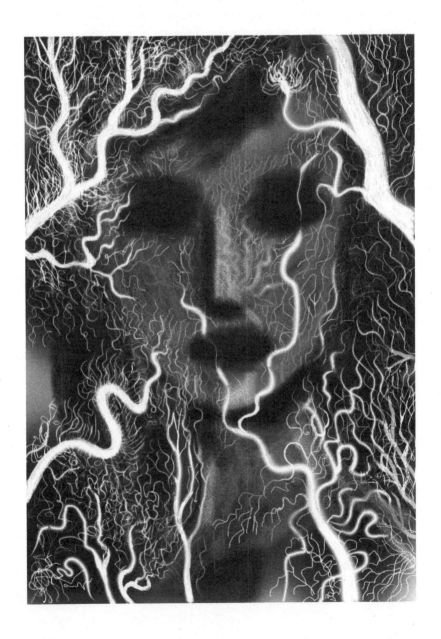

Hlaudi is screaming in one of the dormitories. The patients are terrified. The nurses are running towards him. Blood is pouring from one of his eyes. He is trying to fight off the nurses, but is flailing blindly. The doctor on call is summoned urgently. Hlaudi has taken a spoon from the kitchen and has used it to try and remove his eye. The eye is badly damaged. An ambulance is called and he is taken to the general hospital where the surgeons attempt to save his eye. Too much damage has been done. The eye is surgically removed and Hlaudi returns to the ward. Why has he done this to himself? He cannot give a clear answer other than to say he was told to do it. He had no control he said. He was made to take out his eye. Now he is frightened and angry. He is inconsolable.

All in the mind?

Johan is a successful businessman. He is married with two children. On the surface of things all is well. There is nothing he tells us that can explain the depression that has descended upon him. He has become incapacitated. His colleagues at work have insisted that he take time off. They say he must sort himself out otherwise he will be asked to leave the business he started. His wife is bewildered. She is also afraid. She tells us that his father committed suicide and that her husband has never been able to talk to her about it. She fears he will do the same. She has never seen him in this state. He is transformed. He is inaccessible. He stares at her and the children blankly. They reach out to touch him but he flinches away. He takes no care of himself. He barely speaks. He mutters. He sighs. He does not seem to hear us. "This is not my Johan", the wife cries, "this is not the father of my children. Johan, please talk to us. Tell us what is the matter with you". He looks away.

Is this all merely in his mind?

Marcia has lived with pain for most of her adult life. She had been a lively, energetic young woman. She was a keen and very talented tennis player and her ambition had been to become a professional player. In her final year at school she had strained a ligament in her left leg and was advised to rest for a few weeks. The pain persisted and steadily got worse. It spread to both lower limbs and then to her great dismay, insidiously and remorselessly it engulfed her whole body. She was distraught. She tried everything. Nothing worked. The physiotherapist could not explain why the pain was persisting and spreading. Nor could the general practitioner. Nor could a chiropractor. She became angry when a previous tennis partner suggested that she was exaggerating the pain. She was increasingly desperate. What was to become of her ambitions to become a professional tennis player? What was happening to her? Eventually she consulted an orthopaedic surgeon. He examined her thoroughly and did a number of investigations. He told her there was nothing wrong with her. He said: "it's all in your mind".

All in the mind? Not real? Was she "putting it on", and if so for what purpose?

It is all in the mind, because that is where consciousness resides, but that is not meant when it is said that it is all in the mind. What we usually mean when we say it is all in the mind is that in some deeply strange way that it is not there. It is not real.

When telling me of this encounter Marcia became agitated. She was understandably indignant. If her pain was not real, if it was all in her mind, the explanation could only be that she was making it up, that she was malingering. The implicit allegation was that she was seeking to deceive. This was altogether too much after all the suffering she had been through. Anger and mistrust now compounded her misery. I tried to explain to her, I think without much success, where the surgeon's comments came from.

We are trained to think in an evidence based, biomedical framework. A patient presents with some symptom or another. We take a history and perform an examination and request special investigations in order to seek objective and confirmatory evidence of the diagnosis to explain the symptom. We might prescribe medication not according to a random whim but on the basis of evidence derived from randomized controlled clinical trials. This is all very well but it falls apart in the above circumstances. For Hlaudi and Johan and Marcia there are no objective signs or no special investigations to explain their suffering. To then infer that their symptoms are not real is clearly nonsense. To further infer that the distress arising from these symptoms is not real, and that the symptoms are fabricated is offensive. It is certainly not helpful.

I saw Alicia in the neurology ward. She suffered from epilepsy. She was a bright, surprisingly cheerful young woman in her early twenties. She had coped relatively well with the epilepsy that had developed when she was a child. She was diligent in taking her anti-epileptic medication. She had managed to complete her schooling, gaining sufficiently good grades to consider a course in advertising. The reason why she had been admitted to the neurology ward was that her seizures had mysteriously in the past few months become more frequent. For the first time since the diagnosis was made the epilepsy appeared to be out of control. The reason why I was asked to see her was that there was also something odd about the seizures the staff had observed. The usual stereotyped pattern was not described and the convulsions continued for much longer than normal. There was not the customary shaking but more of a wild and atypical writhing. During this time her eyes were held tightly closed. The incontinence that may accompany such generalized seizures was not observed and there was no self-injurious behaviour. The reflexes were not brisk as usually noted during seizures. When these curious episodes ended she appeared to wake up suddenly, saying: "Where am I? What happened?". More usually after a seizure patients are confused and it takes some minutes to fully regain consciousness. The electroencephalograms showed no indication of recent seizure activity. My colleagues were mystified as to what was going on. Were these real seizures? Was she faking it and if so why?

I told Alicia that there was some uncertainty about the nature of her seizures. There was a change in the pattern and frequency and this was unusual. I asked if I could make some enquiries about what was going on in her life. She said she was struggling. She said she was deeply anxious about embarking on the advertising course. She did not know whether she would cope. She did not know whether she should tell the course supervisors about her epilepsy. She believed that her boyfriend was about to leave her. He said he was scared of the seizures. She thought he was embarrassed to be associated with somebody with epilepsy. There were tensions in her parents' marriage. She feared they were about to become divorced and she blamed herself for the stress her epilepsy might have put on the marriage.

Alicia was not faking these seizures but nor were these seizures due to her epilepsy. The convulsions were not under her voluntary control. The terminology is confused. The word hysteria is of the past and derogatory. In the domain of neurology these episodes would be described as non-epileptic convulsions and in psychiatry a diagnosis of a conversion disorder would probably be made. In this respect a symptom very often of a neurological nature is thought to arise not from a neurological disorder but from psychological and social stressors. The symptom is not intentionally produced and it does not preclude there being a neurological or any other disorder.

I explained this to Alicia in a way that I hoped would make sense to her. She did not appear to have any difficulty in accepting what I said. A referral was made both for her and her parents to see a clinical psychologist. I was told things settled down. The convulsions subsided. She was advised to tell the course supervisors of her epilepsy and to her great relief they told her that that should not in any way prejudice her application. Her parents were able to reassure her that there was no substance to her fears that they were about to separate. The boyfriend went on his way but she told the psychologist that she did not want to be with anybody that was scared or embarrassed by her diagnosis.

Psychiatric problems have physical effects and general medical conditions can have very serious psychiatric consequences but these associations themselves make implicit assumptions of a mind-body dualism. The mind is inherently embodied. There is no mind outside our bodies. Conversely the body can be without mind, as in dementia or a persistent vegetative state following a stroke or a traumatic head injury. The brainstem is intact so the person breathes, the heart beats, but at the higher cortical level there is no activity. There is no consciousness, no mind, only a profound and terrible stillness.

The most obvious and dramatic physical consequence of a psychiatric disorder is suicide. It makes no sense to consider suicide as being all in the mind. Another consequence is anorexia. Anorexia can be life-threatening. It is a deeply mysterious condition. The factors that contribute to its emergence are wide ranging and interactive and include importantly social and cultural influences. That does not make anorexia less dangerous, or ephemerally, all in the mind. It does seem possible that this misunderstanding, or this false assumption that anorexia is somehow psychological rather than a medical disorder contributes to the anguish and the anger that attends this condition. It might also entrench symptoms in order to convince sceptics of the veracity of the patient's predicament.

More commonly psychological factors affect the way a person might cope with a medical disorder. Busisiwe is a vivacious young woman who struggles to accept a diagnosis of systemic lupus erythematosis. It is not possible that this is something that she is going to have to live with and that there is no cure. It is not fair. She just wants to be normal she says, she doesn't want to be a patient. She doesn't want to be bloated with the steroids she will need to take. She doesn't want people fussing over her, pretending not to notice her rashes.

SLE is all the more complicated because of its erratic and unpredictable course. It waxes and wanes. It comes and goes. When the symptoms remit Busisiwe insists that it is all over. There will be no recurrence and she will no longer need to take the treatment. When the rash reappears on her face she is angry and grief-stricken. She rebels. She drops out of school. She begins to use drugs. She becomes promiscuous and she is pregnant at the age of eighteen. Her parents are distraught and helpless. What might have been manageable with difficulty has become increasingly unmanageable. Her future has become bleak.

Khalid is also eighteen and he is also angry. He struggles to accept that he has an insulin dependent diabetes. At one level he understands that without rigorous control of his blood sugars he can become gravely ill. At another level he is disbelieving. He is also defiant. He uses the insulin sporadically. He eats with disregard to sugar. His parents find him comatose in his bedroom. He is rushed to the emergency unit of the local hospital where a diagnosis is made of a diabetic ketoacidosis. He fights with the nurses. He is abusive towards the doctors. This chaotic course continues. Khalid remains deeply resentful of his illness and his adherence to treatment is sporadic. Five years after the diagnosis was first made his left foot is amputated due to an uncontrolled infection. Khalid says he is now a cripple and he is useless and his life is over. Is this all in the mind?

A very wide range of general medical conditions can present with psychiatric symptoms. For this reason every patient undergoes a physical examination on admission to the ward. The great dread is delirium. This can be subtle in that a slightly altered level of consciousness might be difficult to discern, all the more so in a young person who is psychotic and behaviourally disturbed. If missed the consequences can be dire.

Willem was a middle aged man with schizophrenia whom I saw regularly in the out-patient department. He was pleasant and diffident in his manner, and for some time there had been a degree of stability in his illness. When I saw him he was calm and bemused by the anxieties expressed by the staff of the group home where he had lived for years. They said he was not quite himself. There was nothing else. He said he was fine. I reported back to the concerned staff. No, they said, there was something wrong. They knew him well and something in him had changed. I made an appointment to see him in two weeks' time. He said again that there was no problem and that the anxieties of the staff were unfounded. On this occasion, at the conclusion of the meeting, and after getting up from the chair his left foot dragged as he turned to leave the room.

A CT scan showed a large tumour in the frontal cortex of his brain. The staff had been remarkably alert to a subtle shift in his behaviour and did not make the idle assumption that any symptom should be attributed to the schizophrenia. Unfortunately it was too late and Willem died six weeks later.

There are many reasons why people with severe psychiatric

disorders have a reduced life expectancy. One is a bizarre assumption that having been diagnosed with a mental illness persons become disembodied. The mind is not in some separate realm to the body. How mind emerges from matter is a mystery but the neural correlates of consciousness are not.

This confused thinking about the mind in relation to the brain contributes to the stigma associated with mental illnesses. Being intangible and non-substantive, disorders of the mind are perceived as not sharing the gravity of bodily illnesses. It is baffling that the very faculty that makes us who we are in this casual and non-reflective way should be considered to be not quite real.

20

At least it is not going to kill you

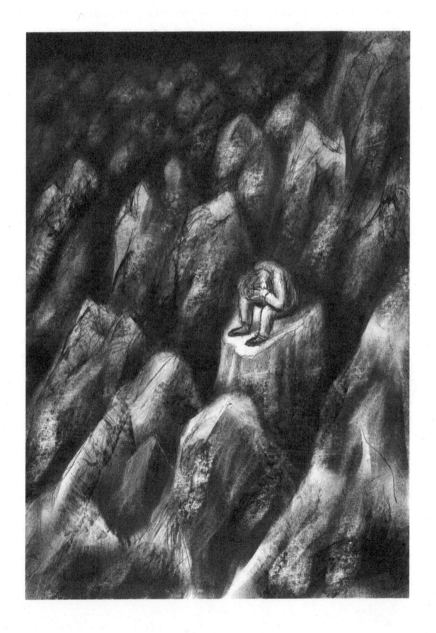

Psychiatric disorders are of less import and less deserving of medical attention because they don't kill you. This is of particular concern in low and middle class countries where resources are limited. Treatment of diseases with the highest mortality rates should be the first priority. Anxiety and depression might be widely prevalent but because these disorders don't kill you they cannot warrant the consideration and the means necessary to save lives. Resource rich first-world countries might be able to afford the luxury of increased spending for mental health services. The rest of the world cannot.

Mortality is a crude and limited indicator of disease severity. Rheumatoid arthritis, and many other muscular-skeletal problems are causes of widespread disability and suffering, as are chronic obstructive airways diseases and a wide range of endocrine and metabolic disorders. These disorders if properly managed don't kill you. That does not make them less serious, either as a cause of suffering or as items of economic cost.

A broader definition of disease severity is the concept of disease burden. A widely used measure is the DALY or estimate of disability adjusted life years. This represents healthy years lost due to disease. It incorporates both mortality and disability and is an estimate of the difference between the current health status and an imagined state of health in which a person might live without disease or disability to old age. The burden is measured in both medical and economic terms. The medical burden is a measure of both morbidity and mortality, morbidity indicating the number of those who are unwell or disabled and mortality the number of people in a population who die prematurely as a result of a specific disease or disability.

The economic burden is direct, involving for example costs of providing medical services, and indirect, involving for example losses to the economy owing to lost productivity. The DALY itself is a limited measure. It does not reflect pain and suffering and makes certain assumptions regarding values or the quality of life. It is uncertain whether or not a premature death is preferable to a life prolonged in suffering. The burden of disease also focuses on the negative, and does not address the important factors that promote wellness and protect against disease and disability.

According to a series of World Health Organization studies the leading cause of disease burden measured in terms of DALY's are cardiovascular disorders. The second leading cause estimated for 2020 is depression. Mortality due to heart diseases might be decreasing owing to improved diagnosis and treatment but disability would then be increasing. There is no hard distinction between what kills you or disables you or causes you suffering.

It does not make any sense that mental illnesses are less important than general medical conditions because they don't kill you, even in terms of the limited but objective measures of the burden of disease. This notion is nevertheless prevalent, especially in areas where conflicts inevitably arise over the appropriate allocation of limited resources, and where these conflicts are driven by ignorance or ill-founded assumptions about the nature of mental illness.

Putting aside these concerns psychiatric disorders are important causes of mortality, particularly in younger people. Suicide is the second most common cause of death in the age group from 15 to 29 years of age. This is a global figure. The statistics will always be imprecise but for those who kill themselves approximately twenty attempt suicide. The great majority occur in low or middle income countries. This is a shameful indicator of the ignorance and hence lack of care provided to those who suffer from mental illnesses.

More common are the more subtle and complicated ways in which mental illnesses contribute to disability and reduced life expectancy. Psychiatric disorders do kill, directly and most dramatically through suicide, but more often indirectly, owing to the very nature of mental illness.

I was especially affected by Timothy's story because we were the same age and were at school together. He was extremely bright and matriculated with distinction. After finishing our schooling we drifted apart. He embarked on a degree in architecture and I studied English and philosophy before medicine. It was to my great dismay that many years later we met again, with him now as my patient.

It was unclear, as it often is, how it all began. There was no obvious family history but again this is often the case. A father or mother might disappear or die prematurely, and it is not known whether or not they or an uncle or aunt or grandparent might have suffered from some form of mental illness. Often shame obscures the truth. Timothy used drugs during his undergraduate years but of course this was not uncommon and his use was not extreme. The drugs would have been described as "soft" which is a meaningless term. Timothy was just doing what many other young people were doing at the time, but for him the consequences were disastrous.

He started to struggle academically and this was mystifying to his parents. There was no doubt that he was intellectually gifted but he seemed increasingly incapable of focusing his attention. This was attributed to the drugs, or perhaps it was rather desperately argued he was too bright and that he was bored by the course. Things got steadily worse and he failed the third year examinations. He refused to return. At about this time he married and started a family.

It was expected that this was just a difficult phase he was going through and it was hoped that maybe the stability of a family might aid the process of regaining control of his life. This was not to be. He became remote from his family. His wife said he was not a father to his children. He declared himself to be an artist but his drawings became increasingly disorganized and inept. Slowly and agonizingly it became apparent to his family that he was ill.

He then abandoned his wife and his young children. He disappeared and then re-emerged insisting that he was now a rock star. He took to the streets, hammering at a broken guitar and singing raucously and without restraint or skill. He was ill-kempt. He began to jabber incoherently. Eventually his appalled, estranged wife made an application for him to be assessed, and after some time he was admitted to our unit, and I became his doctor.

Timothy greeted me amicably and it seemed that he wished to pretend that it was just a chance meeting of two old school friends. There was no problem he said. It was all just a misunderstanding, perhaps a failure on the part of his family to recognize his genius. He was experimenting, he told me, but he did rather begrudgingly acknowledge that he might have gone too far. He was affronted to find himself in a psychiatric hospital. It was ridiculous, he insisted, that he should be punished for bravely going where no other more timid souls might venture.

To my dismay but to the amused delight of the other patients and the nurses he started to sing with abandon to prove the point that he was exceptionally talented. It was not a success. I remember with sadness the puzzlement he showed when it dawned upon him that others did not share his exalted opinion of his singing ability. He became crestfallen. He was confused. He did not seem to know what was going on. Perhaps something was wrong. Perhaps he was ill in some strange way, and perhaps he needed some form of help. He was broken.

Begrudgingly he accepted the need for medication. Things calmed down for a while. He put aside his battered guitar. He resigned himself to the reality that he was not a rock star, and after a few weeks we discharged him from the unit. When I saw him in the out-patient department he was subdued and depressed. What did his life now hold for him without the glorious status of being a star? His movements were slow and lethargic. The tone of his speech was flat. He was making an effort he said, but he indicated that he felt his life was empty.

His wife and children had finally left him. The children now refused to have any contact with him. They told me that they had to get on with their lives, that he had wrought too much havoc, and they could not imagine that any form of reconciliation was ever going to be possible. His wife did make occasional contact with him but there was no longer any intimacy between them. She was understandably angry and she said that she had tried, but that she no longer believed that there was anything that she could do to help him.

He was spending most of his time listlessly with the other residents of the group home. They did not do very much. They smoked. They watched television and they rarely left the home.

Timothy grew bored and restless. It was inevitable that this wan life should become to him an intolerable compromise and that he should again seek the raptures of rock stardom.

So back he came, beating furiously on the guitar that he had retrieved, wailing and shouting and shrieking in some mad belief that his performance was anything other than a noisy and discordant din. After yet another admission he eventually resigned himself to the drab realities of a life that he began to believe had been stricken by his illness.

When we met again in the outpatient clinic he looked unhealthy. He was overweight and he was breathing with difficulty. He was smoking far too much and he did no exercise. He was not looking after himself. He said he didn't care. Smoking was one of the few meagre pleasures in his life.

His difficulties were compounded by the side-effects of the medications he had reluctantly come to accept he needed. Over the years recourse had been taken to the use of increasingly powerful agents to bring him out of his psychotic states, and these medications had inevitably severe and problematic effects on his physical well-being. Although only taken at night one agent was powerfully sedating. Other important side-effect were weight gain and blood lipid or fat disorders. Without doing any exercise, smoking excessively and doing very little with regard to basic health care puts our patients at grave risk of a host of medical risks, including respiratory problems and cardiovascular events, or heart attacks, which are largely responsible for the reduced life expectancy of people living with schizophrenia.

Months later Timothy was struggling to breathe. He told me that he had been diagnosed with chronic obstructive airways disease. He became even more sedentary. The rock star days were over. Now it was an endeavour just to keep going. Showing great determination and strength of character, which was all the remarkable in his depleted circumstances he resolved to stop smoking. It was all too late. His breathlessness grew worse. When I saw him later he seemed much older than his years. It baffled and dismayed me that we were of the same age, and it seemed profoundly unjust that this physical deterioration had been so unfairly wrought upon him by a mental illness for which he could hold no responsibility.

On the next occasion he shuffled into the interview room on crutches. His pallor was grey. He could barely speak. He said he had been diagnosed with an advanced lung cancer. A decision had been made to treat him with radiotherapy. He shrugged. He was resigned. To my distress I formed the impression that he had given up.

Weeks later the manager of the group home asked me to visit him in the general hospital where he had been treated for the cancer. He was bed-bound but he spoke to me warmly and coherently. He said he was unable to move and that this was a mystery to the physicians who were treating him. There was no explanation on medical grounds why he should not have been able to rise from his bed. He did not appear to be depressed. He was calmer and seemed to be more at peace with himself and his circumstances than I had observed for years. He died days later.

Timothy's far too early demise was a consequence of the schizophrenia from which he had suffered for most of his life. The illness did not kill him directly but in many interacting and indirect ways, including his self-injurious behaviour, the effects of medication, a lack of basic self-care, and finally and most importantly the loss I think of the will to live.

It is a nonsense to say that at least mental illness doesn't kill you, both because it can and it does and also because mortality is no measure of the worth and value of life.

21

The cliché of the madness of the world

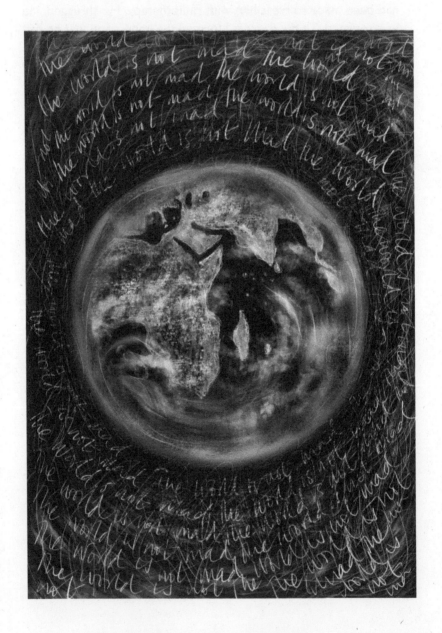

The world is not mad. It is a ridiculous proposition but it is said again and again. Presumably the statement is intended to convey a deep insight into the strangeness and the irrationality of the world in which we live, but the world is not a person and strangeness and irrationality do not equate to madness. It is a glib and fatuous contention and for many of those who suffer from serious mental illness it might very possibly be considered a dismissive cliché.

Mary has lived with schizophrenia for most of her life and so has her mother. They both come to see me in the out-patient department but the mother is managed in private. She accompanies her daughter because the daughter becomes anxious and muddled when she is on her own. The mother does not have confidence that her daughter will tell me the truth of what is happening to her. To some extent she is right. Mary is eager to please. Although she is a woman in her late thirties her manner is childlike. She wishes to reassure me that all is going well and that she is coping and making a great effort not to allow things to get her down.

The mother seems tired and exasperated. "Tell him", she says, "Tell him what happened yesterday". Mary becomes anxious and tearful. I don't think she wants to tell me what happened yesterday. Maybe she is embarrassed. Maybe it has not gone away, whatever it might have been. The mother insists. She is impatient. She is sick of all this she tells me. She is getting older. Who is going to look after Mary when she is no longer capable, and anyway, she tells me, she herself is not well and in no position to help Mary when she suffers these psychotic episodes. She has no support. Both Mary's siblings have long since left home, the one to a city up north and the other to the UK. It seems very probable that they both had fled from a situation that they found suffocating, and that the only way they felt they could survive was to physically separate themselves from their troubled mother and sister.

Mary clearly did not want to discuss the events of the previous day, but the mother says: "How is the doctor supposed to help you if you don't tell him. You can't go on pretending that everything is alright. You are not well". Mary is sobbing now. The mother turns way. This has happened too often. She does not know what to do. Mary will not allow her to leave the room. She needs her mother and her mother cannot help. "It's terrible", she says. It is Albert, one of the residents, or it could be Julian or Thabo or Yusuf or Jacob. Whoever it is on this occasion is tormenting her. "He is trying to hurt me. I know he is. I can see it by the way he is looking at me at the breakfast table, by the way he is holding his knife. He is putting terrible thoughts into my mind. He wants to hurt me. Why is he doing this to me? I have done nothing to him. I thought he was my friend, but now I can see he hates me. He wants to destroy me. It is so unfair. It's terrible. I want to die". Now the mother is in tears. "It is nonsense", she says, "It's all in your mind. It is just not true. You are unwell. It's just your imagination. Nobody wants to hurt you. Everybody likes you. Everybody is trying to help you".

When Mary has eventually left to collect her medication the mother says that on this occasion Mary had started to scream uncontrollably and had had to be removed from the breakfast room. This had caused great distress among the other residents. The manageress had said to Mary's mother that she did not think the situation could continue. It was not fair to the other residents. Unless something was done, and presumably this meant that unless her psychiatrist was able to sort out her medication, she very sadly would have to consider asking Mary to leave. "What am I to do Doctor?. She can't come back to stay with me. I am not well myself. I am not strong, and anyway it's not safe. I know it. It is the neighbours. They are pumping poison through the ceiling of my apartment. They are trying to get me out. Nobody will believe me but it is true. Mary cannot come to stay with me. I won't be able to cope. I will get sick again. Please Doctor, you have got to help us".

This is not the madness of the world. I cannot say to this family, "Oh this is just the way things are. You just need to resign yourselves. The world is mad anyway. There is nothing exceptional in your predicament". Perhaps I might justify such idiotic contentions if I thought it might be therapeutic to change anguish into rage but I think that is fanciful.

One implication of this cliché is that it trivializes mental illness, and in this way fails to acknowledge or blithely dismisses the suffering of patients and their families. Another imputation, and I am not sure if this is made with fully conscious intent, is that there is really no such thing as mental illness. If the world is mad anyway, however ludicrous the notion might be, there is no validity to the phenomenon of mental illness, or in a post-modern context, it is relative to the point of meaninglessness.

Such careless platitudes are not without consequence and do harm. It was difficult for me in the encounter with Mary and her mother to convey to them with confidence that I would be able to help, but mouthing cruel banalities could certainly not be construed as a constructive intervention.

There is a tension between acknowledging the grim reality and the suffering associated with mental illness and the need to be helpful and to be hopeful. Perhaps it is yet another cliché to describe clinical practice as an art but this does to some extent indicate the limits of the biomedical framework and the need to attend to the uniqueness of each presentation. The scientific perspective is both necessary and helpful, but in this encounter there were no fundamental and objectively verifiable strategies that could guide me in how to respond to this mother's plea. It does require some form of a creative balance, being both hopeful and realistic, and there is no knowing whether we get it right, or how often if at all, or what being right might be.

These difficulties cannot distract those involved from addressing the complex nature of mental illness and the problem of delineating its boundaries, but the dismissal of boundaries altogether in the flippant assertion that the world is mad makes no useful or serious contribution.

A linked and equally exasperating cliché that I have had to contend with far too often is the observation that we are all mad. This is delivered as a profound insight, frequently over a glass of wine or on some social occasion where to take issue would cast one as being earnest and boring. Being mad in this sense would appear to be free, to be one's true self, unfettered by social convention, to joyfully discard the constraints of whatever might quite arbitrarily be considered normal.

It is again unclear as to whether the consequences of this have been thoughtfully considered. Perhaps part of my irritation is due to the implication that if we are all mad the notion of mental illness has no validity, and the profession of psychiatry is therefore fraudulent. In this regard psychiatrists are not doctors, seeking to alleviate distress and restore a degree of function in those diagnosed with mental illness, but social policemen, seeking to maintain order, and taking it further, punishing those who stray with incarceration and stupefying medications. Psychiatrists are agents of the state, tasked with maintaining the status quo. Healing, according to this position, is merely bringing the wayward back into the fold. It is fundamentally coercive.

I do not doubt that there are malpractices in psychiatry and in general medicine, and I do not doubt that psychiatry in particular is prone to such malpractices. There are many reasons for this, among which are the absence of any objective signs of mental illness and related to this, the shifting and extending boundaries of what might be considered to constitute mental illness.

Persons with political opinions that are regarded as a threat to the security of the state, or that are simply awkward have been, and no doubt continue to be considered mentally ill in many parts of the world and excluded in different ways from society. This is an egregious and cynical abuse of psychiatry.

In the complaint that the statement that the world is mad or that we are all mad trivializes mental illness I am aware that in using the term madness I am open myself to criticism for a similar offence. The term madness may be interpreted as being careless, loose, vague, dismissive, unscientific and provocative. I would be very disturbed if my use of the word has caused distress to others. It would be entirely contrary to my aims if this use of language were to be regarded in any way as pejorative. I will have failed dismally if the use of the term madness was in any way read to reflect a lack of respect for those who suffer from mental illness, or a lack of regard for the complexity and the inevitable controversies and uncertainties that surround mental illness. I accept that it is possible that the word madness can cause hurt, and we are all therefore obliged to use the term with great care and caution.

The intention is to broaden the context, to take this difficult and contested subject beyond the confines of medicine. The medical perspective is necessary and useful but it is insufficient to address the wide ranging philosophical and ethical, historical and cultural and economic and the many other perspectives that have a bearing in this domain. The notion of a mental illness also confines an often bewildering and frightening experience to a pathology or a deficit. It implies a state of normality or mental health that for many is elusive or indefinable. Particularly with regard to the psychoses the phenomena of a disturbed sense of agency, of an altered consciousness of what might constitute the self raises issues of what it is to be human and conscious that surely reach beyond the objectively verifiable categories of a psychiatric diagnosis.

Mrs. Khumalo seems rather irritable and impatient. We are gathered in a ward round and she has been describing to us the ordeal of getting her son Manto into hospital. A group of medical students are attending. I am required in the interests of the discipline of psychiatry to ask questions that might lead us to one diagnosis or another. Following the conventions of clinical medicine this is necessarily a systematic and ordered process. It is not merely that an impression is gained, or that a few vague and arbitrary questions throw up a random diagnosis. These diagnoses have significant consequences. They might grant access to a disability grant but they can also be stigmatizing. A psychiatric diagnosis is also notorious in that it sticks to one. It is difficult to undo. A diagnosis of tuberculosis for example might be something of the past, a diagnosis of schizophrenia much less so.

The questions are dutifully asked and it becomes clear from the history provided by the mother that her son is probably suffering from schizophrenia.

There are a host of misconceptions attached to this label so I feel obliged to confer this probable diagnosis with hesitant caution. Mrs. Khumalo does not appear to be very interested. Schizophrenia, ukuthwasa, amafufunyane, ukuthakathwa, what does it matter she seems to be suggesting to us. The terms are irrelevant. Her son is sick. He has gone mad. She knows this and that is why she has brought him to the hospital. There is something very wrong and it is our duty to make him better.

The questions we ask, the labels we use and the diagnoses we propose are of much lesser import than the urgency of fixing the problem and getting her son home. She appears to us to be unimpressed by our attempts to be cautious, and it seems quite likely to me that our tentativeness is interpreted as a lack of certainty. Mrs. Khumalo very understandably wants certainty, and that certainty is not about any diagnosis that we might make but that this nightmare will soon be something of the past, and that her son will be restored to her.

The world is not mad. Neither cruelty, injustice and inhumanity, nor mere eccentricity of behaviour, nor the refusal to conform to social convention are symptoms of mental illness. To regard these familiar characteristics of human behaviour as such is demeaning to those who suffer from mental illness.

I am not sure what might be or should be the most appropriate language. Madness is problematic and may cause offence. Mental illness confines a wide and complex range of symptoms and signs of distress to a medical subspeciality. Underpinning whatever terms are used is the need to acknowledge pain and suffering, and not to dismiss these very human experiences with clichés and platitudes.

22

Madness is not a metaphor

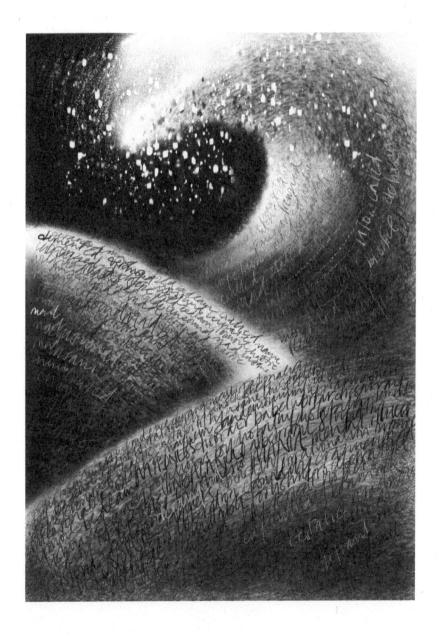

You are mad. You are sick, you are exceptional, you are very brave or stupid. I am mad. I am angry, I am intensely moved, I have been pushed beyond the limits of my endurance. It is mad. It is wonderful, it is extreme, it is profoundly ill-judged. Mad is bad. It is a mad option. In Afrikaans the colloquial term is mal. In French mal means bad. It is good. It is a maddeningly beautiful. I was so mad about her that I was mad with anger and mad with sadness when she turned against me. She was mad to refuse everything that I had to offer her. Mad is fantastic and absurd and nonsensical. A welter of metaphorical associations distorts ideas about mental illness.

Martin is sitting opposite me in one of the out-patient clinic rooms. He is earnest, determined that I should understand. "I am not mad Doctor. It's true". He told me that he was under attack. His assailants were firing bolts of electricity at him causing him great pain and emotional distress. It was a profound injustice he said. He had done nothing to deserve this terrible assault on his body. "It's not fair, doctor. It's not right. They just keep on at me. There is nothing I can do". He is insistent that I believe him, that I accept that what is happening to him is real and not a part of his illness. Nor should I think that the excruciatingly painful bolts are figurative in any way. "It's really happening" he says again and again "It's not what you think it is. I'm not delusional. It's real. You must believe me".

I am not to think that what he is experiencing is as if he is being attacked. It is not as if anything. It is not a metaphor. It is too real. He becomes agitated, I think by his impression that I am seeking to interpret his experience as a mere symptom of something else, an illness. He is driven by a determination that the reality of what is happening to him should be acknowledged. This need seems of greater importance to him that the attacks should stop. Interpreting his anguish as delusional and treating it as such for him would be a repudiation of something personally meaningful. Being believed was the overriding priority.

This need I think is not sufficiently recognized in standard clinical practice and there are problematic consequences. A patient confiding in these deeply strange experiences would be likely to feel disbelieved and therefore dismissed as mad or delusional. Any hope for developing some form of trusting therapeutic relationship is then undermined. This in itself might seem a rather abstract or romantic concept that is of little practical import. A therapeutic alliance might sound right, and ought to be integral to an aspirational standard of best clinical practice. In the grim and time constrained routines of a busy and chaotic admissions unit such an alliance is nevertheless considered to be unrealistic. This is wrong. Non-adherence to treatment leads to poor outcomes and early relapse and readmission rates. Believing that you are believed lays a foundation of trust that increases the likelihood of adherence to treatment, but also something beyond that, and something less measurable, that you are not irredeemably other, that you are acknowledged and not invalidated.

The capacity to abstract might itself seem rather an abstract nebulous quality. It is perhaps difficult to think of it as a fundamental strategy for survival, as being essential to coping in the quotidian world. A failure of abstracting ability, in association with a constellation of other rather vaguely defined functions including goal formation, sequencing and problem solving form part of the neurocognitive domain of deficits in schizophrenia. These contribute significantly to the disability of the disorder and to poor prognoses, and remain relatively resistant to treatment. These impairments are not specific to schizophrenia and are encountered in other severe psychiatric disorders such as the dementias. Carers might be familiar with the confusion and wearying exasperation of an elderly family member, because of sequencing problems, failing to put on his socks before his shoes, or being unable to perform the most basic and comforting tasks such as making a cup of tea, of not buttering the bread before putting it in the toaster. The relatively complex cognitive faculties underlying these apparently simple tasks are taken for granted until things fall apart, until one becomes incapacitated, perhaps more obviously in states of dementia and more insidiously in schizophrenia. The part of the brain subserving this abstracting function is known as the dorso-lateral prefrontal cortex, a term that is of course of utter irrelevance to Martin and the exhausted carers of their demented family members.

Treating madness as a metaphor burdens Martin in different ways. What is happening to him is denied. It is not real. It is a symptom. It is a symptom of an illness that means what is happening is not really happening. It is enough to make you mad, or certainly angry. This is further complicated by the notion that this illness is not an illness at all. It is a metaphor. The metaphor itself is confused by a plethora of contradictory meanings. It is extreme, exceptional. It is evil. It is calamitous.

Martin told me: "I try to find a word, a barrier or protection...to rid myself of these connections induced in my body... I am bombarded by too many people, too many psychic forces... the outside world, my enemies invade my private world...it's terrible...so many nights I have been under attack".

There is no metaphorical space in these utterances, no protective distance. He is bombarded. He is invaded. It is terrifying because it is immediate, vivid. It is so intensely real to him that he seeks to protect himself. He does not have the space or the capacity to console himself that this is not really happening to him, that it is just a terrible dream or that it is confined to his imagination. Intriguingly his defensive strategy is language. He tries to find a word, a symbol to create some distance, a barrier for himself against the invasion.

In the more severe forms of the schizophrenia spectrum patients become mute. I have never encountered Martin in such a state of stupor but I remember Petrus clearly. He had been admitted to the unit as a matter of urgency, having withdrawn into a profoundly silent psychotic world during the preceding week. In the past few days he had stopped eating and then to the great distress of his family he stopped taking any fluids. They knew that if this persisted it could become a medical emergency, as dehydration could rapidly lead to kidney failure. Perhaps most unnervingly was the absence of any visible sign of distress. He was completely and profoundly unresponsive. He gazed through me. In his world I was not there. I don't think that at that time for him there was an external world. He had become engulfed by it.

Martin had at least found some precarious protection, some distance in finding the words to articulate his experience. Petrus had sunk beyond this. He was lost to us. He sat completely still in his chair, seemingly unperturbed by the dismay of those around him, remote, catatonic, utterly confounded by his internal turmoil.

"When I'm sick the machine comes on... there is no barrier...I was too much into this thing to question it...it would drive me completely insane...it's a man's worst nightmare, this remote brain control...there's no escaping it...".

This was Xolani after he had emerged from a catatonic state that was similar in many ways to that of Petrus'. Like Martin he had sought some form of barrier, but as the psychosis developed there was no escape. Like Petrus he was too much into it to question it, to even find a language to articulate it. In these depths it is just terrifyingly happening. There are no metaphorical spaces to provide some refuge. There is no alternative reality. The wretched machine controls everything. Its pervasive force overwhelms his defences. It is a nightmare but it is not a nightmare. It is really happening. As he emerges he finds some space. He needs a metaphorical explanation for the bewildering experience he has been through. He wants me to understand. There is no meaningful signal. There is no pattern, nothing that he can latch onto, no rescue raft in the cruel sea, no clarity, only noise, only a blur. He infers I think that the remote brain control is an immersive experience, that all senses are overwhelmed and that he was drowning. He is describing to me very probably the experience in which Petrus seemed to be so hopelessly trapped.

"You make me mad". "It is a mad world". We use these metaphors to lay emphasis or to expand on what we wish to convey. It is inevitable, but metaphor diminishes madness.

23

The romance of madness

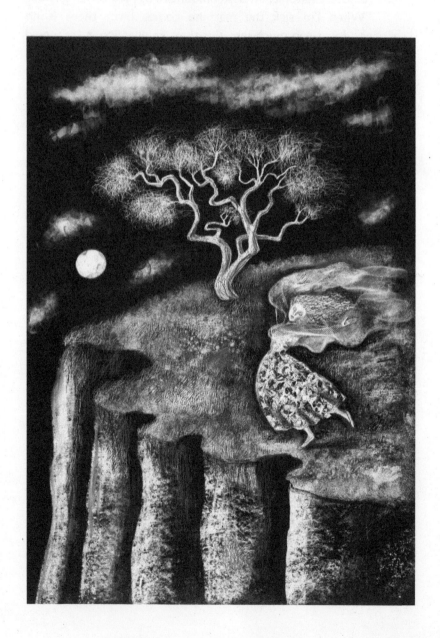

Madness is freedom. Madness is liberating. To be creative you need a little madness. Normality is confining. It is boring. It is grey. It is insipid. To impose normality is to deprive persons of their right to be how they choose to be. It is to shackle them, to chain them to convention. It is what the men in white coats seek to do, brandishing their syringes filled with sedating drugs. Psychiatry is inherently oppressive. Doctors and nurses work in collaboration with pharmaceutical companies and with the state to impose conformity, to induce passivity and to profit from what they call mental illness but what is in reality a heroic defiance of mediocrity.

There is an understandable need or wish to romanticize madness. It would provide at least some comfort but it would be false. I can think of no patient I have known who has in any way believed their madness to be either liberating or creative.

It is conceivable that the disinhibition, increased energy and divergent ways of thinking might dispose to a degree of creativity, but those are not defining features of madness. There is certainly no evidence that mental illness is a requisite for creative genius and the vast majority of those who show exceptional abilities have no history of madness, as the vast majority of those who suffer from various forms of mental illness show no signs of a special creativity. It might just be argued that there is a correlation between creativity and mild and some moderate forms of mental illness but this does not apply to the psychoses.

Perhaps the most obvious association is with mania. Mania fills you with energy. It vitalizes you. It makes everything possible but it does not. It might make everything seem possible, but that is illusory, and it frequently ends in tears.

Gavin only came to see me in the out-patient department when he was in trouble, which was often. He was a charming, handsome man but on this occasion he seemed tired and depressed and his appearance was dishevelled. He was in pain. He hobbled awkwardly into the room on crutches. He had fractured both ankles, doing something he said was "mad". He had fallen from a window ledge, trying to get into a girlfriend's apartment. He said it was a crazy thing to have attempted, but that he had been manic and believed that it was possible. He had been a fool he said and now he felt humiliated. As had happened on so many occasions he had stopped the mood stabilizing medications I had prescribed. He believed that he did not need them. He believed they took something away from him, and he said, as he had said before so many times that he believed he could control his mania. I wished he could. It was ruining his life.

Previously he had been able to somehow bounce back from the damaging consequences of his manic escapades. He would laugh at the craziness of it. He would construe his recklessness as exuberance but now he said he was getting tired and he was feeling older. It was no longer exciting. He had lost too much. His wife had finally left him, angry and exasperated by what she regarded as his irresponsible and feckless behaviour. His children did not want to see him. They said they were teased at school because their father was "mad". He had lost his job as an advertising executive. What he had regarded as brilliant initiatives were dismissed by his colleagues as outlandish, and his manner towards them became increasingly hostile and contemptuous until he was asked to leave. Now his girlfriend had told him that she no longer wanted to see him. What she had considered initially to be high spirits she now regarded as "sick and stupid". He tried to smile but he was dejected and forlorn. Maybe at some stage in the past he had been able to romanticize his manic episodes, but now that was impossible and he regarded his illness as a curse.

Felix had been admitted the previous evening following an urgent application made by his father. He was a very large man and he was in a rage. It was one of the few occasions that I became aware that the nurses were intimidated by a patient. He was belligerent and volatile. He was also highly intelligent and he was entitled, making constant demands and threatening the nursing staff and the other patients with violence.

His father had contacted me a few days earlier. He was in tears. His son had assaulted him. An argument had started over a business decision. The son was a partner in the family's very successful estate agency. The son was clearly manic, and had informed his father of a proposal that the father believed would be financially ruinous. The father had told his son that he thought it was a very bad decision, and that his judgement was impaired because he was ill. This had provoked the son to assault his elderly father, leading to his involuntary admission to the hospital. His fury was fuelled by his refusal to acknowledge that anything was the matter with him. It was his father who was stupid and preventing him from making a vast fortune. Everybody was stupid. Nobody understood how brilliant and rich and powerful he was. He did not belong in a hospital. We were holding him unlawfully. He would sue the health department. He would sue us all. He had very important friends in very high places and he would soon get out of the hospital and do what he had to do and we would all be in a lot of trouble. This ranting went on for hours and exhausted everybody. His mania expressed itself in an arrogance that made it difficult to sympathize with him. It was difficult not to be affected by the contempt and disdain he showed towards us.

When I saw him again after he had been discharged he was a different person. He was abject. It was pitiful. He sat slumped in a chair and sighed and said that he had ruined everything. What most upset him was that his daughter had said she wanted nothing more to do with him. She was tired and angry and humiliated by his outrageous behaviour when he was manic. On this occasion, prior to the assault on his father he had clumsily attempted to make a sexual pass at one of her schoolfriends. The friend was terrified. The daughter could not go on apologizing for her father. He was being totally irresponsible. Why did he always stop taking his medication? He knew what would happen. She had lost all sympathy. He had wanted to say how sorry he was but she was refusing all contact.

Felix had now sunk into a deep depression. He was listless. He could not work. He could not make decisions and the business was in a crisis. He had lost all motivation. He was a talented musician, and playing the piano had in the past been a source of great pleasure for him. Now this was inconceivable. What was the point? Nothing was going to help. There was no romance in this predicament, nor had there ever been.

There is a long and familiar list of writers and poets who have suffered from depression with its attendant maladies of alcohol abuse and suicide. In this association there seems to be an assumption of causality, the direction of which is unclear. Is one driven into a state of depression by being more aware of the true nature of the world, and feeling a need to articulate this in some creative form, or does being depressed make us more creative, as if that is some sort of compensation, or could change things? I think the association between creativity and madness is for the most part romantic. There might be some link between creativity and of being of an unquiet and troubled mind, but that is not madness.

One of the most incapacitating features of a severe depression is a loss of energy and volition. You can do nothing. You want to do nothing. You are in a state of paralysis. There is no light and no shade. There is no colour. You are deprived of the very elements that are necessary to engage in any form of creative activity. Not only do you not have the energy but you don't see any purpose in re-imagining or reconfiguring the world to make it a more interesting or a better place. It is all futile and hopeless. Alcohol might seem to provide some way of coping with this, but after a transitory and illusory lifting of the spirits this only entrenches the emptiness and the helplessness. This is not conducive to creativity.

It is possible that in states of recovery one might be motivated to try to make some sense of the experience of depression in poetry or music or in any other art form. I struggle to recall any such creative response, but then of course my involvement is very partial. I don't get to see the bright side. More often there is an understandable reluctance to return to that darkness.

Finding any kind of romance in schizophrenia is even more improbable. It might be imagined that seeing things in such a different, albeit distorted way might dispose to creativity. Again in my experience, for the most part limited to psychotic disorders it does not. It disposes to fear and avoidance.

The association of madness and creativity throughout history seem to be embedded in the popular imagination. Virginia Woolf, Sylvia Plath, Hemingway, Schumann, Van Gogh are usually included in a familiar list, but there is no reason to believe that the association in these individuals and many others works in the same way. Their madness, and I doubt if that is the right way of describing their troubled states of mind, cannot be assumed to be shared and is specific to themselves. In all probability Van Gogh would have used or not used or suppressed his troubled spirits to make his art in quite a different way to Hemingway or Woolf. It is merely a fairly loose association. In this respect madness seems to be more equivalent with being exceptional, or highly original, or at least not normal. Those are positive attributes. That is not madness. That is not something that can in any way be imagined as an illness. Madness does not enhance creativity. It is more likely to destroy it. It would be nice to think otherwise, it might provide at least some consolation, but in madness there is no romance.

24

Madness and the theatre

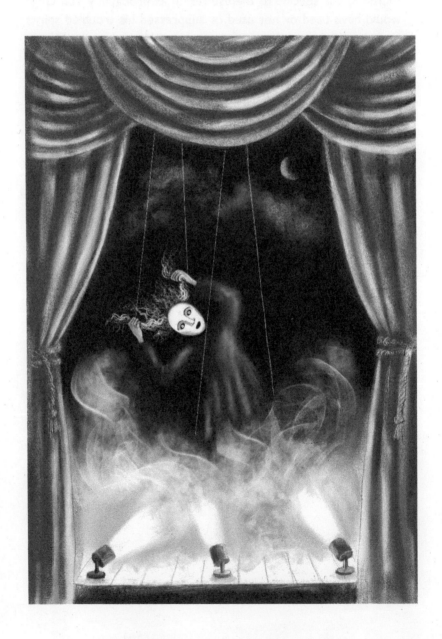

A friend who is a lecturer in theatre studies at the university asked me to talk to her students. They were planning to put on a play that in some part involved madness and she told me that she wanted to do this in a way that was authentic and respectful. I was impressed and agreed very willingly to meet with the students to give them at least some idea of the reality of serious mental illness. I had become exasperated by the banal and offensive stereotypes of madness so frequently and carelessly portrayed in theatre and film.

We met in one of the rehearsal rooms on the campus. The students were eager and thoughtful and asked interesting and intelligent questions. I told them about my work in the admission unit of the hospital and I attempted to demonstrate some of the core features of psychosis and more specifically schizophrenia.

I remember being quite pleased with my performance of a formal thought disorder. This is probably the most difficult symptom to imitate. It is nonsense to think that patients can with ease pretend to be mad. I can remember only one occasion when a patient sought to deceive us and he was unable to sustain it for longer than twenty four hours and the context of his admission made it clear that he was malingering. The patients are under more or less constant surveillance and it is not possible to consistently sustain the simulation of psychotic symptoms, and in particular a formal thought disorder for that period of time. I have never witnessed a remotely plausible portrayal of a formal thought disorder in any play or film.

I performed thought blocking and derailments and loosening of associations and I naively thought that I might have been effective in persuading the students of the need to be careful and to avoid the pitfalls of melodrama and sensationalism. I was invited to the opening night and I looked forward to the performance, and in particular how the lead actress playing the part of the mad young woman would portray the symptoms of psychosis that I thought we had carefully considered. On the night there was an excited atmosphere of anticipation. The director had a reputation of daring and experimental theatre work. I was unfortunately seated in the front row. The light dimmed and there was darkness and then a loud shriek and a crash and the young woman staggered onto the stage. She was completely naked and covered in faeces. She pulled her hair. She rubbed herself. She stormed about yelling and moaning. I suppose it could be said that it was a powerful performance. It had nothing to do with schizophrenia.

I have only once encountered a naked patient covered in their own faeces. This was David, a middle aged portly man who when he was well was mild-mannered and extremely intelligent and articulate. On this occasion he was raving. He stood in the middle of the ward brandishing a chair with which he was trying to hit me. He was enraged, incoherent, grotesque in his nakedness and madness. The other patients were horrified. They cowered behind the tables in the dining room where this miserable and humiliating scene was being enacted. This was not something that would be presented in a theatre or on film or in an opera. This was too grim and ugly, it was too awful.

More recently I attended a performance by a group of professional actors. Again the subject was madness. Again I had been consulted and assurances had been given regarding respect and authenticity and again my tentative contributions were utterly and it appeared quite joyfully dismissed. The cast frolicked about in blissful abandon. The women shrieked and took off their clothes. The men masturbated with crazed determination. One character seemed to consider that this was all insufficiently mad and had stuffed a giant plastic phallus into his pants. Such was the energetic frenzy of his performance that the phallus became dislodged and the ridiculous object was flung onto the floor. This had a deflationary effect. The cast seemed momentarily to be embarrassed. The actor scrambled to reinsert the ludicrous encumberment back into his pants. The audience laughed. The performance thereafter seemed more muted, more stilted, as if the actors had become self-conscious and were unable to retrieve the liberating disinhibition of their caricatures of madness. It was dispiriting, but I suppose not disillusioning. It had happened so often before and I was not going to make any difference despite my earnest attempts.

This disregard of the reality of mental illness, this disdain of the very phenomena that ostensibly are sought to be portrayed is difficult to fathom. It is exasperating and hurtful to those profoundly affected in particular by psychotic disorders, and it is usually this group that are depicted in these lurid ways. Watching somebody have a panic attack is just not titillating or exciting or sufficiently dramatic. These representations also seem exploitative. The suffering of others is fodder for the amusement of the audience, and for the evocation of pity and fear and the consolation that one is not in such a way afflicted. This circus of clichés and caricatures affords vicarious pleasures but also does harm. It is seldom that we read textbooks or scientific articles to inform ourselves about mental illness. Whether intentionally or not we become informed by accounts in literature and film and theatre. We rarely bother to determine whether or not these representations are truthful. Of greater concern is the quality of the performances, or of the production, and whether we were moved or not, or sufficiently entertained.

Agatha Christie's The Mousetrap is acclaimed as the longest running play in the history of the west end of London. It has probably reached hundreds of thousands . The dramatic tension arises from the mystery surrounding the identity of the murderer who must be one of a small group of contenders. At the climax of the performance the murderer is identified by a policeman. This policeman who appears to work as a psychiatrist on the side declares the murderer to be "obviously mad" before he is led away to be sedated and incarcerated. The perpetrator is quite obviously not mad, having planned the murders with great skill and forethought, and with understandable motivation. It is difficult not to think that many of the thousands who have attended this play will not have formed an impression that the criteria for madness must include the capacity for deceit and the committal of evil acts.

It is possibly naïve to think that the arts in general have any sort of responsibility, and in particular a responsibility to educate. The arts are just a form of human activity. It may seem rather pompous to assume there should be any obligation to fulfil any function at all. The arts reflect just one aspect of the exuberance of the market place, a response to the random flows of supply and demand, of fashion or the vagaries of intellectual discourse. One person seeks distraction, another to be informed, another excitement. We are all happily free to make our choices, and it is only in non-democratic or totalitarian systems where what we read and see and hear are determined for us, and this would be regarded not as art but indoctrination. This in itself is something of a caricature, but sometimes it can be helpful to consider a problem in terms of its opposing extremes, if only to find a feasible middle ground or compromise.

So on the one side of the ring we have a joyful, no holds barred free for all, with no strings or duties attached, where every spectator or consumer, user or punter can surely find what they want. On the other side is the grim and rather stern and sanctimonious and cautious contender for something more serious, more careful and responsible. It should be no surprise as to whom the baying crowds are most likely to support. It is no contest.

In this ridiculous scenario there is a question about the importance and the need for the arts in general, and flowing from that, what might be considered good or serious art, what criteria might be used to draw those conclusions, and what in any case might constitute an artistic activity. Another way of considering these polarities might be a tension between cynicism and idealism. The one goes with the other, and there can be no moralistic argument about what art should or not do, or with what is should concern itself. It seems to be more a question of finding spaces, and finding ways of enabling us to think and feel in different, hopefully more imaginative and creative and therefore more helpful ways.

I am perplexed by the different experiences I have when attending a theatrical production and what it might be that elicits these various responses. On one occasion I am bored, irritated, wishing I was somewhere else, and on another engrossed, stimulated, provoked into setting in motion my own train of thoughts. In the one circumstance the proscenium arch seems rigid and alienating, in the other it is disappears. In one production

I am a spectator, in another a participant. In trying to understand my confused responses it seems that being a mere spectator induces an unease, that being passive means being helpless or superfluous to whatever might be happening beyond the proscenium arch. In this situation I don't know what the point is of being there. There are no spaces to rethink or reimagine or to reflect. We are required to laugh or cry, or to be angry or awed. In these kinds of production we are also players, under direction, following a script, responding to cues, until or unless we become restless or disenchanted and disengage.

Another way is to cultivate the space. The book, the film or the play or opera is a sort of proposal, a means, not an end in itself to look beyond, or to look differently at the world, so that circumstances do not seem to impose themselves upon us but provide opportunities to think and feel and behave differently, and possibly to be more free. The representations of madness in theatre can reinforce stereotypes and compound alienation and exclusion or imaginatively and profoundly change accustomed and uncritical ways of thinking. I don't think it is naïve or idealistic to believe that as harm can be done the arts or humanities can also be of great value in changing perceptions about mental illness. With changed perceptions comes the hope of better understanding, and therefore improved care and inclusion. With these possibly rather lofty and ambitious thoughts in mind I attended yet another performance of a well-known opera. It included what had then come to seem an almost obligatory mad scene.

A grimly predictable portrayal was imposed on the audience. The lighting was dim and figures moved about in silhouette, seeking, I suppose to create an atmosphere of a nether world, a world of lost, abandoned souls. Figures in white gowns moved randomly about the stage like wraiths, animated at intervals by the familiar shrieks and jerks. It was, I think intended to be horrifying or harrowing, but it was more like a pantomime. The persistence of these falsifying caricatures continues to confound me. It might be merely wishful to assume that there is any serious intention to portray mental illness in a realistic or respectful manner. Something else is going on, and it seems possible that madness is being presented as a metaphor, or as a means of escape from a rational and a bleak reality.

In this respect madness is imagined as liberating. Being mad you can be free to express your deeper self, to give vent to your thrilling and dangerous passions. This most often and conventionally seem to involve sex and violence. This is trite and superficial but is also demeaning. If an artistic performance seeks to be taken seriously, if we take the trouble to go to the theatre in the expectation that we might learn something, or be provoked into thinking about something in different ways, these thoughtless distortions are likely to lead to cynicism and a disenchantment with any notion of the potential value and importance of the arts. Theatre serves merely to distract and entertain. It is frivolous. It can make no useful contribution to the real world. Medicine and the arts are two different worlds.

The morning after this dismal experience I set out to write what turned out to be a short opera or cantata with the title: "Madness: Songs of Hope and Despair". Anger and exasperation do not seem to be particularly worthy motivating factors, and perhaps my attendance at that theatrical event was more of a precipitant of something I had wanted to do for some time. Certainly a central motivation was to create something that was authentic. At that stage I had no clear idea what that something was, or what form it should take other than that is should stand in emphatic contrast to the false and exploitative representations I had previously encountered.

Another, in some way related motivation arose from another frustration concerning the nature of the scientific perspective. Central to this are the necessary and valuable principles of objectivity, experimentation, verification and replication. These scientific methods have been of enormous benefit and provide the sound basis of modern medicine. A scientific foundation separates medicine from mere quackery. An objective stance is fundamental, but it seemed increasingly to me that it was not enough, and that valuable information was being lost or neglected by not including the subjective perspective.

Persons experiencing psychotic symptoms are not mere objects but subjects. Describing the terror of one's thoughts being stolen by a machine might validly be described as a persecutory delusion but that seems insufficient. Merely ticking the boxes of a checklist of psychotic symptoms is an impoverished way of comprehending the rich and informative complexity of psychotic worlds. This objectivizing stance neglects the experience of psychosis. It pays no heed to the meanings a person might attach to their symptoms, and to personal strategies of recovery. It seems excessively reductive to assume that because something is not quantifiable it is not real or meaningful.

A central idea was therefore that the voices of the patients themselves should be used. Confidentiality could be assured without too much difficulty by changing names and avoiding specific accounts that could identify individuals. I asked the permission of my patients. Without exception they agreed enthusiastically. They did not seem overly concerned about the confidentiality issues. They said they wanted their stories to be told.

I had made previous attempts to describe first person narratives, but certainly in the mainstream journals little priority is accorded to qualitative studies, and my verbatim accounts seemed to me bland and prosaic. Literal records of patients' psychotic experiences somehow did little justice to the strangeness and at times the surprising beauty of their vivid, intensely lived, mad worlds. It seemed more possible that this might be articulated by moving beyond the conventions of theatre and integrating words with music and images, and so a collaborative project emerged.

In addition to the voices of the patients it was important to include the other voices that contribute to the process of assessment and management in the acute phases of a psychotic illness, including the nurses, the doctor, the family, the lover. A neuroscientist, a traditional healer and a priest also sing songs that reflect the various and at times conflicting perspectives that form part of this turbulent process. A chorus is made up both of patients and the nurses seeking to comfort them. The libretto tries to communicate the confusion and the fear and ambivalence of the patients and also some of the anxieties and uncertainties of those seeking to help them. Both the music and the projected images aim to express the shifts in coherence and clarity and relative calm to chaos and disharmony and discordance. The natural inclination to find patterns or to construct a meaningful narrative are deliberately disorganized. We sought to dislocate the senses and then establish fleeting moments of coherence to imagine madness.

There is no nakedness in the performance, no masturbation, no screaming and manic prancing about the stage, only a determined respectful austerity. The intention is both to describe in an as authentic way possible the wide variation in the expression of psychosis, but also to evoke the sense of a mind in turmoil, to attempt to create a sense of what it must be like to be inside, to be there.

Madness: Songs of Hope and Despair was first performed at the World Psychiatric Conference in Cape Town in December 2016. There was acclaim. It was gratifying. Melodrama is superfluous and unnecessary.

I don't know if it will make any difference, but we tried.

25

Art and madness

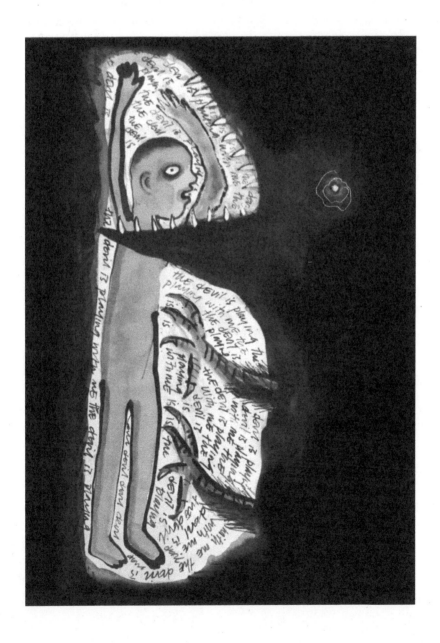

I have known Jonathan for years. He has a long turbulent history associated with the hospital. Recently in the out-patient clinic he told me with some pride that he had been admitted on over thirty occasions. It had been some sort of battle he said. He had been determined to demonstrate most importantly to himself that he was stronger than the illness. He would come in, get better, be discharged and then to the dismay of all around him, including family and friends and ourselves, he would stop the medication and relapse and need to be readmitted yet again. Now he said he was getting older. He was tired of this. He had lost too much. He was divorced and had become alienated from his children. He was unemployed and in poor health. He felt he had also lost his self-esteem and his confidence that he would in some way beat this illness and regain control of his life. He was not depressed but he seemed wearily despondent. He had now chosen to continue with the treatment and when I saw him he told me that he had not been readmitted for the past year. It had been the longest period of remission since his first admission in his early twenties.

I felt a cautious elation. It was not too late. Despite the many losses there was still a future. I suppose there is a reflex need for optimism, that the situation should never be considered to be beyond hope, and in Jonathan's remission there was a genuine sense of achievement, and even in his middle age the possibility of a new beginning.

Jonathan had been a talented artist. When he was well he made delicate, exquisitely crafted ink drawings, some of which he had given me and which I had proudly put up on the walls of my office. When he was unwell the nature of his art changed. He became more prolific but the precision and clarity was lost. Lines became scrambled and entangled, the colours were lurid and over the images he had compulsively scribbled reams of indecipherable prose and poetry. There was no sign at all of the graphic skill and the almost cold formality of the works he had produced when he was well. He produced these mad works it seemed in a frenzy, and foisted them on me with enthusiasm. On one admission he decided to transform his bed in the dormitory of the admission unit into an installation. He collected branches and bits of wire and string and other random objects that he found on the grounds of the hospital, and constructed an elaborate canopy over the bed. It was a ramshackle untidy mess and it required considerable agility on his part to simply get access to the bed. I was deeply impressed that the nursing staff and the cleaners allowed this. The other patients were bemused but despite their disorganized behaviour made no attempt in any way to interfere with this delicate and bizarre construction. There seemed to be some shared acknowledgement that this was a project of his, a work in progress, and that however incoherent, it was important for him and in some way necessary.

The different, quite distinct ways of expressing himself seemed to reflect in an eloquent way his shifting states of mind. It was not simply that when he was well his art was good and when he was sick his art was bad, or not art at all, just incoherent ravings and scribblings. This elaborate, intricate chaotic installation that he had constructed with such painstaking care in the ward did suggest to us a quite desperate determination to give a three dimensional form to something that was menacing and that could otherwise overwhelm him. He seemed compelled. The task was urgent.

The finely executed drawings he created when he was well seemed to serve another function, to be necessary in a different way. There were in these images another kind of need, a careful imposition of order, of precision, of the clear demarcation of spaces. It was as if there were two different strategies of dealing with his madness. When ill in hospital the spontaneous uninhibited process of giving form to inner turmoil with the hope of gaining control was in tension with the formal mastery he displayed when he was well, a determination, having regained control, to maintain it, to keep at bay the fragmented disorder of psychosis.

Sitting together in the out-patient clinic we reflected on these past events and turned with some hesitation to the future. Despite his air of inertia and lassitude I felt the need to be, if not naively optimistic, at least positive. Circumstances had changed. There was no reason now to think that the past should repeat itself. At last there was a degree of stability. I think I urged him to take pride in what he had achieved in coming to terms, albeit belatedly with his illness, and having now created the possibility of being free of the hospital, and the dismal and surely soul destroying routine of repeated relapses and readmissions. Jonathan was composed and thoughtful but there was an apprehension beneath the surface. This routine was not just a routine but had also been a struggle, and it had been a significant and profound part of most of his adult life. In a way his struggle with his madness over the many years was how he had come to see himself, it was part of his identity and now he wondered how he might adjust to this new world of relative order and calm, without the drama of the madness that he had come to believe was part of him.

We talked about purpose and direction, about finding new meanings and different ways of getting through the day and the rest of one's life. Making art had also been part of his identity. Now there was an opportunity to work on his art without the disruption of his admissions to hospital. He could make use of his past experiences. He could creatively transform the misfortune and misery of so much that had happened to him into something possibly eloquent and helpful both to himself and to others. Making art is making a mark, a way of defining oneself, and simultaneously reaching beyond oneself, both marking the paper or the canvas and going through the surface to something beyond that is open and free. I imagined in this way that making art was an act of generosity and of hope, and for Jonathan, burdened as he was by the past, possibly some sort of liberation.

Jonathan looked at me as if from far away. He was quiet and then he sighed and said no, he did not think that he could do that. It was not a feasible option. It was not the way forward. He implied, in a polite way that I just did not know what he was up against, how difficult it had been for him and how difficult it continued to be. The struggle was not over. I asked him why not. He had not lost his skills. He had much to communicate that could be of great help to myself in forming some understanding of his plight, but also to others in a similar position to his own. More importantly he could possibly through art give some form to the chaos: he might transform something distressingly without structure or any discernible significance into something of value. He responded almost vehemently. I cannot remember the exact words he used but it was clear to me that he regarded returning to making art would not be good for him, that in some way it was dangerous. He explained this with some difficulty but said that in order to make art, and this had been a pleasure for him, he had needed to lose himself. Engaging himself in the process took him away from himself, and nothing else mattered. Yet there had been a cost, and now he considered that cost too great. There was too high a risk of everything breaking down again, of going backwards. He said that madness was in a way losing oneself. There had been an ambivalence about this. In the past there had been an almost joyful abandonment of the struggle to be sane, and he had been able to regard his psychotic episodes as adventurous journeys. Now he believed too much damage had been done in the process. He had lost too much and it was irrevocable. He was tired. He was getting older. What he wanted now more than anything else was some degree of peace and stability. But he knew that was fragile. It would always be. Making art, losing himself was too dangerous. It would bring him too close to the edge, or overcome him, and that was something that now filled him with dread.

There was a sadness in this. In one way I should have been relieved by his new determination to stay well, but in this caution there was a compromise. In choosing to become himself, not to lose himself in his madness he had had to put aside a vital part of himself. It seemed that in the process of making art one could either find oneself or lose oneself. His sense of self was too uncertain. Now, and for the rest of his life he said he needed to be careful because he wanted at least some peace of mind, and in this there was a wistful resignation.

The schizophrenia that Jonathan had struggled with for much of his life may be conceptualized as a disorder of the self. Defining the self is problematic and subject to a wide range of variables, including social and cultural factors. Being conscious of oneself, a degree of unity and stability, and internal and external worlds being separate are nevertheless fairly consistent features. In psychotic states this edifice breaks down. The sense of self, or the integrity of the self fragments, and the external world irrupts into the internal essentially private world. In this respect there is an anguish or a crisis that is of an existential nature. Who am I in the world? Is the mad self or the sane self the true self, or is there a true self? I think Jonathan had found himself in this distressing quandary and he was becoming exhausted by it. The task was now just to get through the days. Not only was the sense of self precarious but so was external reality. There was no continuity, no stability. At any time, and certainly in his turbulent past the outside world could break down the feeble barriers and invade his inner world. What he had now achieved was fragile and precarious. Becoming an artist again was too hazardous. In this awkward state it is understandable that not only the self but the external world can seem unstable and insubstantial and that playing with it, or any other artistic reimagining of it could jeopardize a delicate balance.

There is a confusion in this. To believe that one needs to be a little mad to be an artist I think is a romantic fiction, but art can create spaces for different realities and so can madness. For somebody living with a psychotic illness there are no such safe spaces. It is too much of a risk, it threatens to disrupt whatever continuities there might be, and this is an indication of the potential dangerousness of what otherwise might be a sensuous immersion in the process of making art.

The predicament that preoccupies Jonathan is characteristic of schizophrenia but in other respects it is unusual. Some of the most disabling aspects of the schizophrenia spectrum are the neurocognitive deficits. These include impairments in the ability to abstract, or to imagine. To imagine is to be able to consider other possibilities, to be free of an obdurate given state of affairs. It might be considered as a basic requirement for being able to act on the world, to be an agent and not a passenger. This fails in persistent psychotic states. Many of our patients, to the greater distress of their families perhaps than themselves drift through their lives. I have tried repeatedly to persuade them, if not to make art, to at least record what they have been through after emerging from a breakdown. I have had little or no success, and that is why Jonathan is unusual. I do not think this is because my patients are unwilling to oblige me, or that they might be afraid. I think it is because they cannot.

The cantata, Madness: Songs of Hope and Despair was conceptualized as an attempt to give a voice to those suffering from severe mental illnesses. The question arises as to why a psychiatrist should presume to do this, and not the patients themselves, and their families and communities. For the reasons I have attempted to articulate this was not possible. Perhaps the difficulty can be described broadly as an inability to find the necessary symbolic space. Using the utterances of my patients themselves and describing their stories was at least one way of being authentic and showing the necessary respect. For the same reasons we would have liked to use the art works of our patients for the project. Some were included but regrettably few. We were attempting to get into the psychotic experience, to imagine and also to communicate what it might be like. The very nature of the condition precluded us for the most part from using our patients' works.

In this there is a problem that I find perplexing. Dr. Hans Prinzhorn a German psychiatrist in the early part of the twentieth century encouraged his patients to make art, and he also collected the very various forms of art, including paintings drawings and collages made elsewhere by patients in psychiatric hospitals throughout much of Europe. These extraordinary works have been widely published and presented across the world, and remain on permanent exhibition in the Psychiatric Institute of the University of Heidelberg in Germany. The images movingly and eloquently convey the inner worlds of these patients. What has changed? Why almost a hundred years later has it been so difficult for us to find works of equivalent beauty and expressive power. There are I suppose a number of possible explanations: the art tutor might have encouraged a more conventional representational style in the belief that that might be therapeutic, and medication might have played some part. It is also possible that our patients today inhabit a different world in which there is a plethora of given images in a wide range of media, and that this might close down the spaces, even in the refracted worlds of the patients in our hospital, for making art that is furiously personal and profound and intensely meaningful.

I had previously tried to describe the subjective experiences of madness in more academically oriented articles but the results seemed bland. For the cantata, integrating the libretto with music and with images, at times coherent and at other times disorganized, brought the possibility of conveying more vividly and more forcefully the turbulence of psychotic states of mind. Fiona Moodie's art work for the project created a sense of these shifting states of terror and stillness, of disorder and calm eloquently and powerfully and more effectively than the work of any patient I have encountered. Hers is a work of art. It is reaching out, imagining, wondering. Otherwise there is nothing, only silence and empty spaces. I don't think that that is helpful.

I recently found myself wandering around a modern art gallery, trying to understand why I should be feeling so dispirited. Perhaps there was too much of it, perhaps I was in the wrong mood, but the works somehow seemed superfluous, attenuated, wilfully obscure and vapid. My impression was of a display of self-preoccupation, an almost solipsistic disregard for the confused world we inhabit in common. I felt as if I was the mere spectator of a wan parade of introverted miseries. The works were accompanied by explanatory texts of dense jargon, replete with "explorations, interrogations, discourses, narratives and tropes". Any notion of wonder or any sense of a need to communicate with clarity or of caring deeply about a shared world I suspect would have been regarded as sentimental and irrelevant. Perhaps I was also vaguely antagonized by the hallowed atmosphere of these large antiseptic spaces, as if in denial of the banalities of fashion and the market place that drove the whole contrived process.

Perhaps I was also searching for the raw honesty and intensity and high risk of madness. The complex and confused and at time contradictory nature of Jonathan's artistic endeavours moved me profoundly, I think because they represented an urgent search and a yearning for meaning, a way of surviving and of being in the world. I don't know what criteria are used to decide what might constitute good or significant art, but in some way what is valuable is the sense that it is necessary and authentic, exciting, maybe unsettling and possibly dangerous.

26

Madness and machines

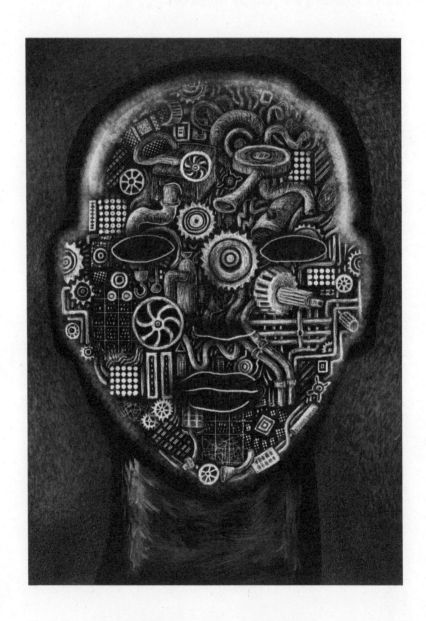

"It's my own brain that does it...it's like an electrical machine that switches on...when I'm well the machine has no control over me...when I'm ill the machine switches on...when you are well you've got control...you bring it on yourself...you think it's your subconscious and then this mechanism is triggered...if you are sitting in a chair and you want to get up before your time, you can't...it's hell." Johannes, describing experiences that led him to an attempt to end his life.

We are in the out-patient clinic and Johannes is explaining to me what had happened. His brain had been hijacked by a machine. Now he had recovered and he spoke with great insight and eloquence about this terrifying experience.

I think he is speaking with insight because I have no idea what it must be like to feel that your brain is controlled by a machine. There is insight, or an indication of recovery in that he associates the experience with being ill. The events are recalled with great clarity. There is no escape in forgetfulness. The experience is vivid. He seems to want me to understand. When he is ill there is no barrier, there is no distance, no capacity for abstraction that might enable him to interpret what is happening to him as a possible symptom of illness. He is so immersed in the experience that there is no space to question or doubt it. There is no getting away. The nightmare is not simply that he has lost control, which might be something that many of us have experienced to some extent for short periods of time. In moments of high emotion, in states of grief or intense fear we might experience a fleeting sensation of having no control, or of the need and struggle to maintain control. What had happened to Johannes appeared to be of a different quality. Not only had he lost control but that control had been usurped by a machine.

He could not in any way attribute what was happening to him as something internal, some aberration which perhaps through force of will he might overcome. Any notion of personal agency had been cruelly and inexplicably surrendered to an external device, to remote control. There seems to me to be something particularly menacing about this experience of remoteness. This overwhelmingly powerful adversarial force was not close or tangible yet it was intrusive and manipulative. It was mystifyingly not discernible to him. It had no shape. There were no outlines. There seemed to be no substance to it.

Whatever it was it was all the more sinister because he could not grasp it, he could not protect himself. He did not know what it was, and because he did not know what it was he could not devise strategies to defend himself. His psychosis had rendered him helpless.

It is imaginable, and again fleetingly, that we might feel that we are under the control, or unduly influenced by another, but this is "as if", it is metaphorical. It does not equate to the concrete anguished conviction Johannes describes. Being under the control not of a person but of a machine is all the more menacing and degradingly an affront to human dignity.

This indiscernibility, this lack of any familiar element to which one might begin to attach meaning is described as a "hell". The malevolent machinery is relentless. It has switched off all meaningful signals, all familiar patterns and any hope of escape. It is difficult to understand what might have been happening to Johannes in this psychotic and nightmarish state of being: it is surely not too difficult to understand the desperation that led him to an attempt to end his life.

I had just taken up a post as a junior consultant when I first encountered David. I thought he might have been the superintendent of the hospital, or that he held some senior administrative position in the department. He had a dignified, urbane, detached demeanour. He was dressed immaculately. He was wearing a tweed jacket and a tie, his flannel trousers were ironed, and his shoes were polished. He stood alone on the lawn, his hands clasped behind his back, gazing across the river and up towards the eastern buttress of the mountain. He seemed preoccupied but calm. Perhaps what was most striking about him was his stillness. I was often to see him in the same position, always alone, always absorbed in himself, always gazing outward. It was unimaginable to me that he was a patient of the hospital. I was naïve. I did not know that he had been a patient for longer than any other, and that he was gravely ill. What was I expecting: torn filthy clothes, swivel eyes, wild hair, a raving lunatic?

The next time I saw David he was in the hospital clinic. At first I did not recognize him. He was emaciated. He was severely dehydrated. He appeared to be terrified. I thought he was close to death. The nurses were desperately trying to give him fluids and feed him but he was resisting them with a strange ferocity.

On that occasion he survived. He recovered and was eventually returned to his ward. I found him in his familiar position, restored to himself, composed, apparently intact.

It would never go away he said. He was just waiting for it to start again and he did not know whether he would have the strength to cope with it. He was getting older and weaker. He was tired of it all. I had the impression that he was also tired of having to explain himself. Nobody really understood. Nobody could really help.

When he became ill, when he lost guard, the machine would come on, he told me. At first it was insidious. He felt a vague disquiet, a sense of unreality, an uneasy and growing awareness that he was not quite in control of himself. This became more intense and eventually overwhelming. He could no longer resist it. He no longer had the strength. The machine had got to him, again. It was in total control. What surprised him, he said, was that he was surprised. When he was well it seemed impossible to him that this would happen again. It was inconceivable. It made no sense. It was too cruel. Perhaps, he mused this was just wishful thinking. Now he knew better. It would never go way, not completely. That was the last image I recall of David, standing alone, apparently impassive, gazing up at the mountain and towards the setting sun, waiting I suppose, for it all to come raging back and engulf him.

However hesitantly it might have begun, the control this machine exerted over him rapidly increased in its pervasive power. Initially it was just an almost dreamlike sense of disorientation, then a growing, sickening awareness that the machine was gaining control of his thoughts and actions. His helplessness filled him with dread. The machine bored relentlessly into his world, into the most intimate aspects of his life, and eventually into his body and his mind and soul. He became incapacitated. The machine controlled him entirely. It controlled his ability to swallow, to feed himself, to breathe and to survive.

He was no longer himself but a function of this wretched malevolent apparatus.

The horror of it, the absurdity and the monstrous injustice of it was that this thing was being controlled by a homosexual couple living in London. He had never met these people. He did not know who they were or why they were inflicting this on him. He just knew with certainty that it was this couple that were controlling the machine that was controlling him. Perhaps it was just a random act of cruelty, perhaps it was to amuse themselves in some callous way. He could not explain it, but what he knew with a fatalistic certainty was that it was real and that it had become unbearable.

David disappeared from the hospital a few weeks after this meeting. There had been no signs of a relapse. He had been his quiet, polite and reserved self. It seemed that at least for the time being he had regained some peace of mind. Now abruptly he was gone. There had been no indication that the machine was beginning yet again to exert its terrible control. He had never left the grounds before and we were all apprehensive.

The next morning I was informed by the hospital administration that the police had found his body washed ashore on one of the beaches on the other side of the city. There seemed to me something so utterly forlorn in the image of his crumpled, inert and always solitary figure, now dishevelled in death, beneath the glittering and impassive apartment blocks of the Atlantic seaboard. I do not know whether it had been due to the machine, and whether David on this occasion had chosen not to tell us because it was hopeless, or whether it was not the machine but his own decision to finally take control by choosing to end his life. I would like to think of this as an act of defiance but it was probably and more simply driven by despair.

Machines and more recently specifically computers loom largely in the content of our patients' delusions. This is shaped to a great extent by cultural and probably socio-economic factors. Believing one's mind is being controlled by a computer is vastly more common in a middle class urban population, and that very often corresponds with being white in our persistently racially preoccupied world. Our young black patients from rural backgrounds are far more likely to attribute their distress to witchcraft or the displeasure of the ancestors. It seems very probable, and there was some evidence of this emerging recently in our wards, that with urbanization the wrath of the ancestors or the evils of witchcraft would be replaced by the cold and possibly more sinister malevolence of machines.

The prevailing theme has been the persecutory delusion of being under the control of a machine of some kind, but with recent and dramatic technological advances machines enter the world of psychosis in a very different way.

Machines are being created that are so intelligent that they are developing the capacity to learn or think independently. Mimicking human intelligence these machines are possibly beginning to surpass human intelligence.

It is not unforeseeable, and it is poignant that at some point in the future our much vaunted consciousness will be a mere function of an algorithm devised by a machine that is without consciousness, but is vastly more intelligent than ourselves, and that we will never know.

Another implication of these advances is a possibility that in having minds of their own these machines will develop the capacity for madness.

It might provide a curiously informative perspective on our human madness to speculate on how a machine might go mad. A machine somehow seems unlikely to complain that is being controlled by another machine. It is improbable that a machines would complain of being bewitched. They are unlikely to complain about hallucinations. They are unlikely to complain. They are more likely to go awry.

That might seem of little consequence. The machine merely no longer functions, or functions less efficiently. It is neither here nor there. It is simply a dud, mad, useless machine. This fails to take into account the extent to which machines have crept into our humdrum, quotidian lives. It might be an extreme position to claim that machines control our lives, not in any metaphorical or insane way, but in the way of an increasingly and insidious dependence upon which we possibly choose not to reflect too much because of the clear and dramatic benefits. Technology has transformed our world, and it could only be a gloomy pessimist or a luddite or doomsayer to dispute that this is not for the greater good. Yet those who have the knowledge and the expertise acknowledge that no programme is entirely secure. A hacker with malicious intent can hack into any system, and in this way, for example, powerfully disrupt food and water and power supplies and create havoc.

This does not necessarily require evil intent. It might merely require a fault, a glitch in an immensely complicated programme, a machine gone haywire. It seems increasingly more probable that a nuclear holocaust would be the outcome not of a battle between great powers but of human error or an errant algorithm.

This scenario is to some extent analogous to the human brain and its malfunctions. Being the most complicated thing in the known universe the brain is in all likelihood more prone to error, however slight that might be. The problem arises in that due to the very complexity of the system an error however trivial can have chaotic consequences. An apparently minor genetic variant, in isolation or perhaps acting in concert with some non-specific adversity in childhood or later exposure to cannabis triggers a cascade of events that eventually manifest as schizophrenia.

A mathematical error in the engineering of a critical vault leads to the collapse of the cathedral. The higher the spire, the closer it reaches to heaven, the more precarious it becomes and the greater the risk becomes that the whole yearning edifice will come crashing down to earth. A broken string, a jarring note can change a symphony into a cacophony. A disconnection, or a disorganization of neurochemical transmission in a critical part of our brain may lead to the collapse of the infinitely complex and delicate construction of what we regard as ourselves and our sanity. We are it seems ill at ease with this contingency, this embodiment of ourselves. It cannot be that our consciousness, or what we believe to be the essence of who we are and what is intrinsic to our humanity could be so prone to chance and error. This might be a factor in the fear of madness, and the consequent stigma and the exclusion of those who suffer from mental illness.

We are afraid of our vulnerability. We are afraid of our being in part mere machines, things, bodies, and that fear is compounded by the knowledge that machines can and often do malfunction. This of course applies to any form of illness and is not confined to madness. It is understandable. It is surely not ridiculous and pathetic and it is a reflection of a very human and fear of unavoidable death.

What is rather ridiculous and pathetic is that with the advances of technology we come to believe we will be able to achieve immortality. Whatever the means, whether we are frozen or the contents of our consciousness are uploaded into the blue skies of cyberspace, there is always going to be some bored and distracted technician who might momentarily fail to maintain sufficiently precisely the temperature, or some software fault that brings the whole proud enterprise down to earth and to ashes. There appears to be no escaping our fragile dependency, and to think otherwise is illusory. The mind cannot escape the brain. We are bound to the machinery of ourselves.

Being bound does not entail being confined. While there might be a tension or some uncertainty as to who or what is in control, I do know that I do not feel as if I am a function of an algorithm, and that this is irreducible and uncontestable, whether or not at some other level of analysis it is illusory.

When our patients tell us they believe they are under the control of a machine it seems possible that they are saying that in some way they are no longer under the illusion that they are in control. However frightening that might be it is not madness.

Being utterly out of control is perhaps intolerable, and we choose to believe that there is a degree of control over the circumstances of our lives, whether that is ourselves or a machine or god or fate.

*

Perhaps we are just machines anyway, with a degree of superfluous self-consciousness that we believe to be transcendent, granting us humanity. The question then arises whether in the process of evolution we are to become more or less like machines.

A teacher in my undergraduate years sought to explain the workings of the central nervous system by drawing a box with an arrow entering into it at one end and another emerging from it at the other end. This represented the sensory input and the motor output. It became more complicated with another box or perhaps it was a circle above the first box, representing higher control centres which regulated what the output should be if there were a multiplicity of inputs. This seemed ludicrously simplistic at the time but it has become intriguing in its ramifications. What if the capacity of this regulatory function became engulfed by an excess of inputs? Presumably the function would be referred upward to a yet higher and more sophisticated regulatory centre, but what if at that level the system became again overwhelmed. Would the excess of signals, the surfeit of inputs or information lose significance and become mere noise?

We live in a world increasingly preoccupied with information, or data. We attach value to the accumulation of more and more information. We worship at the altar of big data. We believe that this will grant us greater control over the circumstances of our lives, or enable us to reach beyond ourselves. We need more and more, we become hungry for more information, and in the process there is the spectre of us becoming bloated, rendered catatonic with an excess of information, gazing in a stupor upon our screens, increasingly incapable of thought or action, drowning back into helplessness. How to process the escalating torrent of information available to us in a useful way is not clear, but the predicament is a way of imagining madness.

27

Psychopathy and psychosis

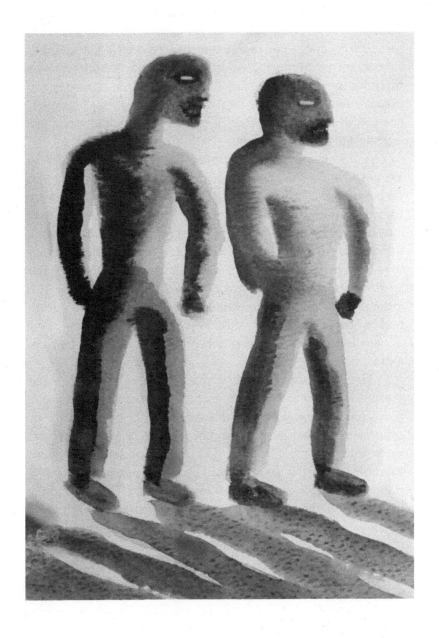

Psychopathy is not psychosis. The confusion of these two terms has contributed significantly to the burden of stigma. In the broadest possible terms psychosis refers to what might be described as a serious mental illness, or madness, and this includes the schizophrenia spectrum disorders, the more extreme expressions of the bipolar disorders and other neuropsychiatric illnesses, most commonly the dementias. Psychopathy is a particular form of a personality disorder. As such it is enduring in its course rather than episodic and it is not associated with psychotic symptoms including thought disorders, delusions and hallucinations. Psychosis is regarded as an illness. Psychopathy is not and this itself is a source of much confusion and moral and legal debate and controversy.

A violent act is reported in the daily news. It is of such an extreme nature that notions of evil are invoked. The act was perpetrated in a "psychotic frenzy", its cruelty and callousness are named "psychopathic". Both terms in this context loosely and interchangeably define an extreme degree. The act is of such a heinous nature, it is so lacking in any human quality that it can only have been perpetrated by a madman. Madness in this sense is not an illness. It is a form of behaviour beyond the human pale. It is incomprehensible. It is intolerable, it is unimaginable that a normal person could behave in this way. There has to be some explanation of this terrifying otherness, and all too often the explanation is madness.

This is "psycho" territory, the domain of fiction, film and theatre, intended to thrill with horror. The extra syllables are of little consequence. Whether it is psychotic or psychopathic or even psychological is of lesser import than it being "psycho", deranged, monstrous, bestial. The notion of something being psychological in this context itself evokes a certain unease. It is mysterious, uncontained and essentially private. It is beyond the reassurance of an objective or physical verifiability and therefore all the more unfathomable and frightening.

In this morning's newspaper there is a report of a young man who has been declared– a psychopath. The very nature of his crimes, the sheer gratuitous violence of his behaviour has led to this conclusion. It appears as if it is the action itself, rather than the mental state invokes the epithet or the diagnosis or the non-diagnosis. The judge asks whether this "psychosis" is due to genetic or environmental factors. The young man's father is in prison following a conviction of murder. It is possibly careless misreporting, but the terms psychosis and psychopathy are used randomly in the report. It is assumed that it does not matter but it does. In the legal framework psychopathy is not an illness and the perpetrator is therefore considered criminally responsible for his or her actions. The consequence is in all likelihood a lengthy prison sentence given the extreme nature of the offence that has given rise to the notion of psychopathy. Psychosis is regarded as an illness and as such there is a high degree of possibility that whoever might have committed the act will not be considered to be criminally responsible, and therefore be held in a hospital rather than a prison.

Mr. Viljoen was a patient of mine many years ago. I remember him as a rather timid, sad and intelligent elderly man who had spent a large part of his adult life in the forensic unit of the hospital. He described the circumstances leading to his admission. It was so many years ago that he said his memory of the events preceding the tragedy was hazy. He was working as an accountant for a successful business in the city. He nevertheless recalled with clarity working one morning on a series of accounts with his manager. An entry was made by this unfortunate man of an account number that included a sequence of three sixes. The realization then dawned upon Mr. Viljoen that his employer was in fact the devil. As a god-fearing Christian he then concluded that it was his duty to rid the world of this evil person. He was not of a violent disposition and lacked physical strength so conspired with his nephew to kill the manager. This respected and prominent person in the community was thereupon hit on the head with a brick and died of the injury.

Both Mr. Viljoen and his nephew were charged with murder. Mr. Viljoen was indignant. Rather than being treated as a criminal he should be hailed as a hero he said. He had destroyed the devil. He had saved the world. In the opinion of a forensic psychiatrist during the course of the trial he was considered to be delusional and as a consequence not criminally responsible for his actions. His nephew was not considered to be mentally ill. It is not known whether the notion of psychopathy was invoked at the time but he was considered to have acted cynically and with intent, probably motivated by the large amount of money that his uncle had promised him. These events took place prior to independence, at a time when capital punishment was on the statute books. The young man was found guilty of murder and hanged. This caused outrage in the community. Two family members had conspired to commit the homicidal act. As a result one was cared for in a hospital and the other was dead. One was judged psychotic and the other treated as a psychopath, with the most dire consequences. This was considered to be a great injustice. That life or death decisions should hinge upon something as vague and abstract as a diagnosis of psychosis was regarded as a travesty.

Hendrik Verwoerd the intellectual founder of apartheid was assassinated by Dmitri Tsafendas who insisted he had been acting on the instructions of a tapeworm within his body. Tsafendas was found to be not criminally responsible. As some sort of compromise he spent most of the rest of his life in prison and died eventually in a psychiatric hospital. This again caused outrage, particularly among the worshippers of Verwoerd. It was far too soft a way of dealing with a heinous crime. The tapeworm business was absurd, it was held, and anyway, regardless of whether the tapeworm or the man was ultimately responsible Tsafendas should have been severely punished. Conversely, for those in vehement opposition to the policies of apartheid, the attribution of the murder to madness robbed it of its political import.

Bartho was recently admitted to the unit after he had stabbed his friend in the neck with a kitchen knife. He also said that this was his duty. They were both in hell and this was a way of saving his friend. He told us that his last clear memory before everything became confused was the knife which was under some form of external control moving towards his friend's neck. He was dumbfounded. This was happening and it was not happening. He was a gentle person. Stabbing his friends was not in his nature. The knife in the neck of his friend he said was not "poetic". Now he was getting better he believed his "schizophrenic parts" were coming together, but he found being in the high care unit difficult because it was "incoherent".

Again it might not seem evident why this young man should have been admitted to a psychiatric hospital rather than be charged with attempted murder. A possible key is in his curious use of the word "poetic". This suggested to us that this was a psychosis. It would be very unlikely that a psychopath would tell us that that stabbing his friend in the neck lacked poetry, nor that he found the ward to be devoid of coherence. A more probable psychopathic position was that his friend was somehow asking for it and that he did not deserve to be in the ward amongst mad people.

The terms are not mutually exclusive. Psychopathy does not protect against psychosis. Younis has been admitted on numerous occasions, usually following acts of fairly extreme violence. This violence has in turn been precipitated by the use of "Tik" or methamphetamines. Younis knows the likely consequences of his methamphetamine use. He does not seem to care. He does not seem to have learned anything from his previous admissions. We convene a family meeting. An angry weariness hangs heavily over us. The mother is in tears. The family is devoutly Muslim. The son's delinquent behaviour has brought shame upon them. They have been ostracized by the community. The brother is hostile and impatient. On this most recent occasion Younis had tried to throttle him. When he was now asked why, Younis said he had thought his brother was "the king of calamity". He said it was all because of the Tik that had made him "crazy". He shrugged and laughed. It was no big deal he said, his brother had come to no harm and now he had recovered it was time to go home. The mother wept and said nothing. The brother said: "he chooses to be like this. He knows what he is doing. He knows what will happen when he uses the Tik. He enjoys it. He doesn't care. You are going to discharge him and it will be alright for a while and then he will start again and there will be violence. He is destroying our family".

In the out-patient clinic I ask Younis why he continues this behaviour. Again he laughs. He is nonchalant. He blames his family. He says they no longer trust him. They cage him in, he complains. They treat him as if there is something wrong with him, or as if he is a child. They grant him no freedom. He gets bored. "What is there to do, doctor? Tik makes you strong. "It is wild", he tells me with relish. It all seems self-evident to him. He has come to live with the dire consequences, or not to be concerned nor deterred.

He is back in the unit a month later, roaring, berserk and exultant, his own king of calamity. "Hey Doctor! What did I tell you? It's mad man, it's wild!" he shouts across the ward. He is chaotic and elated. He had yet again stopped his medication. It seemed he did not understand the point of it, the grim struggle to be merely normal, the need to appease his family. He was bored and frustrated and angry. He had managed to obtain the keys to the family car and roamed up the coast, not having any clear idea about where he was going or what he wanted to do. The details were vague but he somehow got involved in an altercation with a stranger. He had assaulted this person and when the police were called he said that he was our patient. He was not charged but brought back to the unit. When he greeted me he showed no remorse. It had been a big adventure.

Younis did show many of the features of psychopathy in his lack of concern for others, most especially his family, and in his failure to learn from his experiences and his careless disregard for the consequences of his actions. Yet I found myself surprised by a degree of sympathy for him. He was in an unenviable predicament. He was middle-aged and solitary and unemployable. He had alienated himself from his family and his community. He was fully aware of the disgrace he had wrought upon them. His life he saw was empty and only occupied with the struggle to contain his bipolar illness and stay out of hospital. This sapped his energy and demoralized him. It was not beyond understanding that he would rebel against these circumstances and take flight into mania, regardless of the predictable aftermath.

This conflict is not uncommon amongst people living with in particular bipolar disorders and there is much debate about what is described as the comorbidity. The nature of the association of personality disorders with bipolar disorders is uncertain and the controversies are about whether the one group is integral to the other or whether or not the one predisposes or is a consequence of the other. The difficulties might arise in part from the nature of psychiatric diagnoses and in particular the hazy construct of personality disorders. There is something inherently problematic in making a diagnosis of a personality disorder that is not considered to be a mental illness, and more specifically not an illness in a medico-legal sense, in that somebody with a diagnosis of a personality disorder is considered responsible for his or her actions. A further complication or uncertainly arising from this is what to do. A diagnosis implies a problem that requires a solution. The treatment of personality disorders is controversial and uncertain, and this concerns among many other issues whether treatment is either beneficial or even warranted.

It is not clear in what way the diagnosis of a personality disorder is useful or helpful. The problems are compounded by the pejorative associations of the diagnosis or the construct. Particularly with regard to psychopathy or the anti-social personality disorders the implication is that the behaviours that prompted this assessment are morally reprehensible and the character of the person diagnosed in this way is deeply flawed and beyond help. With regard to the newspaper report mentioned above, the recommendation to the court was that the perpetrator was dangerous, that he was unlikely to benefit from rehabilitation, was likely to reoffend on release and that therefore he should be given a lengthy prison sentence.

Not infrequently in our unit, when called upon to assess a patient on admission, and usually in the context of an act of violence, the registrar would conclude in the absence of any clear psychotic symptoms that the patient was "just a psychopath". This was dismissive. The message was that there was nothing for us to do. He, or more rarely she belonged elsewhere and this was usually prison. I rarely encountered a patient in our unit with a diagnosis of a personality disorder who was not profoundly damaged by life circumstances. These extreme behaviours did not arise from nowhere. The usual trajectory was from a broken home, an absent or abusive father, a neglectful mother, a total absence of any form of support or nurturing and as a consequence a profound lack of self-esteem and a grim descent into drug abuse, gangsterism and criminality. These patients, and that is how they were described while in the unit, provoked an anger and a moral indignation that too often deflected attention away from the tragedy of these abject histories.

There are of course exceptions but I struggle to recall any in my own clinical experience. A deeply moving and harrowing account is given in a memoir by the mother of one of the young men involved in the Columbine high school killings in the United States. She describes a loving, supportive, relatively privileged, and she uses the word carefully, normal family. There were no clear antecedents to an act of extreme and utterly callous brutality. The mother agonizes over these events in painful detail. She struggles but she is unable to explain her son's behaviour. The killings are terrifyingly unfathomable. This is another kind of psychopathy.

The difficulties in the diagnostic construct of personality disorders relate to the problem of the notion of personality itself. This supposedly describes a relatively stable and enduring way of being in the world and relating to others. This is of a doubtful validity. The way we are is probably more random and contingent than we would like to think. I do not know how I would be without the good fortune and the many chances that have been afforded me. I do not know if I would be the person I am, and I doubt it, if I had been born into impoverished circumstances, abused by my parents, leaving school early and having no prospect of a job, and living without any self-respect and without hope.

28

Fear

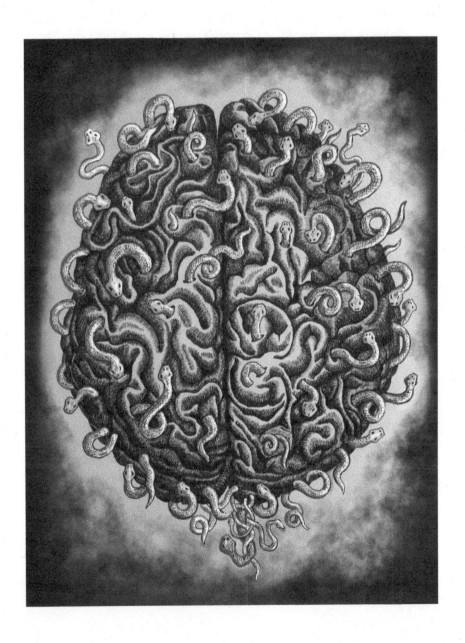

Fear pervades madness. Being mad we fear the world. Being in the world we believe to be sane and ordered we are fearful of madness.

Wynand has disappeared. It is now three weeks since he left the boarding house where he has lived following his discharge from our unit about a year ago. His mother is in my office. She is in tears. "Do something Doctor. You have got to find him". There have been various sightings of him. He has been seen rummaging in refuse bins. He is described as gaunt, dishevelled, raving to himself. At every attempt to apprehend him he has fled. "Do something Doctor! He needs help. He needs to be in hospital. I can't stand this. He is going to die. You have to do something".

The manager of the boarding house reported that he had probably stopped taking his medication about a month earlier. The problem is compounded because he has tuberculosis and it is almost certain that he has also stopped his TB medication. It is winter and cold and it is difficult to imagine that he will survive much longer if he is not found. He frightens people. It is more likely that they will close their doors than help him. Occasionally a call is made to the hospital to report that he has been seen. By the time the police arrive he has again disappeared. The police are reluctant to accord this a priority. There are other more grave crises to which they have to respond. This after all is not a criminal matter, they tell me.

The mother is distraught and inconsolable. She is understandably afraid that her son might die. The people in the community are afraid. He is roaming the streets and he is unpredictable and they think he might be dangerous. I do not know his current state of mind, but it is difficult not to think that he is not afraid. It is usually fear that drives this behaviour, either a concrete fear of an imagined danger or something more diffuse and inescapable, of the threat of danger being everywhere, of there being no refuge.

I am afraid. I cannot console or reassure the mother. I am afraid that her fears might be justified and we might not find him and that he will die. He is extremely vulnerable and he is unable to look after himself. He might die of exposure in the cold, his disorganized behaviour might provoke a homicidal assault, he might succumb to the tuberculosis. Anything is possible and nothing is certain.

Andries is wailing and howling and screaming in the ward, causing great distress to the other patients. "Oh my god, oh my god, oh my god" he cries. He is inconsolable and it is a struggle to understand what might be the cause of his torment. One part of it seems to be that he believes that he has to leave, and by keeping him we are only making his predicament more intolerable. Eventually a nurse manages to coax him into a quiet corner and gain some understanding beyond the mostly incoherent moaning and shrieking of what is happening to him. It still does not make much sense but it becomes apparent that he believes his family has been killed, or that he has killed his family. He knows and accepts that the community will kill him in revenge. The only option is for him to kill himself, either to pre-empt the horror of his own impending murder or to punish himself for his dreadful crime. We are cruelly making everything worse for him by confining him to the ward. We don't understand. We are not helping him. On the contrary, we are merely hindering him from doing what he has to do. He has no choice. He is doomed.

It seemed to me that the worst kind of fear, the most intense and the most intolerable was the fear that had no form or shape or meaning. These patients were utterly immersed in their fear. They could provide no explanation of it, they had no understanding of its source and they certainly had no idea what to do about it. Fear rendered them helpless, incapable of action.

The nurses described Mandla crawling around the edges of the ward, groaning in terror. They asked him what the matter was but he just muttered incoherently and wept and moaned and sighed. He gnawed at his fingers and blood dripped in bright streams from his mouth. The other patients were horrified. Everybody wanted to help. "What is it Mandla, what's going on. There is nothing here. There is no danger. Why are you so afraid? What are you seeing that we cannot see?" He cast his eyes about in panic and confusion. Then eventually, almost to himself, unsure, he muttered, "the snakes, the snakes are coming at me". It seemed that he was desperate for something, anything to account for the terror that was overwhelming him. The snakes might have been quite random, but they provided some kind of an explanation. They were a beginning at least. He knew about snakes. Snakes were out there in the world. He had seen snakes before and snakes were a recurring theme in his cultural, mythical world. You could also do something about a snake, like hitting it on the head. Slowly, falteringly Mandla calmed himself and regained his composure. Later he said, bemused, "What snakes?"

Anxiety, and also fear we can for the most part understand. These states of mind can be considered appropriate and serve a function. A degree of anxiety for example can be useful in motivating us to prepare for an exam. If we cannot swim it is helpful and quite possibly life-saving to be afraid of water. The problem arises when states of fear and anxiety are not appropriate, or utterly disproportionate, or there is no context to make sense of these powerful and potentially chaotic feelings. Fear and anxiety can then feed upon themselves. The problem escalates and panic and terror ensue.

We could have no idea what triggered the extreme response we observed in Mandla. Some spark was ignited, some switch was pulled, there was some idea, there was some neurochemical turbulence that suddenly and wildly spun out of control and overwhelmed our young patient. I tried to imagine it, Mandla, his fist crushed into his bleeding mouth, staring in paralyzed horror at something vast and evil towering above him and swaying menacingly, something undefined that could have been a snake or a writhing mass of snakes, maybe hissing, a tongue, or maybe many flickering, vast fangs flashing, gleaming hateful eyes intent on his destruction. I could not imagine it. It is not possible to enter into another's mind, but we could make inferences from the behaviour we observed, and I think we were all distressed by the mad and intense distress we witnessed that afternoon in the admission unit.

The neurobiology of fear is to some extent understood. A threat in some form is perceived, and in very broad terms two systems are activated, the one rapid and more or less unconscious, and mediated at lower levels of the central nervous system, the other slower and conscious and mediated at higher levels.

A decision whether to fight or to take flight makes sense in terms of a very basic need to survive, but the various cognitive and emotional and other factors that shape that response are complex and cannot simply be assumed to be the most effective or efficient in that specific context. Fear becomes pathological when this system goes haywire. The very mechanisms intended to protect turn awry, and we become incapacitated. An innocuous event is misconstrued as menacing.

This in itself can be due to a host of factors, including past experience and a current disposition of mind. Being fearful, being on guard we become more fearful, more wary, more inclined to perceive danger. Lower brain centres are activated and the body goes in to a state of high alert. Adrenaline flows through the system. Our hearts beat faster, our breathing is shallow and rapid, we might become dizzy and nauseous. The more immediate, visceral, intensely powerful emotional, possibly blunter response, rather than informing an appropriate course of action can overwhelm the slower more elaborately calibrated evaluative system. We become paralyzed with fear. We lose a sense of control. We lose focus. The fear response is ratcheted up, and panic ensues. Our thoughts are distorted and we become disorganized by fear. In this frenzied state of mind we cannot respond to reason. We become inconsolable. Mandla could not hear us. He was overwhelmed by terror. All proportion was lost. All was noise and menace.

Last night, taking the dogs outside into the garden I misjudged a step in the dark and I fell. I found myself lying on my back, gazing up at the stars, momentarily disoriented. I thought, very briefly that I might have done myself harm, but quickly reassured myself that I could move all my limbs. I was alright I told myself, but my body did not seem to heed this. I began to shake violently. I found it difficult to breathe, my heart seemed to be beating dangerously fast and a curious deeply unpleasant electrical sensation suffused my whole body.

This must have lasted a few seconds but during that time I felt I was out of control, and it was that, rather than any fear of having done myself harm that scared me most. My body seemed to have developed a mind of its own. My attempts to reason with myself that there was no danger, that it was just a careless accident, and that there was no cause for alarm seemed for that short while feeble and inadequate. My sense of myself had become disorganized: one self was telling me that that I was alright and that I was in control and another more embodied self was sending me very clear signals that I was most emphatically not alright. I was in the grip of a violent wholly disproportionate physical response over which my conscious rational self seemed for those frightening moments to have no control.

Anxiety and fear are necessarily and inevitably part of our lives. The problem then might arise less than from the nature of the stimulus itself and the perceived danger than the inappropriateness or the disproportion of the response, and the wrongful or misconstrued interpretation of the context. Mandla appeared to be in great fear, and it seemed possible that he formed the idea of the snake or of those many snakes to account for this fear, or at least to start the process of mitigating the fear by giving it some form. I soon forgot about my wildly disproportionate response to a minor fall. It seemed ridiculous to me. It was unimaginable that Mandla would ever be able to consider his fears ridiculous.

We could not reason with Mandla while he was in the throes of terror. He was inaccessible to us. In this circumstance the most practical and the quickest way of helping him and alleviating his distress was to use medication. A simple benzodiazepine is an effective way of diminishing the incapacitating distress, enabling one to regain a degree of control and restore at least some sense of proportion. Only then might it become possible to use reason to dismantle the looming towers of fear and terror, to put things hopefully into some sort of perspective and to restore at least a semblance of calm.

A young medical student made a particular impression on me during the various ward rounds and seminars they are required to attend. She was inquisitive and bright and thoughtful, and at some stage I found the time to ask her whether, given her clear interest in the subject she would consider specializing in psychiatry once she had completed her undergraduate studies. She said she had given this some thought but had decided that it would not be suitable for her. She did not think she would be able to cope. I was surprised and asked why she should think in that way as she appeared to be a remarkably mature and confident young woman. She said she was fearful. But is that not just part of being a medical student, or a doctor, I argued. You cannot not be anxious if you have any imagination.

It is a source of amusement to senior doctors to observe students in whatever speciality they might be engaged, believing that a chest pain signals imminent cardiac arrest, a mere cough treatment resistant tuberculosis. When we qualify and become doctors a fear that we will miss a diagnosis, that we will make a surgical error or that we will not be able to help seems an inevitability.

"No", she said, "it's not that". She seemed to struggle to articulate what she wished to say. "Perhaps it's got something to do with my young age, but it's too close. I find myself at times identifying with the young patients on the ward. I become frightened that this might happen to me. I find myself avoiding these encounters and that is not helpful. I don't think I could be a psychiatrist".

I am also at times fearful, but not to the extent that I have considered turning back as I cross the river to enter the hospital, and rather flee into the mountains. It is less the fear of not being able to help I think than the fear of becoming insane. The loss of the feeling of being in some control, however precarious that might be, and of the sense of the world having some meaning or stability has filled me on many occasions with dread. Turning away from this, turning back cannot either help or dispel the fear, and perpetuates the exclusion that seems to be so much part of the suffering of madness. We can all help, and one way might be, if not to overcome our fears, to at least resist the temptation to turn away, and to be there and listen and in this way at least to contain the fear by giving it some form and meaning, restoring a degree of proportion and hopefully bringing some calm and a peace of mind.

29

Anxiety, psychiatry in disarray and a celebrity circus

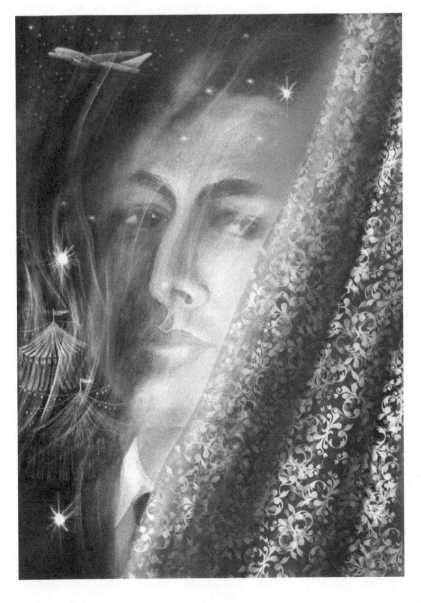

On the 7 November 2010 a beautiful and glamorous couple arrive in Cape Town on their honeymoon. He is a wealthy businessman from Bristol in the United Kingdom and she is an engineer of Indian origin resident in Sweden. In October they had celebrated their marriage in a three day Hindu wedding attended by five hundred guests in Mumbai in India, and had left shortly thereafter for South Africa. They take a domestic flight to the Kruger National Park where they stay in a luxury lodge for four days, returning to Cape Town International airport on the 12 November. There they engage the services of a taxi driver to take them to the five star Cape Grace Hotel. They retain this driver as a tour guide and that evening he drives them through the city to the Strand on the False Bay coast where they have a light meal.

On the way back to the hotel the wife is reported by the husband to say she wants to see "the real South Africa". The driver takes them into Gugulettu, a township on the outskirts of the city notorious for its high crime rate. Shortly after turning off the main road two armed men hijack the taxi. After driving a short distance the taxi driver is thrown from the vehicle. The husband is robbed of his wallet, his watch and a mobile phone, and after driving onward for about twenty minutes he is also thrown from the car. On the morning of the 14 November in Lingelethu West the young wife is found dead on the back seat of the abandoned taxi. She has suffered a single gunshot wound to the neck. The body is removed to a city mortuary where this gunshot wound, having severed an artery, is confirmed as the cause of her death. There is no sign of a sexual assault. On the 17 November her body is released by the South African authorities and she is returned to the United Kingdom, accompanied by the husband.

The murder makes global headlines. In the UK the Daily Mail's website runs the story under the headline: "Honeymoon horror: newlywed Briton's wife is killed after robbers hijack them in taxi". The high rate of crime in South Africa again receives international attention. On the 20 November the taxi driver is arrested. Reports begin to emerge that the killing had been planned, that it was not just another random hijacking that had gone terribly wrong. The driver reports that he had been paid

R15,000 for the murder. On the 7 December the husband, Shrien Dewani is arrested in Bristol under a South African warrant on suspicion of conspiring to murder his wife Anni. On the 8 December Mr. Dewani appears in a City of Westminster Magistrates Court. He is remanded in custody as South Africa prepares for his extradition. It proves to be a long and fraught process.

In arrests made soon after the murder, hijackers Mziwanadoda Qwabe and Xolile Mnengeni and hotel receptionist Monde Mbolombo admit to their involvement in what they initially claim was an unintentionally fatal robbery and kidnapping. Confronting the likelihood of life in prison they later change their account of the events to allege that the crime had been a premeditated murder at the behest of Anni's husband Shrien Dewani. The taxi driver Zola Tonga initially claims to have been an innocent victim. Faced with the evidence against him implicating his involvement by the co-conspirators, he then also changes his account, and alleges that the husband was the instigator of his wife's murder. All those implicated at this point in the killing of Anni Dewani have lied to the Court. It is hardly credible that the case against her husband should be based on the testimonies of these clearly unreliable key witnesses.

In December 2010 British police question a German male escort or prostitute named Leopold Leisser. He calls himself the German Master. He claims to have been in regular contact with Shrien Dewani for months before the crime. He tells the authorities that their encounters involve sado-masochistic sex. Dewani reportedly has to lick his boots. The German Master is to be the next key witness in the case for prosecution.

Plea bargains are offered to the accused conspirators in exchange for future testimony in legal proceedings. Zola Tonga pleads guilty to murder in December 2010 and is sentenced to 18 years in prison. Mziwanadoda Qwabe pleads guilty to murder and is sentenced to 25 years in prison. Xolile Mnengeni is convicted on charges of murder and is sentenced to life in prison. Monde Mbolombo admits his involvement in the crime but is offered immunity in exchange for testimony against the others alleged to have been involved in the crime. In July 2014 a medical parole application is made on behalf of Mnengeni who is reported to be terminally ill owing to a brain tumour. Parole is denied and he dies in prison in October 2014. Leopold Leisser the German Master is found hanging in his Birmingham apartment in September 2016. His suicide is attributed to stress relating to the adverse publicity arising from his involvement in the case against Shrien Dewani.

On the 8 February Shrien Dewani's legal team file papers setting out the grounds on which extradition to South Africa is to be opposed. He is said to be too ill to be extradited. The nature of his illness is vaguely described as a "stress-related condition". In February he is admitted to the Bristol Royal Infirmary. A provisional diagnosis is made of a post-traumatic stress disorder (PTSD). There is an unconfirmed report of an attempted suicide. Anxiety and depression emerge as key factors in this sequence of events. His condition appears to deteriorate and in April he is compulsorily detained under the Mental Health Act 1983 at Fromeside Clinic in Bristol. In May the extradition hearing begins at Breimarsh Magistrates Court in London.

Dewani's barrister Clare Montgomery QC argues that the extradition proceedings are hanging over her client "like the sword of Damocles" and that he needs a period of calm to recover from the symptoms of anxiety and depression, and to prepare himself for extradition. She argues that a twelve month period under medical treatment would increase the speed of her client's recovery, rather than jeopardizing it by sending him to South Africa. He is reported to be making a slow recovery. One damaging factor is said to be his "constant awareness of the court proceedings". The Court is informed by his psychiatrist that the symptoms are of a moderate to severe degree and that he continues to pose a suicide risk. The Court also hears that Mr. Dewani "is unable to give an account of himself, possibly because he cannot remember", which is a curious supposition given that intrusive memories are a central feature of a post-traumatic stress disorder. The section order in terms of the Mental Health Act 1983 is renewed.

The state of Mr. Dewani's mental health becomes

increasingly central to the repeated postponements of his extradition to South Africa to face the charges of the murder of his wife. Initially the symptoms are described as an "acute stress disorder" and a "depressive adjustment disorder". This is revised to a post-traumatic stress disorder and a "clinical" depressive disorder. His counsel describes difficulties in communication with her client and tells the Court that his continuing ill-health prevents her from taking instructions from him. These are not characteristic features of either anxiety or depression.

It is further submitted on behalf of Mr. Dewani that: "If it is true-and it plainly is the case- that Mr. Dewani is seriously mentally ill, and he were sent back to a prison system that simply cannot cope with that level of mental illness, that is a violation of articles 3 and 4 of the European Convention of Human Rights which prohibits inhuman or degrading treatment". The trial of Shrien Dewani for murder becomes a trial of South African prison services. It also becomes a challenge to South African medical services.

In a report by two eminent British psychiatrists submitted on behalf of Mr. Dewani it is stated that: "This risk would be unacceptable in the absence of proper and adequate management of his illnesses. The prognosis for recovery depends on whether Mr. Dewani can receive treatment. If he cannot then the prognosis is poor...travel to South Africa would greatly enhance his distress and cause him substantial further psychological harm. It may result in him killing himself...the problem with extraditing him now is that even with the best possible psychiatric facilities in South Africa it will be very difficult to get him to a state where he is fit to plead'. The report concludes that that "there is no doubt that Mr. Dewani suffers from a severe and incapacitating mental illness. He is not faking the symptoms. There is currently a real and significant risk of suicide. That risk will increase if he is extradited to South Africa".

The High Court in England temporarily halts Dewani's extradition on the grounds of poor mental health. The Court rules that it would be "unjust and inappropriate" to send him to South Africa immediately, but rejects claims that he should not be extradited on the grounds of human rights. It declares that in the interests of justice he should be extradited "as soon as he is fit". Ashok Hindocha, the uncle of Anni Dewani says after the hearing that the family desperately needs answers. He says: "I don't know how much longer the family members can take the pressure psychologically".

In addition to concerns raised about Dewani's mental health, doubts are expressed on behalf of Mr. Dewani in regard to the likelihood of a fair trial in South Africa. The South African Police Chief General Bheki Cele says: "A monkey came all the way from London to have his wife murdered here...he thought we South Africans were stupid when he came all the way to kill his wife in our country. He lied to himself".

In March 2014 the High Court in England finally rejects all grounds to appeal against extradition and denies Dewani the chance to take the case to the appeal court. The Court accepted the validity of an undertaking on behalf of the Government of South Africa that if Dewani is not fit to stand trial within eighteen months he should be returned to the UK. With regard to the forthcoming case in South Africa the Hindocha family say: "We need it...South Africa needs it...the world needs it...everybody wants to know what happened to Anni...everybody is seeking justice for her".

Shrien Dewani is extradited to South Africa on the 7 April. He arrives in Cape Town international airport on the 8 April on a chartered flight accompanied by a doctor and nurse and a bevy of officials. He is arrested and immediately taken to court where he is charged with five offences: conspiracy to commit kidnapping, robbery with aggravating circumstances, kidnapping, the murder of his wife and obstructing the administration of justice. He pleads not guilty to all charges and is remanded to Valkenberg Hospital for the assessment and treatment of his psychiatric problems. He arrives in a cavalcade of vehicles with the international press in attendance. It is a circus. Shrien Dewani grotesquely is a celebrity. He is also now my patient.

Given this history and the global attention being paid to the saga, it was of critical importance but also difficult to keep a determinedly open mind, and to be impartial and rigorous in our assessment. I could not ignore but I could not allow myself to be swayed by the opinions of our respected and esteemed colleagues in the United Kingdom. Our multidisciplinary team interviewed him and observed him and over the weeks and months that he was with us and evaluated him with I think the greatest care possible. I began to form an opinion but made a strenuous effort to not allow my thinking to influence my colleagues. Nevertheless a consensus did begin to emerge.

I cannot describe in any detail my encounters with Mr. Dewani in regard of the professional code respecting confidentiality in the doctor-patient relationship. I can however summarize a report I submitted to the Court as this is in the public domain. With the support of the multidisciplinary team I developed the opinion that Mr. Dewani was not suffering from any form of mental illness and that he should therefore be discharged from our unit.

In the report I wrote: "At the time of admission Mr. Dewani presented as being calm, alert and cooperative. His manner was confident and self-assured. He showed no features of anxiety and depression. He denied suicidal thoughts...he insisted that his intention was to appear in court to face the charges against him and that he wanted no further delay in the proceedings. Owing to the low risk he presented he was transferred to a medium secure unit. During the following weeks his confident demeanour diminished. He appeared more anxious, particularly during more formal interviews, and at times showed hypervigilant behaviour, flinching dramatically in response to the routine noises of a busy ward. He was distracted by these external stimuli but was able to rapidly regain the focus of attention. The occasional symptoms of anxiety, tearfulness and depression were considered understandable in the context of his failed appeal against extradition and the pending court appearance. At other times, in interactions with the occupational therapist and the clinical psychologist, or when unaware of being observed by the nursing staff he appeared more calm...The medication prescribed in the UK was gradually withdrawn owing to the unclear benefit and side-effects including irritability and anxiety, impaired concentration and biochemical abnormalities. At the time of writing Mr. Dewani is on no regular medication. The anxiolytic prescribed on an as required basis at the time of his admission has not been used..."

I reported that a consensus had developed amongst the members of the multidisciplinary team that Mr. Dewani was not depressed. With regard to the diagnosis of a post-traumatic stress disorder I stated that while it was acknowledged that Mr. Dewani did appear to meet the standard criteria for this diagnosis the context should be taken into account, in that the symptoms of anxiety could more probably be accounted for by his predicament at the time rather than past events. The avoidance displayed could be less an inability to recall past traumatic events than an understandable anxiety with regard to needing to appear in court to account for circumstances leading him to be charged with the murder of his wife. For these reasons the diagnosis of a post-traumatic stress disorder was set aside. I reported: "At the time of writing the opinion is that Mr. Dewani is not suffering from a mental illness. It is recommended that Mr. Dewani should be discharged from this unit. Further hospitalization is unlikely to benefit him and on the contrary is more likely to have the adverse effect of reinforcing the avoidant behaviour that has developed subsequent to the events of November 2010".

On the 6 October 2014, after a delay of over three years following the charges of murder against him, the trial finally commences in the Western Cape High Court. Under cross examination the key witnesses who alleged Mr. Dewani's involvement contradict their previous statements and each other on most of the key elements of the "murder for hire" story. The testimony of the German Master is judged to be irrelevant. Mr. Dewani's sexuality was not considered to be on trial. On the 24 November after the closure of the case for the prosecution Mr. Dewani's counsel argues for the case to be dismissed, citing a lack of credible evidence linking his client to the crime. On the 8 December this application is granted. Mr. Dewani is acquitted of all charges against him. He boards a flight for the UK.

The presiding Judge Traverso says in Court that the evidence of the three criminals already convicted of murder was "so improbable, with so many lies and inconsistencies you cannot see where the lies ended and the truth begins". South African National Prosecuting Authority spokesman Nathi Ncube expresses disappointment with the outcome but says the decision of the court will be respected and that there will not be an appeal. He says: "It is unfortunate that Mr. Dewani has been acquitted because we believe that he was involved. The court did not find that he was innocent. The court could not rely on the evidence given by three witnesses who themselves had been convicted of the crime". The Hindocha family say they have been failed by the justice system. Their desperate need for the answer to what happened to Anni Dewani on the night of 13 November 2010 remains unanswered.

I cannot help. I don't know. I never asked Shrien Dewani whether or not he was involved in the murder of his wife. It was not my business. My task was to assess whether or not he was ill, and treat him if necessary so that he could appear in court to face the charges against him. I also believe that had I asked him it would almost certainly have had a negative impact on whatever relationship I had with him. I did not want to jeopardize anything that might further delay him appearing in court.

To this day I feel angered and exasperated by the outcome. I think South Africa and in particular the criminal justice system shamefully failed the Hindocha family.

It is difficult for me not to feel that I also failed the family, and that the profession of psychiatry had wrongfully been involved and that the confusion of psychiatric diagnoses had complicated this tragic course of events. I believe that I am one of very many who share with the family of Anni Dewani a perception of justice having been thwarted, and an anger at the role played by psychiatry in what I believe many thought to be the obstruction of the administration of justice. In amongst all the noise and clamour surrounding these events the focus seems to have become blurred or lost. A young woman was brutally murdered. A life full of hope and beauty and promise is lost. I cannot imagine what anguish this has caused the family, and must surely continue to afflict them.

30

The problem with depression

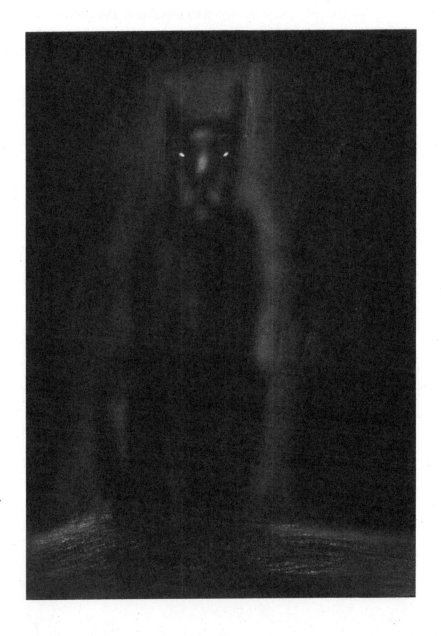

The problem with depression is to some extent the vocabulary of depression. Depression is part of life. It is inevitable. In many ways it represents the burden of self-consciousness. Not to feel depressed at times is not to be quite alive, as it would be not to feel joyful or sad or apprehensive.

The difficulty arises in regard to thresholds and contexts. It might be understandable, and regarded with a degree of sympathy if at times one might become depressed while pondering the futility of life given the certainty of death. But this might also be regarded as ridiculous and self-indulgent if it persisted, to the exclusion of any other emotion that might mitigate such a gloomy appraisal and make life worth living. Depression in the context of loss and bereavement is appropriate and necessary. It is an integral part of the process of recovery and restitution. A degree of depression in times of adversity is understandable. Waking in the morning with sunlight bursting through the bedroom window and feeling an utter exhausting dread is altogether another matter.

Depression as an illness does not seem quite to be depression, at least not in the way the word is most commonly used. Depression in the quotidian use of the word is relatively benign. In its malignant forms it seems to be something qualitatively different. It is very often less understandable in terms of the context, and it is of a different degree and of a different nature. It is another, different beast.

"I can't understand it", Hannes said to me. We were meeting for the first time in the out-patient clinic. He sat slumped in the chair. He was ill-kempt and his speech was slow and monotonous. "There is no reason for me to be this way. Nothing has gone wrong. There is no particular crisis. There is no major problem at work. There are no difficulties at home. I have a supportive wife. I am embarrassed. I feel ashamed. I just can't seem to pull myself together. I feel hopeless. I am hopeless. This has come from nowhere".

There did not seem to be any identifiable stressors. He was a reasonably successful, middle aged business man. Apart from a raised blood pressure he was relatively healthy. The only clue was that something similar had happened to his father who had committed suicide when Hannes was in his late teens. "I coped with it somehow" he told me in regard to this. "I just got on with things. I have always regarded myself as a strong person. That's why I find this so difficult to cope with. It's not me".

He described an insidious onset. Perhaps the first indication was a difficulty in concentrating at work. Tasks that he was used to performing easily now had become onerous. He had struggled for the first time to sleep through the night. He was finding himself waking in the early hours of the morning filled with a trepidation that he could not fathom. He had no appetite and had lost a considerable amount of weight. His libido was extinguished. The worst he said was an overwhelming, enervating fatigue, and a profoundly distressing loss of interest and pleasure in all the things that had previously sustained him. He said there was no longer colour in his life. All was grey. There was no variation in tone or pitch in the world around him. All senses were dulled. There was only a bleak and pervasive emptiness.

He had previously been an enthusiastic gardener but now he said he simply could not be bothered. It was too much of an effort. His wife described him gazing upon the ruin of the once immaculate garden in blank disinterest. When she attempted to encourage him to do some work in the garden, hoping that some simple pleasurable task might kindle the process of recovery his response was irritable and impatient. She simply didn't understand, he had told her, and insisted that she leave him alone. His small children were bewildered: their loving father had become absent. The wife became angry and frightened and confused. She said she felt that there was something very wrong but she had no idea what it might be or where she should turn for help. It had to be something physical, she said, to account the extent of his decline. An assessment of depression did not make much sense to her. There was no reason for him to be depressed, she said, and anyway depression was psychological, and therefore could not explain the dramatic physical deterioration that was so evident to her and to me.

Another part of the problem of depression arises from this dualist way of thinking. Depression has grave physical consequences, most obviously suicide. Defined as being psychological, particularly in a materialist culture depression is perceived to be of less import than a diagnosis of a general medical condition. In my experience patients are acutely aware of this implicitly dismissive attitude, and this failure of understanding compounds the sense of shame and isolation and hopelessness they describe.

Consequences less dramatic than suicide are also potentially dangerous. Hannes had stopped his anti-hypertensive medication. Again he said he couldn't be bothered. He denied suicidal intent but he did say that he thought his life was not worth living. He did not mind if he had a stroke or a heart attack or if he just happened to die. It was some sort of solution. Perhaps it would be better for his family, a relief of the burden of having to look after him. Yes, he reflected in the presence of his appalled wife, although he was not going to kill himself, he did not have the energy anyway, perhaps he would be better off dead than alive.

People who are severely depressed don't look after themselves in the most basic way. They don't have the energy and they don't care. People living with severe psychiatric disorders have a reduced life expectancy of between ten and twenty years. A high proportion of deaths are due to cardiovascular problems. In depressed states, people do not bother to exercise, they have no motivation and no energy. They do not take their medication. They smoke. They use alcohol and other drugs, either because they do not care or out of a desperate need to escape, however briefly, from the dark entrapment of their depressed worlds.

Alcohol is a depressant psychoactive substance. It exerts its transiently mood elevating effects by depressing higher inhibitory centres in the brain. It is understandable that one might seek escape by resorting to this easily available and apparently extremely effective agent. Use and misuse are compounded by the phenomenon of tolerance. More and more of the substance has to be used to achieve the same effect. A downward spiral develops into a vortex. Increasing amounts of alcohol are consumed with diminished and then no pleasure in an increasingly desperate attempt to quell the mounting depression and despair, or at least to numb the pain. A complex web of psychological and physical and social problems ensues, closing the trap. Social isolation, physical ailments, depression and alcohol itself are all risk factors for suicide, either in overt or less direct forms. Escape is no longer imagined as possible. There is no hope and the only avenue is descent to oblivion, which is imagined as some sort of escape.

I tried and failed to help a colleague who was also a friend. There had been a number of difficulties but nothing that in the early stages seemed insurmountable. He had used alcohol for as long as I had known him, perhaps excessively but not in a way that I thought was out of control. Then he suffered perhaps a major disappointment in that a funding proposal was rejected. He seemed to lose direction, or make too much of this setback, and gave up seeking funding from other sources. He began to drink more heavily and his partner complained. She said he became morose and apathetic. His work performance declined and his colleagues began to express concern. He was living in another city at the time and I went to visit him. Initially he seemed to be his old self. He expressed pleasure in seeing me and I thought and hoped that the fears had been exaggerated. He prepared a meal and suggested that we have a drink together to celebrate my visit. It felt churlish to refuse and I worried that I might alienate him. There was a fairly animated conversation initially but he was drinking steadily and then he seemed to lose concentration. It was evening and getting dark but he did not seem to register. We sat together in the gloom and his conversation became increasingly rambling and disjointed and then incoherent. I switched the lights on and he faced me in silence and immobile, as if confounded by something that he could not articulate and that had overwhelmed him. I somehow got him to bed and left the next day. A fortnight later he put a gun to his head and ended his life. We sought to console ourselves that by that stage there was nothing we could have done to stop him, but the sense of guilt and failure was inescapable. It is one of the consequences of such a malignant trajectory, the helplessness of those trying to help.

Bastiaan said he did not need help. I saw him in the out-patient department at the request of his friends. He was HIV positive and he was depressed. He had given up. He said there was nothing to live for. He had stopped eating. He did not wash himself and he was refusing anti-retroviral medication. He had alienated himself from his family, he had lost his job and his friends had become exasperated by his apparent refusal to help himself and his rejection of hope. He dismissed the proposal of anti-depressant medication as he did the anti-retrovirals. It was pointless he said. There was nothing to be done. In his way of thinking the situation was clear and it was hopeless. It is so often a tangled, complex story, but it seemed clear to us that his depression, and the decisions and the behaviour that flowed from it would eventually lead to his death. A difficult and ethically complicated aspect of the treatment of a severe depression is the hopelessness that is part of the depression so often leads to the rejection of treatment, or any other means of mitigating the burden of suffering.

Extreme forms of depression may develop a psychotic intensity. In schizophrenic states the content of delusions tends to be mystifying incongruent. A person might describe being pursued by unknown assailants intent on killing him, but appear to be nonchalant. In a severe depression a person might describe the same experience but say the persecution is right and proper. He or she is so irredeemably bad and guilty that they deserve to die.

A schoolteacher I met in one of the community clinics had a vivid memory of his depression that had required an emergency admission many years previously. It was difficult for me to imagine, he seemed so well and informed and insightful. He had fully recovered and had returned to work as a secondary school teacher. He was clearly respected by his colleagues and he was happily married with two teenage children. I had seen him regularly over a period of about six months and thought I had got to know him fairly well, so I suggested on one encounter that he might consider a trial period without medication. He declined, saying that the memory of that depressive episode was so terrible that he did not want to put himself at any risk of a relapse.

Another few months passed before he told me that he had discussed the issue with is wife and his family, and the decision given the stability of his mood over the past at least ten years was to embark on a cautious withdrawal. I organized a very gradual programme of reducing and stopping the anti-depressant medication and made an appointment to see him in a month's time. He dutifully kept the appointment, but when he entered the interview room he appeared to be dishevelled and perplexed. I worriedly asked him how he was doing but he did not answer for a while, and then whispered to me: "Doctor are you carrying a gun?". I said no, of course not, and asked why was he was asking this strange question. He said: "I am a dog. I'm just a dirty dog and you must shoot me".

He did recover, as he had done previously, but there was to be no further attempts at withdrawal. It did mean though, sadly that the depression was something that he was going to have to live with, that it was not some sort of aberration, and that it was in some way part of him. There was to be no cure, no putting that dreadful experience behind him forever, but an acceptance, perhaps a resignation that this malevolent dog which he had momentarily become would be always lurking at the periphery of his otherwise bright life.

The problem with depression and the language used to describe its wide range of expression is also in the way it should then be managed. Severe and less severe give some indication of a continuum but are inadequate terms. Nevertheless on one side of the spectrum there seems to be a syndrome more related to adverse life circumstances, and on the other side, a syndrome less associated with external circumstances and having more the nature of an illness. There is an apparent paradox in the way these two forms respond to treatment and particularly pharmacological treatment in that the more severe forms of depression are more responsive to treatment. It is perhaps understandable that socio-economic ills, or bereavement are unlikely to be ameliorated by a chemical agent, whereas the more severe forms of depression, which seem more probably to have a biological basis should be more likely to respond. Treating the hardships of life with an anti-depressant medication does not seem helpful and is more likely to be harmful. It is unlikely to be effective. It fails to acknowledge difficult and complex life circumstances, offering rather a simplistic, paternalistic pharmacological sop, and can undermine the necessary and more constructive process of developing the resources to cope with adversity as best as possible.

What is certainly not helpful is to be dismissive, and this takes many at times covert forms, and may be well intentioned. "Don't worry, it's not so bad" "it will be alright, it will pass with time", "the same thing happened to me and I got over it" are likely to be heard as mere noise by a depressed person, or confirmation of a failure to understand.

Finding the right balance can be difficult. It is rarely one thing or the other but in whatever form it takes depression is a grim reality. There is a tension between acknowledging suffering and seeking to suppress its various manifestations. The woman in the clinic whose husband had been abusive and had deserted her and who now fretted how she might support her family for the month did not expect me to take her problems away.

Another, incapacitated and tormented with fatigue, a total absence of volition and afflicted with thoughts of suicide will more probably seek any form of help, or possibly not, if in the depths of depression the situation is perceived as hopeless.

31

The illusory thrill of mania

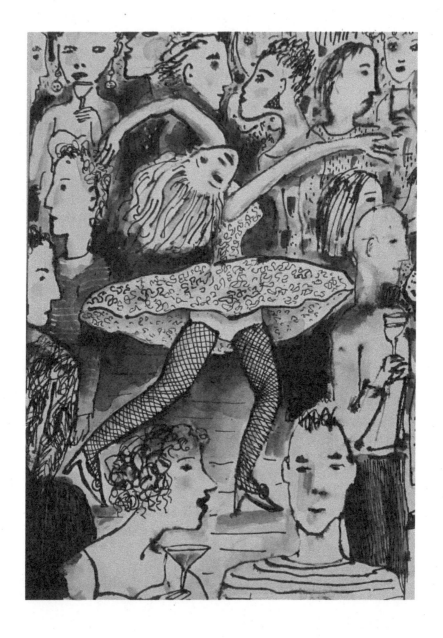

I have never encountered someone in the joyful throes of a manic state. By the time of the admission it is over. We have to cope with the aftermath, the appalled family, the shame and the anger. But even at the high pitch of the mania I am not sure of the joyfulness of it. More often our patients have described feeling out of control and being frightened. It is not an exuberant, liberating epiphanous state they say, in retrospect. It is more a joyless frenzy.

Pieter sits slumped in a chair in the out –patient department. He had recently been discharged after yet another relapse of a bipolar illness. At the time of his admission he was manic. He was not full of joy. He was not on top of the world. He was hostile, irritable and extremely aggressive. He was violent towards the nursing staff who tried to calm him. His language was abusive and obscene and racist. I had known him for years. This was completely uncharacteristic. His manner was usually cautious and considerate. His attitude towards me seemed curiously formal at times, as if he needed to keep me at a distance. This was perhaps understandable given that I had known a side of him that he struggled to acknowledge and which he sought to hide from the world. He had been an extremely successful businessman. It is quite possible but merely speculative that part of the success had owed something to an energy of incipient mania that had subsequently spun out of control. Now everything was in ruins.

He was bankrupt. His wife had left him. His friends had fled. His reputation was destroyed and in his world this also meant his future. He was particularly distressed by his daughter's refusal to have any contact with him. She was angry and she said she had lost all patience. This had happened too many times before. Following a previous episode he had apologized to her and promised to take the medication. It came to nothing. He stopped the treatment and very soon things began to take a predictable and frightening course. He made reckless business decisions. He drank heavily and perhaps the worst for her was that he made embarrassingly inappropriate sexual advances to her friends. She was ashamed of him. Trying to explain that this was part of an illness meant little to her. He knew he had a bipolar disorder she said. He knew what would happen when he stopped the treatment. She could not look after him. He was her father but he had failed her. She had to get on with her own life she said, and it would be best if she now cut off all contact with him.

Sitting opposite me Pieter seemed exhausted and defeated. He did not make any excuse for what had happened. He did not seek to blame the illness. I asked about the future and he just heaved a weary sigh. He could see no future. There was little that I could say that would not have seemed to him insufferably trite. This was not a depressive phase of a bipolar illness. It was the understandable and familiar aftermath of a manic episode. Given his perception of the hopelessness of the situation I was compelled to ask him about suicide. He appeared to ponder this option for some time and then said no, he did not have the energy. He then said with some bitterness that it would be some sort of solution for his business colleagues, and his lost friends and family. He was trapped, and it did seem to me that a more likely event would be for him, seeing no future to again stop the treatment and take flight into a despairing mania.

A similar tired, exasperated and angry response was described to me by the mother of Thembakosi. Again she had been through this too many times. She had tried so hard. She had been hopeful so many times. And so many times she had had her hopes dashed. But she was his mother and she had to stay with him. There was nobody else. He had alienated all other members of his family and all his friends. The first episode was while he was at university. He was an exceptionally bright student. In retrospect he was probably veering into mania, and it seemed possibly that this was in part due to academic pressures as he was about to write his final exams for a degree in commerce.

For no apparent reason Thembakosi assaulted a fellow student. At the time of his admission thereafter to our unit he was clearly manic, but by this time he had been expelled from the university. A tribunal was held and I managed to persuade the university authorities to allow him to write the final examinations although he remained barred from attending lectures. He passed and everybody was happy and relieved. Whether to celebrate his success, or possibly because he could not accept the diagnosis Thembakosi stopped the treatment and relapsed and he was back in the unit within months. This sequence of events went on for years. After yet another admission he would sit facing me in the out-patient department and say earnestly: "Doctor I have learned my lesson. I can see what damage this has done to my life and how much suffering this has caused my family. It will never happen again". I did not doubt his determination but it was not to be. Months later I received a call from his mother. I am sorry, she said as if she herself had somehow failed me. She sounded exhausted, beyond anger now, as if all her strength in keeping the family together had finally been depleted.

On this occasion Thembakosi had become bored with the human resources position his father had managed to find for him. He had developed the quite brilliant notion that he could make a lot more money gambling than he could working in a job that he found unfulfilling. In one night he lost a fortune. He somehow managed to get access to his parents' credit cards and used all their money. He continues to pay off the debt. The mother said: "He is my son. I can't turn my back on him", but the father just stared into the distance, absent, as if there was nothing further that could be said. The family, Thembakosi, his parents, his sister and his ex-wife and their young child seemed at that moment to be broken. Again I formed the impression that it was a great struggle for him to be well, to be a responsible son and husband and father and worker, and that at times these demands became insuperable, and like an alcoholic reaching for the next drink, he succumbed to the joyless abandonment of this struggle.

These manic episodes are expressed in many different ways, and the differences between men and women are often marked. For men aggression and violent behaviour often associated with drunkenness were common precipitants to admission to our unit. Violence provokes violence and the effects are enduring. Enraged by his mother's entreaties to stop his excessive drinking, Stefanus in a manic fury attacked her. The father could not restrain him. He hit his son, repeatedly in a desperate attempt to subdue him. We met the family after Stefanus had been admitted. They were all appalled by what had happened. This time it was not: "This is not my son". It was "This is not our family". I think such manic episodes have a more devastating effect on families than any other form of mental illness.

Inappropriate sexual behaviour seems to be a more common expression of mania among women. A dismayed mother described her daughter's behaviour at a party hosted by her brothers. She was drinking heavily and nobody could stop her. But it was not just drunkenness the mother said. She herself seemed reluctant to describe the events, and it was clear that the whole family had been profoundly embarrassed by the young woman's disinhibited behaviour. It was not flirtatious or amusing in any way, the mother said, it was lewd. The party had been ruined. Her dismay was compounded by her sons' subsequent refusal to have any further contact with their sister. It did not matter that she was manic, that she was ill in a way that might have been difficult for a young person to understand. They were ashamed of her.

Parties, and especially wedding celebrations can be fraught affairs for persons of a manic disposition. I attended the wedding of a friend whose sister was known to be struggling with a bipolar disorder. The sister began to dance wildly after the marriage ceremony. She hauled elderly and bewildered men to their feet and frolicked about them in an increasingly hectic and lascivious manner. This being a wedding celebration there was initially much goodwill. She was just having a good time. She was just being wild and unconventional, we wished to believe, but this gradually shifted to unease. To my dismay she then headed for me. She cavorted about me and then grabbed me towards her, pushing herself against me. "Help me", she whispered urgently, "Help me. Stop me. I am out of control. You have to help me". Perhaps at some point there was for her a blissful moment of sheer exuberance, but it was ephemeral, and my memory is of a beautiful young woman trapped in joyless agitation.

It might seem impoverished or churlish to describe the excitement of mania as illusory. There is an extensive literature about the association of genius with mental illness, in particular mania. Conventional ways of thinking and seeing and hearing are blown away by the liberating and exhilarating force of a manic episode. The corollary is that it is profoundly unimaginative if not destructive to attempt to control or subdue this potentially creative force. Doctors and nurses possibly unwittingly are perceived as the agents of political economic and cultural control, imposing conformity and submission to authority. If only people with mania were allowed to roam free, unfettered by convention or medication, the world would be a brighter and more exciting place. This seems to be a romantic, wishful position, and I doubt that those suffering from bipolar disorders or their families or communities would subscribe to it. It does nevertheless seem very possible that those who have lived through these extreme states of turmoil and who have developed strategies of coping might have a wider more imaginative sense of being in the world, and something valuable to communicate. Whether this might be considered fortunate, or a blessed endowment of any kind is another matter.

Johannes said to me: "Mania is a selfish illness. I want the mania. I miss it but I cannot cope with what it has done to my family. I cannot afford it. Not any longer".

I have never been manic. I don't know what it is like and I cannot imagine what it is like.

It might then seem presumptuous to describe the possible thrill of mania as illusory. But the patients I have encountered either in the throes of a mania or in its aftermath have described no joy. They have nevertheless described an intense ambivalence both about the nature of the experience and how it should be managed. For the most part it is accepted that it is not possible to live in this way, and that damage is incurred. But at the same time, with this acceptance something is lost. Something is sacrificed. Treatment represents some form of compromise, as if some important part of oneself is being suppressed. Achieving the balance of holding the energy, the exhilarating sense that all things are possible, and preventing the ensuing chaos and disorganization is exasperatingly difficult and elusive.

32

The allure of intoxication

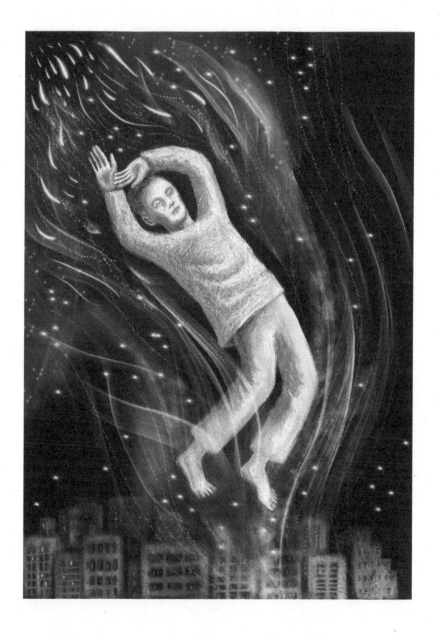

"I don't understand it. How could you do this? How could you do this to your family? How could you do this to yourself? I don't know what to say. Honestly, I don't know what to do. I'm finished".

The mother sighs and stares ahead, angry, looking at nothing.

Xolisi sits slumped in his chair, his legs splayed, his eyes downcast in a posture of defiant nonchalance. The occupational therapist fidgets and stifles a yawn. The students look away from both mother and son, embarrassed by the mother's distress. The silence is oppressive. There is nothing I can say to console her or to reassure her. I think it is probably important that she speak and that we listen but I am not sure that it will help her and I am a little bit more sure that it is not going to make any difference. This has happened before and it is going to happen again. Xolisi will get better. We will discharge him and within a few months he will be back and we will listen again to the mother vent her fury and exasperation.

She has to deal with this on her own. The father is absent. The community has shunned her. When intoxicated Xolisi has been violent and he has stolen from the neighbours to obtain the drugs he uses that make him mad. The mother's anger is compounded by shame. To add to her woes she is poverty stricken. Xolisi is her only child. He is unemployable. She asks whether at least she can apply for a disability grant. The social worker is stern. Xolisi is not sick or disabled she says, in that he brings this problem on himself. If he did not use the drugs he could go out and find work. He must take responsibility. He does not qualify for a disability grant. The mother sighs wearily, defeated. I turn to Xolisi, attempting to prompt a response. He refuses. He has also heard this all before. He has been through this time and time again and he is telling us that there is nothing for him to say. The occupational therapist excuses herself. She says she has another meeting to attend but I think she is bored. If it is not Xolisi it is Thabo or Jan or Yusuf. It's the same old sad predictable story. We are going around in circles and nothing is learned.

It is a struggle not to become resigned–or angry, to imagine Xolisi not as just another member of a lost and aimless tribe of young and hopeless men. I try to imagine him, crouched in some dark and empty space, the wind tearing at the frail wrought iron shelter, the loneliness, outside the menace of poverty and deprivation, craving for that moment of bliss, that rapturous escape. The lighting of the pipe, the rattle of the crystals against the glass, the luxurious inhalation of the fumes are familiar but also thrilling. He becomes transformed. Nothing matters, not for this wonderful moment when he can imagine he can do anything, that things are not as they are and that he is free.

Intoxication is not a form of madness. It is a transient, self – limiting phenomenon arising from the effects of whatever psychoactive substance has been used. These effects are broadly categorized as being stimulant or depressant or hallucinogenic in the derangement of perceptions. The apparent stimulating effect of alcohol is illusory. Alcohol is a depressant. The euphoria sometimes associated with its use is due to the depressant action on the higher inhibitory centres of the brain. There seems to be something rather sad in the observation that the most evolved and highly developed parts of ourselves are negative or inhibitory, in limiting ourselves, and it is perhaps a factor in our persisting use of a drug that is so obviously harmful. We imagine, in a state of happy intoxication, that we are more ourselves.

Intoxicated people do not come to our unit. If there is extremely disturbed behaviour they might be admitted to a casualty unit where they cause much havoc and anger among the nursing and medical staff. This is not an uncommon occurrence, particularly over the weekends, and it is potentially dangerous and it is also complicated. The danger of course can be due to the drunken disruption of emergency care, but it can also be due to less obvious causes. An assumption cannot be made that the disorganized behaviour is due solely to intoxication. People when they are drunk and disinhibited do stupid and dangerous things. They fight and fall over. The casualty staff, very often harassed and overworked in the chaos of medical and surgical emergencies therefore have to be on alert to the potentially lethal effects of head injuries. These injuries might not be immediately obvious. A closed head injury might have no external sign. An assumption might very easily be made that the altered level of consciousness is due to intoxication and hours later the person is found dead due to a rupture of a blood vessel within the brain.

The situation can also be complicated in that it might not be straightforward clinically to distinguish an intoxicated state from a psychosis. A psychosis implies a clear consciousness, differentiating it from delirium. But defining and identifying an altered level of consciousness is itself fraught with difficulty. Broadly and perhaps rather simplistically clear consciousness may be inferred by the ability to focus, sustain and shift attention appropriately. This can be very difficult to determine in a floridly psychotic state, and of course one does not preclude the other, as for head injuries and intoxication. Psychosis does not protect against intoxication. On the contrary, it seemed to me very often that our patients intoxicated themselves to escape the burden of their psychoses.

The matter is further complicated by the fact that intoxication might induce a psychosis. In this circumstance the intoxicated state is not limited to the time in which the psycho-active substance exerts its effects on the brain, but shades into a persistent psychosis independent of the direct effects of the substance, but considered to be causally related. This is perhaps most marked with regard to cannabis or dagga. It is this induced psychosis that brings Xolisi back to our unit time and time again.

Exposure to cannabis increases the risk of developing a psychosis, more specifically schizophrenia, two to threefold. The increased risk is associated with the amount of exposure and the concentration of the psycho-active ingredients, and the exposure is particularly hazardous before the age of approximately fifteen years of age. At this stage the brain undergoes a number of subtle and complex changes, including a process described as synaptic pruning, whereby unnecessary or unused neuronal connections are discarded or edited out. This is also the stage when young people are most likely to start using cannabis, if only in the spirit of experimentation. The theory is that it is this disorganization of neuronal connections, owing both to a genetic vulnerability and environmental factors including exposure to cannabis, that form the neurobiological basis of schizophrenia. It is therefore quite mad, or it constitutes a high risk if having a family history of schizophrenia one voluntarily exposes oneself at a young age to cannabis. Yet this happened too frequently in our unit, and it seemed all the more tragic as arising out of ignorance or a false and romantic notion of the innocuous allure of intoxication.

Another hazardous consequence of this allure is of course addiction, a phenomenon which although related is distinct from intoxication. One can be intoxicated without becoming addicted and one can be addicted to a substance without being intoxicated. Some of the elements of the clinical syndrome of addiction include a feeling of compulsion to use the substance despite its harmful consequences, a priority accorded to the use, a stereotyped or routine pattern of use, withdrawal symptoms and the phenomenon of tolerance whereby more and more of the substance is required to gain the same effect.

A disease or medical or biological model has been proposed to account for the at times quite mystifying self-destructive phenomenon of addiction. According to this way of thinking the problem arises from a distortion or derangement of the natural and fundamental processes that ensure survival. Eating and drinking and sexual activity are associated with pleasurable feelings or rewards that encourage the repetition of these behaviours that in turn enable us to continue living and encourage procreation. The allure of intoxication and the associated problem of addiction provides a false reward that does not ensure health and survival but is more likely to do great harm.

There seems to be something rather simplistic or reductive in this, certainly if it excludes any form of personal agency or responsibility. Being adult or responsible or behaving in a civilized manner, however vague or problematic these constructs might be, include some sense of being able to inhibit through the higher centres of the central nervous system impulses that arise in the lower centres. As much as we might need to eat and drink and have sex in order to live and ensure the survival of our species we also need to control these impulses according to the context in which these activities might occur. What might be healthy and gratifying in one circumstance might be shameful and grotesquely inappropriate, if not criminal in another.

Given some of the uncertainties regarding the notion of free will and with it a problematic doubt regarding personal responsibility, in our quotidian,-daily lives there needs to be at least some sense that we have a degree of control. Eating can be a pleasurable activity but we do not therefore gorge ourselves to death. Sexual activity can be joyful and enhance life, but to claim an addiction to sex seems more probably a cynical manoeuvre to avoid responsibility for one's actions. To pathologize this behaviour, to invoke the concept of a disease is to exempt the individual from responsibility and this has grave personal but also social consequences. It would surely be regarded as preposterous for a person accused of rape to seek exoneration on the basis that he had no control over his action owing to a problem of addiction to sex. There is little doubt that addiction to alcohol has a familial or genetic predisposition, but that is what it is, a biological vulnerability rather than a genetic determination or fate. Addiction to alcohol and other substances such as the opioids is a tragic condition, and trying to make sense of it in order to be helpful is not promoted by simplistic models or facile solutions. The medical model in its reductive form is inadequate, as would be any alternative model that failed to take into account the physical components of this extremely complex phenomenon.

Some years ago while recovering from a serious back operation I was prescribed morphine. This had a most memorable and blissful effect. I think it was on the fifth day after the surgery that I recall having to make a very conscious and determined effort not to request any further doses of the opioid. A degree of pain was preferable to what seemed to me a very real possibility of becoming addicted. As has been described so often, it was not so much that the pain was dramatically diminished but that it did not matter very much. It also seemed possible that this mysterious nonchalance could have been extended to the problem of addiction, that it might not matter too much as long as I was guaranteed a regular supply of the morphine.

At the time of writing it is estimated that in the USA tens of thousands of young people are dying every year due to opioid addiction, the majority due to prescription opioids, and the numbers are escalating. More are dying than at the peak of the HIV/AIDS epidemic. There is an urgent need to make sense of this in order for public health authorities to make useful and valid recommendations, yet this in the present day appears to be elusive. I don't know what various factors stopped me from demanding more morphine that day following the surgery, but some part of it must surely have been an understanding of the grave consequences of this apparently simple and apparently harmless act. Far too many are less fortunate.

The allure is powerful and its nature is complex. Many social and economic and psychological factors must surely contribute, and it would be inappropriate to generalize from one particular story. There nevertheless does seem a degree of ambivalence, or even a paradox in many of the events we encountered in our unit. In one respect it seemed that the allure of intoxication and its extension into madness was that things then did not matter too much, that the burden of consciousness was diminished. Given the dire circumstances in which many of our patients lived this altered state was likely to be extremely seductive. In another, contrary respect the allure seemed to arise from a sense that it made our patients feel more themselves, that this intoxicated and mad self was the true self, unfeterred, unconfined by social constraints or by medication, liberated and intoxicated by the illusory belief that one was all powerful and that everything was possible.

We said goodbye to Xolisi on a Friday afternoon. His mother had come to collect him. He made a little speech. He thanked us for helping him and he said that he now was well and that he felt strong enough to face the challenges that he knew awaited him beyond the hospital walls. He said that he had learned an important lesson and that he would never use drugs again. I did not doubt that Xolisi was sincere in this and that he was determined to stop the drugs and never return to our hospital. I also did not doubt that he would return, and that we would again sit down together, his mother angry and dejected, Xolisi dumbfounded, and ourselves trying against the odds to maintain yet again some frail hope.

33

Madness as a disorder of consciousness

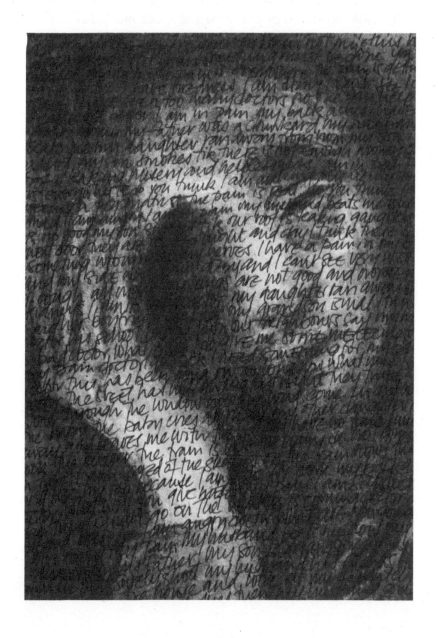

"They know what I am thinking...it is horrible...they know everything about me...how can I protect myself". Damian.

"I am not ill...it's just a phase I am going through...the doctors stole my organs for black magic...I need a herbalist to clean my blood, not a doctor...I am working with the devil...I see the visible souls... they just stand and watch me...I have to kill myself because I am too afraid...I am fighting to take control of my mind". Hoosain.

"You are absolutely under control...if you don't cooperate it's hell...I have no privacy...I couldn't take it". Arnoldus, following a suicide attempt.

Although these utterances are in some ways disorganized and inconsistent there are in addition to the anguish certain shared themes. There is a loss of autonomy, or the sense of being in control. The feeling of the self as being differentiated from the external world and being able to act on the world appears to have become profoundly disrupted. Definitions of consciousness are various and problematic, but generally include at least in part the intactness of these faculties, and it is in this respect that madness or more specifically the psychoses may be considered as a disorder of a particularly human consciousness.

There is a loss of privacy, of the self being separate and therefore protected from the external world. It is described as being terrifying to the extent that suicide is considered as an escape. I am told it is a kind of hell. Things happen that should not happen in a familiar and customary world or in a shared reality. One's most vital functions, of breathing and of the heart beating are under external and absolute command. There seems to be a losing battle for control of the mind, and in this a part of the horror must be the exquisite and paradoxical consciousness of the disorder of consciousness, of being mindful of losing one's mind.

Part of the problem of consciousness is that it may be conceptualized at different levels, and at the more basic levels its functions are more clear that at the higher levels. I need to be aware of hunger to eat to sustain myself. I need to be conscious of danger in order to decide whether to take flight or to fight. I also need to have some sense of agency, or a capacity to act on the world to keep myself alive. These are not particularly human faculties, and consciousness in this respect is fairly simply an evolved capacity to increase the chances of survival. A higher more human consciousness is certainly more complex, and in terms of its need quite possibly unfathomable.

There is a certain poignancy in that the purpose of what might be considered as our greatest endowment, our essentially human consciousness is not at all clear to us. We do not need this higher level consciousness to stay alive. It enables us to seek meaning, or to contemplate the possibility of meaninglessness, or of god, and to acquire knowledge, but that does not make us stronger or better, or live much longer or transcend our mortality. On the contrary our human consciousness can at times seem burdensome. Much time and effort is expended in either altering or subduing our consciousness with alcohol or in other forms of intoxication, or we might seek to annihilate it altogether in acts of suicide.

If a higher level particularly human reflective self-consciousness is difficult to define, and its function in the grand scheme of things obscure, how it might arise from mere matter poses yet another enigma. Some argue that having to use our consciousness to explain our consciousness makes the problem intractable. Others propose that we simply do not have and will never have the capacity, being human, to make sense of it. Others consider that it is merely a matter of time, that it is a problem that can be solved such as the nature of life on earth or the origins of the universe. The argument is not that these mysteries might drive us mad, but that it is these very elusive and very human qualities that become deranged in psychotic states.

I ask my patients when they are recovering and regaining a degree of insight what they think might have gone wrong, what might have caused them to become mad. Perhaps the most frequent response is: "I think too much". Consciousness is perceived as a burden that at times can become intolerable. Something that is quite enormous and grants us the dignity of our humanity has been gained but at a loss. Being self-aware, being conscious of ourselves as separate from the world has enabled us to acquire a vast amount of knowledge and gain mastery to a great extent of our circumstances. That this might lead to eventual self-destruction is not of immediate concern. But having taken that fateful step, in Adam's making the choice to accept the apple from Eve and with it the capacity for knowledge and self-consciousness we became banished in the Fall from the garden of Eden. We lost our innocence. In becoming aware of ourselves we gained the capacity for shame. We lost forever the capacity for a voluptuous immersion in the oneness of the world, for many quite possibly a desirable unconsciousness, a deep and tranquil sleep, or the solace of not knowing. That is what I think my patients were telling me. "It is all too much. My consciousness is too much for me".

A loss of insight is a core feature of psychosis. Psychotic states might then be interpreted as a shutting down of insight into our separateness, or a refusal of consciousness. This combination of an intense self-awareness and the conviction that one is not in control is a cruel paradox of the psychoses, and in particular schizophrenia. I am agonizingly aware that I am not separate from the world, that I am no longer I.

Mpho says he wants or needs a circumcision. He tells us that he is not interested whether or not this is done in a cultural way with all the attendant rituals. He is determinedly pragmatic. He needs the circumcision to give him the strength to kill his enemies who are tormenting him. He is being mutilated. His brain is being devoured by dogs that are set upon him by his persecutors across the river. The only way for him to survive is for him to gain the necessary strength to destroy his enemies. He is desperate and alone. He is at the mercy of his tormentors with their devouring dogs. He is terrifyingly conscious of his predicament but this consciousness does not help him to resolve the crisis. He cannot help himself. He is afflicted with the awareness of his helplessness and desperately seeks our assistance in organizing the circumcision he insists he needs. He says nobody can understand what he is going through, and of course he is right.

To describe what he might be experiencing as persecutory delusions, although valid in one sense seems pitifully inadequate. The objectively identified psychopathology is in a profoundly different realm to the felt horror of believing that your brain is being devoured by dogs. Consciousness is inherently subjective and in that respect private and inaccessible and in some essential way unknowable. I can only with difficulty imagine what it must be like to have my brain eaten by dogs, but I can't really. It cannot even be a faint approximation. We are in two separate worlds and this is what he bewails. Nobody can possibly understand. If only this minor procedure of removing the foreskin from his penis could be performed he could begin to sort out his problems himself. He is tormented and also estranged from others and the sense of a shared world by the mystifying contents of his disturbed consciousness.

Somewhere along the way this has to dealt with, but in the midst of the crisis the first priority is to get him out of this horrifying space, to create some distance between him and the dogs. I don't think it would be very helpful to him to engage at this point in some form of psychotherapy as to what it might feel like to have your brain devoured by dogs. One can only begin to imagine that it is horrifying. Pity is not going to stop it.

Bernard is bright and articulate and indignant. He is under the control of an artificial intelligence device that in turn is controlled by the ANC in collaboration with international intelligence agencies including the FBI. This conspiracy against him has developed because of his work as a developmental officer for the DA, the opposition party to the ANC. The device that has been installed in his brain controls every function, including the most intimate and private. It forces him to have erections and to masturbate in public. This was profoundly humiliating to him and intolerable and he had been admitted to our unit following a suicide attempt.

An integral component of consciousness is a sense of autonomy and of free will, or at least the feeling that one is free to choose how one might act. The distinction is pertinent in the light of evidence casting some doubt on whether this might be an illusion. Based initially on electrophysiological studies, signals of brain activity are observable prior to the conscious decision to perform a simple action. This has been interpreted in many ways and does raise interesting questions about the freedom of will and hence the nature of consciousness and what it might mean to be human. Whether or not we are free in this empirical, objective sense does not detract from the feeling of being free to choose how to act in one way or another, or to choose to act or not to act.

There appears to be an unbridgeable gap between the observable, implacable world of objects and our essentially subjective world, however unknowable to others, that grants us the sense of who we are. Being intractably private makes this sense or this feeling or belief no less real, and it is the invasion of this privacy that seems so often to drive suicidal behaviour. It is a grim existential quandary in schizophrenia that in the loss of control and autonomy the perceived recourse of regaining control is self-destruction.

The clinical features of the schizophrenia spectrum are various but share certain core characteristics. The content of delusions or false beliefs often concern notions of thought insertion or withdrawal or of thought broadcasting, the feeling that one's thoughts are known to others. These clusters of symptoms are described as passivity phenomena, and are considered to be of first rank significance in making a diagnosis of schizophrenia. These delusions are associated with various forms of thought disorder which may be described broadly as a loss of the effectiveness of one's utterances, and a loss of awareness of that loss, and auditory hallucinations which represent a misattribution of events generated internally to the external world. The more negative cluster of symptoms, described in this way because they represent absences or deficits, are a loss of volition or a drive to action, a restricted emotional range and responsiveness and social withdrawal. Together these apparently quite disparate features share core elements in the loss of a sense of self, and of the unity of the self and of the self being autonomous. If this subjective sense of self is a core feature of a consciousness, the schizophrenias represent a profound disruption in whatever might be construed as the faculty of human self-consciousness, or whoever we are in the world.

Another feature of this higher level possibly rather vague notion of human consciousness is a sense of unity, both in the moment and over time, and of the awareness of the outside world that is personal and individual, in respect that there is an "I" that is the subject and at the centre of this experience. We presume ourselves to be the lead actors in our constructions and productions. This unity, or the feeling of it becomes threatened or disorganized in psychosis. "They know what I am thinking...it's horrible...how can I protect myself" is an utterance characteristic of the more positive side of the spectrum, in contrast to the confounded, catatonic states on the negative side, in which any sense of self or self-consciousness seems to have become obliterated.

Carel says nothing. He gazes through me. He is not present. He is vacant. It is profoundly disconcerting. I don't know where to begin. It seems impossible that we will ever retrieve him. He is lost to himself, to ourselves and to his family and to the world. Whatever consciousness there might be of himself and everything that surrounds him is to us a baffling mystery.

The lament "I think too much" raises the question as to whether the disorder of consciousness is not a deficit but an excess of consciousness, a loss of balance and filter and proportion, with the result that one becomes overwhelmed and engulfed by the world.

Descartes in the 17th century proposed "I think therefore I am", arguing for reason or thinking as a defining characteristic of human consciousness. My patients were telling me: "I think too much, therefore I am lost to who I am". There is a neurobiological correlate to this. Too much thinking might be interpreted as corresponding to a disorder of connectivity in the brain. In late adolescence a process of "synaptic pruning" takes place. This rather bizarre term describes an editing phase whereby connections between nerve cells or synapses are reduced if redundant or superfluous to the needs of the individual. This editing or refining developmental process should enable us to become more efficient, to focus attention, to develop the capacity for judgment and to plan and to problem solve, the very faculties that become impaired in schizophrenia. It seems that this enormously complex and delicate process becomes disorganized in schizophrenia, presumably as a consequence of an interplay of genetic and environmental factors, and the stage of life at which this occurs corresponds frequently to the time of onset of schizophrenia. Through the loss of an effective filtering there is a surfeit of redundant connections leading to a storm of signals to the higher centres. We are incapacitated, attaching meaning or attributing salience is random, and all becomes noise.

We have much to learn from madness about the nature of human consciousness.

It is a curious paradox that schizophrenia might be imagined as a condition of both being less or too much of whoever we might be. An intricate balance is lost.

34

Madness as a disorder of self

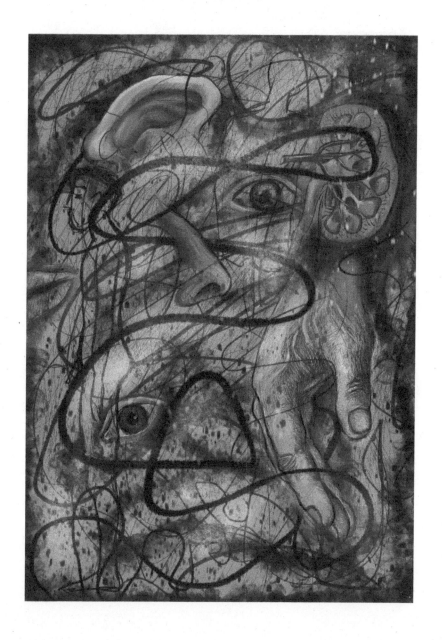

"No that is not me. It's been put there".

"What do you mean?"

"I don't know. Maybe it was some sort of transplant".

"Are you telling us that your face, your nose, your mouth, your ears, that this has all been transplanted?"

"Yes I think so. Maybe."

"Your eyes?"

"Yes my eyes also. All of it".

"What do you mean, all of it."

"Everything. Me."

"Your skin? Your whole body? Your brain?"

"Yes. But not all at the same time. It just happened".

"But then, if everything, absolutely everything has been transplanted in some way, who are you?"

Hoosain gazed vaguely around the room. He seemed bemused by the question, as if it were of no consequence.

He shrugged.

"I don't know", and then as an afterthought, "It doesn't matter".

His posture was of indifference. His tone of voice was flat, on the edge of irritation at my persistent questioning regarding a matter he seemed to consider trite and irrelevant.

Perhaps this is what many of us in the room found disconcerting. His apparent nonchalance challenged our assumptions of the notion of self, of the unity of the self and the notion of self being dear to us. There might at times be conflict, we might on occasion be angry or ashamed of ourselves and particularly in adolescence we might wish that we were not ourselves, but it is profoundly curious to disown oneself. To do so in such an emphatic way, to insist that one is not oneself, both in a physical and a psychological sense, is not merely a bizarre impossibility but compels an anxious questioning about our own confidences in the privacy and unity of the self.

Hoosain was confronted by a curious predicament. He was not himself, and yet he was embodied. The evidence of his physical being was clear to everybody in the room. In an attempt to resolve this apparent contradiction he constructed an elaborate and very strange explanation, that he had been transplanted, except that he quite obviously did not think it was strange. It was nevertheless some sort of answer, because although it was not himself, something resembling himself was evidently there.

Hoosain had been brought to the community clinic by his anxious family and then referred on to our unit. It was perhaps an unusual story in that in this instance there was no dramatic event that precipitated the admission. There had been no crazed behaviour, no violence. He had been a bright, devout and caring young man, but in the few months before he came to us he had drifted away his mother said. He was not himself. He was not present. He was / elsewhere. His family was dismayed and mystified. Nothing dramatic or in any way untoward had happened. There had been no significant or distressing event to account for his changed behaviour. He was described as a rather placid, unassuming young man. He had recently completed his schooling, and if there was any stressful circumstance his mother wondered whether it might be due to some uncertainty as to what direction he might take in life. This was speculative. He had never expressed any concerns to her. He had not confided anything to her. He was rather a private young man and she thought it best to respect this privacy. Now she was profoundly dismayed. She was also angry and frightened. Her son was denying and disowning himself, and in this way his mother and his family.

"What has happened Doctor? Is it me? Is it something I have done? This is not my son. Bring him back to me. My son is sick. You must bring him back to our family".

I don't think that the word "schizophrenia" meant anything to her, or provided any meaningful explanation for the devastating changes that had taken place in her absent yet present son. Yet one way of understanding schizophrenia or more specifically the psychopathology or the experience of schizophrenia is to imagine it as a disorder of the self or of self-consciousness. The notion of self is fluid and various across time and culture but broadly includes in some way concepts of unity, privacy and autonomy, or some belief at least that we might be in control of our thoughts and actions. It is these very feelings or beliefs or assumptions that become disorganized in schizophrenia. One is no longer in control of one's thoughts. There is a machine manipulated by alien and persecutory forces that control every thought and action. There is no privacy. Thoughts are broadcast to all and sundry. Although my thinking and my mood and behaviour might change to some extent over time and in different situations I have a fundamental sense of a self that is continuous and unitary. I am my own, until such time that I myself might become afflicted with such a profoundly and dreaded altered state of being.

Hoosain has lost all that. He is dispersed, fragmented, arbitrarily and ineffectually reconstituted in random bits and pieces. He is broken in another way also. There is no correspondence or unity of thinking and feeling. If I were to believe that somebody had stolen my thoughts I would be very angry. If I were to conclude that my friends were my enemies and hell bent on trying to kill me I would be very distressed and very frightened. Hoosain is neither angry nor afraid. He seems blank, perhaps, although I am not sure this is my own imputation, baffled by the extraordinary events that have overtaken him.

Given the depth and pervasiveness of these deranged states it is difficult to imagine how we could possibly hope to put him back together again.

Sometimes I have found myself dreaming whimsically of being an orthopaedic surgeon. A simple X-ray could identify the broken part. A relatively simple procedure could reset the fracture and the problem would be solved. Of course nothing is that simple but in this domain of psychosis we do not even understand clearly what is broken in order to fix it. It is difficult, or it seems utterly inadequate to attribute these profoundly disturbing experiences of a disordered self to a dysregulation of dopamine transmission or any other neurobiological fault.

Perhaps the high value attached to the self in the frenzied narcissism of the present day is unusual, and amplified by social media and other technological advances. The extent to which this might translate into a greater sense of confidence in the self, or in the sense of being in control of one's circumstances is unclear. A paradox seems to have arisen in that the high accord attached to the self appears to be associated with an increase in misery and insecurity, if the relatively recent increase in self – harm, depression and suicide among young people may be considered indicators of this disturbing trend. We do not so happily put ourselves on display. We gaze upon the enviable ways in which others present themselves and wonder and worry how we could possibly compete. A false, virtual world holds us in thrall. The self presented to this ephemeral community becomes increasingly fictional, and it seems plausible that a disjunction between whatever might be regarded as the true or authentic self and the virtual self is a part of this distress. Possibly imagined as self-affirming this grim charade appears to have the opposite effect, certainly among the vulnerable, and vulnerability and a lack of self –confidence may be regarded almost as defining characteristics of young adolescents, those most engaged in the tangled webs of the social media.

Ambivalence about the value or the priority accorded to the self is evident in other domains. We seek to lose ourselves in dance or meditation. We abandon ourselves in the hopeful bliss of sexual intimacy. We unburden ourselves of the consciousness of ourselves in alcohol and the misuse of other psychoactive substances. We aspire to transcend ourselves in the worship of the divine, and most definitively and tragically we destroy ourselves in acts of suicide. It does not seem to be without question that we regard our self-consciousness as an unreserved blessing.

The value attached to the self in relation to the community has some pertinence to varying outcomes in schizophrenia across cultures. Rather unexpectedly, given limited resources, outcomes in developing countries have been shown in some studies to be superior to those in developed, better resourced countries. There are a number of possible explanations for these anomalous findings. It is conceivable that in highly individualist materialistic societies a person disabled by mental illness would be ostracized as worthless because he or she is unproductive. Conversely, in a less formal economy someone living with a serious mental illness might be accorded a degree of dignity in performing unskilled but valued work, for example in taking care of young children in an extended family. Another possible factor is that psychotic symptoms in traditional contexts may be granted meaning and are therefore socially and culturally validated. Hearing voices might be interpreted as receiving messages from the ancestors. The person is then more likely to be granted a certain status and included in the community, rather than being excluded and alienated for demonstrating symptoms of mere madness. Another factor might be the importance attached to the self in western cultures, in that the breakdown of the self in psychotic states might be expected to have a more devastating impact than in more communalist societies characterized by a greater value being invested in the community rather than the individual.

I have observed these differences in our hospital. Among the more advantaged families, and this often but not always correlate with being white there seems to be an extra burden of disgrace. This is of course deeply felt by our patients. Perhaps there is a greater degree of indignation and injustice. How could this happen to us? How could it be that our relative good fortune, our material wealth, our caring and conventional middle class world has not provided an adequate bulwark against this strange illness? Implicit in this is a perhaps understandable need for some sort of explanation. This takes many forms but often it is that something or someone is at fault, that there has been some sort of moral failing and this madness is the consequence. The troubled self is further burdened with shame and guilt.

It is wrong and unhelpful to engage in crude generalizations, but perhaps among the more disadvantaged families there is more a sense of anxiety, and sometimes of fear. "Will he be able to work? Will he be able to support himself? What will happen if he goes mad again? We are at work. There is nobody to look after him at home. The last time this happened he destroyed everything. He can do terrible harm to himself. What can we do?"

Part of the difficulty is possibly my own sense of the burden of expectation. Again it would be wrong to associate inappropriate expectations or even entitlement with any particular group, and most often I found the families of my patients quite extraordinarily understanding and accepting of the difficulties in treating symptoms and predicting outcomes. But there were some encounters when parents, and it was most often the father, became angry and impatient. However understandable this might have been, however worried I myself might have been at the failure of progress, this expectation of a rapid resolution of all symptoms or of a cure complicated and quite possibly undermined the faltering process of recovery.

That the self is private and unique is a tenuous assumption. If grand socio-economic and political polarities have any validity, in the capitalist supposedly individualist West, mass marketing seeks to impose a uniformity of need. We are persuaded that we need the newest motorcar or the smartest smart phone to define our worth. We happily "share" our private worlds with strangers on the internet. In one of the few countries in the world still prepared to call itself communist a "social credit system" is proposed. Big data systems are to be deployed to reward citizens who are deemed to be good because they are loyal and obedient party members or patriots and to punish those who might be of unsound political persuasions. Rewards might take the form of employment opportunities, or better access to services. Punishment, because the rating and rankings are to be made public is likely to be social exclusion. Worth is defined not as being a good consumer but as being a good citizen. On opposite sides of the world, in two opposing social and political systems the notion of the self as private and having some sort of agency and value is undermined or abolished, and that of course has nothing to do with schizophrenia.

"You should not be ashamed of being a homosexual. Everybody is talking about it. They know what you are because of the way that you talk and the way that you walk. You should just accept it".

I am taken aback, as are the students who are with me in the cramped interview room of the out-patient department. Jacob appears to be admonishing me.

"You were always the odd one out at school. Everybody seemed to know what was going on except yourself. He said he didn't care but you know he was hurting. I said it was nobody's business but you begged to differ. You said it was wrong. I said I didn't think so but she was laughing behind your back. You see".

He paused, and stared at me meaningfully, as if seeking confirmation that I could indeed see, but I couldn't. I was struggling to make sense of his utterances. One of the young medical students was attempting to stifle laughter. The consultant was being accused by his patient of being a repressed homosexual. Jacob was staring at me impatiently, and then he embarked on a further tirade of confused sexuality, innuendo and fragmented but vivid memories. I felt myself being swept up in the current of this, trying to hold on in the turbulence to at least something that might make sense.

It then occurred to me that the problem was his random use of the personal pronoun. "I", "you", "he" and "she" were being used interchangeably. He was not referring to myself but himself when he said one should not be ashamed of one's sexuality. He was showing features of a formal thought disorder characteristic of schizophrenia but perhaps of greater significance was the particular nature of that disorder. His shifting use of the personal pronoun seemed to be an expression of his shifting sense of self. His self was disorganized. There was no stable "I", no unity or continuity of self. He was floundering. There was no anchor, no stable perspective. He was being buffeted by random events. As in in an Escher etching, he was going up stairs that were going down, he was looking out of a window at an image of himself looking back at himself. All was to and fro and inside out and up and down. It was exhausting just listening to him, just trying to understand. I cannot imagine what it must have been like for him, being on the inside.

Jacob's illness was intractable. Over the many years that I knew him there was no significant change. His curious thought disorder persisted. At least I began to understand what might be underpinning it, although I can't imagine that made much difference to him.

We managed to put Hoosain back together again. It seemed to me deeply mysterious that through the manipulation of a few neurotransmitters his body could be restored to itself.

I asked him before the discharge what he made of it, how could every part of himself be transplanted and reimplanted. He laughed and said he must have been mad. He didn't attend the follow-up appointment. I don't know what happened to him and can only hope that he remained intact.

Schizophrenia might be imagined as a disorder of self, but that calls into question the nature of self, and a host of assumptions regarding the unity and the autonomy of the self that might be more contingent and precarious than we are inclined to accept.

35

Bring back my son

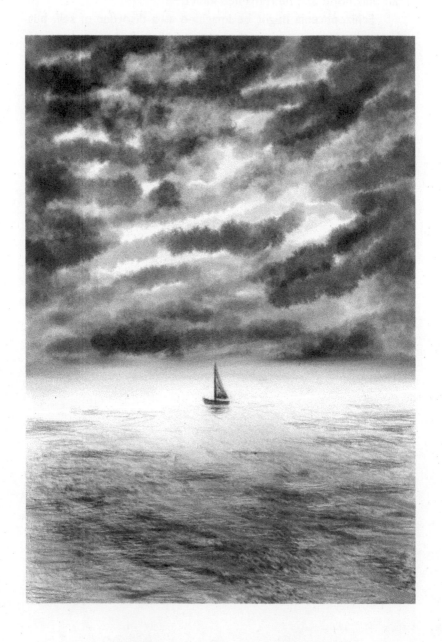

To be hopeful is fundamental to living with and coping with schizophrenia, but very often this is a struggle in itself. It is something we need to say and also to believe, but on many occasions the words have seemed hollow to me, utterances of a blind faith. I listen to myself insisting to a weary family that there must always be a hope, that the very uncertainty of the course of schizophrenia gives some cause for hope and I sense their tired disbelief and resignation. But to give up hope is untenable.

There is a dismally familiar trajectory culminating in the plea: "Doctor bring back my son," bring back my husband, my wife, my daughter, bring back that person whom I care for and now who seems so far away and so changed.

Jannes was a bright, good looking confident young man. There was no sign of what was to happen. There was no family history of mental illness. There were no problems at birth and no delay in the developmental milestones. He grew up in a happy secure and stable household. He flourished at school and enjoyed playing rugby and cricket. Tentatively, cautiously his parents began to entertain high hopes for his future.

Even in retrospect it is difficult to identify the point at which things began to fall apart. In his middle teens he began occasionally to use drugs. Initially this caused no great alarm. His parents reflected that this is what young people did. It was an experiment. He was exploring, and in any event it was only cannabis, a soft drug, nothing dangerous like heroin. Everybody was doing it. It was some sort of adolescent rite of passage.

But he became withdrawn. He no longer seemed to care about his appearance. He seemed to be less self-assured. Previously of a cheerful disposition he became cautious, wary, sullen. His increasingly troubled parents attributed this to adolescence. Other parents described the same behaviours in their children, seeking to reassure. Jannes drifted away. He stopped playing sport. His teachers reported that his school work began to deteriorate. His parents confronted him. "What is going on? What is the matter? Talk to us."

"There is nothing wrong with me. Leave me alone" he retorted, irritable, almost hostile. He spent increasing amounts of time locked in his bedroom. He stopped attending school. His parents did not believe that at this stage he was using drugs and so could no longer attribute this to his frightening decline. The situation deteriorated. He hardly spoke to his parents or to his younger sister. When he did he seemed vague, distant. He did not wash. He did not comb his hair. The situation was becoming intolerable.

Eventually one fateful evening the parents and the daughter were uneasily having a meal while Jannes had retreated to his room. They heard a scream and the sound of breaking glass. Rushing into the room they found their son, cowering in a corner, covered in blood from a shattered mirror. He appeared to be terrified. He said it was the voices, the incessant voices that were tormenting him and the cameras in the mirror that were monitoring his every movement. His distraught parents attempted to calm him. They somehow managed to get him to the casualty unit of the local hospital. The harried casualty officer asked about drugs. The parents confirmed that he had used but they thought that was something of the past. The doctor concluded that parents of adolescent children often did not know what they were up to and attributed the psychotic episode to substance abuse. He prescribed benzodiazepines and sent the family home. For a short while there an awkward calm. The medication appeared to make him tranquil but he seemed to have lost all spontaneity. He was distracted, remote. The family struggled on, frightened and mystified.

It was only after a further dramatic event that he was admitted to our unit. He had again withdrawn to his room and his mother hovering anxiously outside the door listened to him muttering and cursing. She was fearful. She forced her way into the room and shouted at him: "What is the matter with you?" "The voices, the voices" he screamed at her, "it's the cameras. Don't you understand? Don't you people know what's going on?" "That's nonsense, you are taking nonsense. You are sick", she retorted, terrified and exhausted. He lunged at her, his hands about her throat. Hearing the commotion the father ran to the room and managed to drag his enraged son away from his wife.

He told us afterwards in the ward round that the attack had been ferocious. It was as if his son was possessed by some demonic strength. The mother said she believed her son at that time had wanted to kill her.

This takes place on the Wednesday afternoon ward round. The clinical team is attending, registrars or specialists in training, clinical psychologists, the social worker and the occupational therapist, the medical and nursing students and myself. The father and mother and daughter seem huddled together, as if these events had isolated them from a world that was no longer familiar or secure. The mother is crying. Rather absurdly, she apologizes. The psychologist offers a tissue. The daughter watches her mother anxiously. The father appears stoical, or tries to be. For a while there is silence. I worry if this is the right way to help the family, a group of strangers bearing witness to their anguish. But they say they want to go on, they want us to understand what has happened so that maybe we can help.

I ask a rather odd question, but it is often useful in trying to come to some sort of meaningful diagnosis. 'It might be a strange thing to ask, but does it seem to you that in some way your son is a different person, that this is not Jannes?" The mother becomes animated. "Yes" she says emphatically, "yes, certainly. That's right. This is not my son. I want Jannes back. This is not who he is". The father and daughter nod in fierce agreement. So this is not Jannes. But what has happened to him? Where is he, I wonder, when he eventually joins us and gazes upon me with disconcertingly vacant eyes.

Perhaps this is one of the greatest difficulties for the family: he is there and he is not there. He is young. He is healthy. There is no outward indication that he might be profoundly ill. There is no clear understanding about where this illness might be, where in his body or his mind. If it is in his mind this leads to a further set of problems in that there is also no adequate understanding or consensus about what the mind might be. A strict materialist would argue that there is no mind, only matter. If that should be so there is no such thing as a mental illness. It would be an illusion, this absence, this young man being no longer himself.

The diagnosis, of mental illness, of psychosis or of schizophrenia is based on a characteristic cluster of clinical features, including delusions and hallucinations, various forms of thought disorders, social withdrawal, a restriction or blunting of emotions and a loss of volition. It represents a clinical syndrome rather than a diagnosis based on an objectively verifiable biological abnormality. This necessarily conventional description is insufficient, certainly beyond the confines of medicine, in the lived experience of those living with schizophrenia and their families. It gives little account of what is encountered as a calamity.

Again on one of the Wednesday afternoon ward rounds, Jacob's wife is describing the events that led to his admission. She speaks in the present tense, in a soft voice, as if in a trance. "He is on top of me...it is night...his hands are on my neck...I think I am going to die...I push him...away...I run for the door...I collect my children...I run from the house...the children are screaming...they are so afraid...he takes a knife...he comes after me...witch, he says, witch". He was not himself, she told us. He was a gentle man, a pastor in the local church. Now he is better. He is himself again, she says. She doesn't know how he has achieved this recovery but she is grateful.

He is appalled by what happened. He loves his wife. He doesn't want to kill her. That is inconceivable. She is not a witch. We ask him what he makes of it. Why? He is unsure. "It's the past. It's over. Perhaps it was some sort of devil possession. But I must go now. I must continue my pastoral work". Perhaps to placate us, to persuade us that it is safe enough to discharge him he promises to take the medication. There is no option but I don't think any of us share his confidence. He does not know what caused this to happen. He does not consider it to be an illness, certainly not in a biological sense, and so why should he then take the medication. It is more probable that prayer would help him. It was just perhaps some sort of spiritual lapse. The likelihood seems to us is that he will eventually stop the treatment. He will relapse, the symptoms will recur and the lives of his wife and children will again be at risk. We tell both the pastor and his wife of our concerns. She says she will do what she can to ensure that he does take the medication. But she is not sure. She cannot be. She is clearly troubled. What possible sense could be made of her husband being not himself, and now himself again, and how could she ever again be sure.

Beyond the cluster of clinical features described above is what appears to be a profound and pervasive disturbance of personhood, of a familiar way of being in the world, of somehow being oneself. In this respect it might be considered that there is some correspondence with either personality disorders or dementias. The schizophrenia spectrum disorders are fundamentally different. Personality and its disorders are variously described, but an intrinsic characteristic is a degree of continuity. Personalities, and personality disorders do not change significantly after adolescence. These constructs describe relatively habitual ways of thinking and feeling and behaving over time and in different situations. X has a confident, cheerful disposition. Y tends to be moody and introspective. These patterns have a degree of predictability: X and Y are more likely than not to demonstrate these characteristics in a range of circumstances and at different times. This is in dramatic contrast to the stories of Jannes and Jacob. In both what was described by their families was a profoundly disturbing change of personality. They were no longer themselves. This has nothing to do with a "split" in personality. There are no different personalities or selves, but rather a loss of the integrity of the self.

Being no longer oneself is also described in the advances stages of dementia. "Dementia praecox" was used in the nineteenth and early twentieth centuries prior to the adoption of the term schizophrenia and then schizophrenia spectrum disorders. In a similar way families describe a radically changed person, or a lost person, but the two disorders are again fundamentally different and in many different ways. Perhaps the most important, distinguishing feature of the dementias is their relentlessly progressive nature. The initial indication might be forgetfulness, and this is often considered to be a merely benign feature of aging. But as the dementia develops the deterioration is increasingly pervasive. First memory, then all cognitive functions, the capacity for feeling, and being able to behave in an effective and socially responsible manner are cruelly eroded, and progression to death is the certain outcome. This is not schizophrenia, which is broadly conceived of as a neurodevelopmental disorder. The dementias are by definition neurodegenerative disorders. The more characteristic course of the schizophrenia spectrum is a pattern of relapses and remissions. There are wide variations, but for the most part people with schizophrenia become ill, this being precipitated by a range of factors. They get better, to various degrees, and then, most often, and after various periods of time, they become ill again and recover again.

It should not be assumed that delusions indicate schizophrenia, and certainly in the southern African context there needs to be great caution in ascribing a delusional process to beliefs that might be entirely consistent with a person's cultural background. The delusions more consistent with a diagnosis of a delusional disorder tend to more plausible and of a less bizarre nature. Angus insisted his wife was having an affair. She was a very conservative middle aged woman and she found this as preposterous as it was distressing. He resorted to the most ludicrous, contorted arguments to justify his beliefs and he became extremely agitated when challenged. He had threatened her with violence and this had led to the admission. There were no other features to suggest a schizophrenia or anything other than a delusional disorder. This encapsulated delusional was rigid and entrenched. We could not shift it but nevertheless she refused to consider a separation. She thought he was sick and that he needed her. He was her husband she said. She did not say he was not the same man. She did not use the language of asking us to bring him back, but she was angry and sad and bewildered. Eventually a compromise was reached but I was not confident that it could be sustained. He told us, and in a way we were impressed by his honesty, that he continued to believe in the affair, but maybe this was something of the past and perhaps at some stage in the future he could consider forgiving her.

Kobus was not psychotic but the stories he told us had no

basis in his present reality. He had no short term memory. The parts of his brain that subserved this vital function had been destroyed by alcohol. When I asked him what he had done over the weekend he had no idea. To fill the void he took recourse to memories of a more distant happier past. He was helpless, incapacitated by his amnesia, drifting through what remained of his life trapped in a bubble of the perpetual present. He was not deluded. These stories he made up of the past were not fixed in any way but rather desperate strategies to orientate and retrieve himself. He was his old illusory self, living the moment, enjoying too many beers with his mates, out in the bush somewhere, entirely content with his re-imagined circumstances.

There are no such consolations in schizophrenia. There are no such confabulations to grant a degree of respite. Too often there just seemed to be an emptiness with nothing to fill it, and a distraught mother pleading for her son's return.

36

I can't go on like this

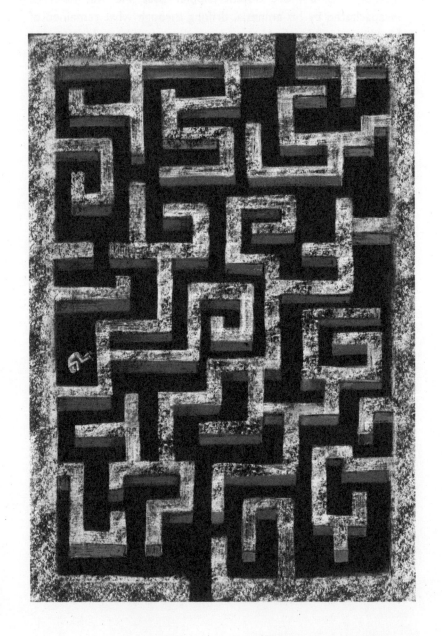

"I can't go on like this. I have had it, Doctor. I don't know what to do now. Where is the end to it? I am on my own. There is nobody I can turn to. Everybody has given up trying to help. Maybe they blame me. They think it is my fault that he is like this. They think I must have done something wrong. His father has gone. He said it is either him or me. How can he expect me to make a choice like that? It is so cruel. It is so selfish. I need him but now he has left and he has got a new girlfriend and he wants nothing to do with us. He says the hospital must sort it out. He says the boy is sick and he is not a doctor or a nurse and it is not his responsibility. And now my daughter is suffering. She is afraid of her brother and she does not understand it is a sort of illness. She is being teased at the school. She says the other children mock her and say that her brother is mad as if it is the whole family that is mad and they think his strange behaviour is funny because they don't have to live with it and they don't know how frightening it can be. She is a bright child but now she is failing in the subjects that she was good at. The teachers say she is not paying attention in class and they get angry with her. How can they understand what we are going through. Now she says she wants to change schools but how will that help. It will be the same thing at another school. It is terrible that she is ashamed of her brother but I can understand it I suppose. She is still too young to know that this is because of an illness but it is difficult anyway because he doesn't look ill. It's not as if he has a broken leg or coughing with tuberculosis or dying of something. He is strong and healthy and so people don't believe he is sick so they don't feel any sympathy for him or for me. If it is not my fault they say it must be his. It is something he has done to himself. Maybe it is the drugs. Maybe he is being punished for something bad that he has done. When I say to them that the doctors have told me it is schizophrenia they say they don't know what that means as if they don't believe there is such a thing and it is perhaps just a word the doctors have invented to cover up for bad behaviour or a mother not knowing how to discipline her child. At the beginning everybody was giving me advice but nothing helped. They said I should go and see a traditional healer. He said it was amafufunyana and that somebody had put a curse on him. I gave him the medicines and we had to do some things but it didn't work. He got worse so I took him back to the healer and then he said perhaps it was ukuthwasa, that he was being called to be a healer but I don't know about those things and then anyway my boy said he would not go back to the healer and nothing came of it. Nothing was helping and I was becoming desperate. Then people said I must just throw him out but how can I do that. He is a child. He is sick. He would not survive. There is nobody else now except me and I don't know how to cope any longer. I know you doctors are trying to help and I know you can't just keep him in hospital forever but what am I supposed to do. It's so sad. He is quite well when he comes out of the hospital but it does not last for very long. He has no friends. Nobody wants to see him. They just see him now as a mad person and they are embarrassed when he tries to approach them. They laugh at him and run away. It is understandable that he gets angry. It is not his fault he says, this illness. He did not ask for it. It is too unfair. Then he starts with the drugs because he is angry and lonely so then the only people who will have anything to do with him are the gangsters. They use his disability grant to get the drugs and they don't care if the drugs make him sick so that he has to go back to hospital. I am so afraid. He is going to get into trouble because of these gangsters and then he is going to end up in prison and then there will really be no hope. I am afraid of these people. They come into the house and they show no respect for me. They know that I am on my own and they will start stealing from me for the drugs and the police will do nothing because they say they have more important things to deal with and anyway it is my son's fault because he invites them into the house. Things are just getting worse and worse and Doctor it is terrible to say this but sometimes I just wish that he was dead. How can a mother say that about her son? It is wrong. I will be punished but it is the truth. Either him or me. I would rather be dead than go on like this. Last night it was just too much. I knew it was going to happen at some point. I knew it was coming. So I locked the door and my daughter was with me. How can one live like that, in fear of your own son? But this time

I was really afraid. He had been behaving strangely all afternoon and I couldn't reach him. He was so angry. He was in a rage but he would not tell me or he couldn't tell me what the matter was. Perhaps it was the drugs. We, my daughter and myself locked ourselves in the bedroom but we couldn't really sleep and in the early hours of the morning he started hammering at the door and screaming things that I did not understand. My daughter started screaming also, she was so afraid. He went on and on. He wouldn't stop even though I was pleading with him through the door to leave us alone. Then he started to kick at the door. It is not a strong door and I knew he was going to break it down. He came into the room and he was ranting at me and he was carrying a knife from the kitchen in his hand. He was mad. He shouted at me "You witch!" There was hatred in his eyes and I thought he was going to kill me. I just screamed his name and said "Leave us, please leave us!" Then he just stood there as if in a daze. My daughter was sobbing in terror. A neighbour must have been woken by all this noise and started hammering at the front door and shouted that the police had been called. My son just stood there shaking, and when the police did come he went with them without complaining or fighting with them. He seemed like a little boy then, bewildered, obedient, no longer the mad dangerous person he had just been. So now he is in hospital and we feel safe for a little while and we can sleep at last but I know you are going to discharge him when he is well enough and this all going to start again. I don't know what to do any longer Doctor. I can't go on like this".

"I can't go on like this. Last night was the worst. It was terrible. I was frightened. I don't know what was going on. I think I nearly killed my mother. How could that have happened. I was out of control. Everything was muddled. I didn't think she was my mother. I thought she was somebody that was pretending to be my mother. I thought she was an imposter and I was angry and frightened. I thought that she was a witch. This suddenly became clear to me. I knew it. I knew that she was why everything was going wrong in my life. I felt I had to do this thing, that I did not have any choice. I took the knife from the kitchen and I went to her bedroom. She had locked the door and this made me even more angry. I was in some sort of uncontrollable rage. It was almost as if some force had taken control over me and was driving me to do these things. I was not myself. Maybe I was possessed. I smashed down the door. I saw that my mother was terrified. So was my little sister. My mother shouted my name. She shouted, "Leave us, please leave us!" I became confused. Perhaps it was her calling my name and seeing my sister being so afraid. I felt horrible. I did not know what was going on again. I was not sure whether this woman who might have been my mother was a witch or not. Nothing was clear or certain. Then maybe I thought something had happened to me, that I had become sick again and that I needed help. In a way it was a relief that the police came. It was too dangerous. I could have killed my mother. How would I have been able to live with that? How can I live with that? I don't understand this illness. The doctors call it schizophrenia but what does that mean. It is not a sickness that I can understand. It is not that I have got an infection or a broken leg or anything like that that the doctors can fix. They say that it is a problem with my brain but I don't get fits. I don't get headaches. I feel quite well. I am healthy. What kind of sickness is this? There were no problems when I was younger. Things were just fine. I am not sure when or how it started. I think it was a problem at school. There never had been a problem but I started to have difficulties in concentrating and I started struggling and the teachers got angry with me. They said I was being lazy. Then my friends began to tease me. They said I was weird. I didn't know what they were talking about but I became unsure of myself and things got worse and then I had no friends and people were laughing at me and calling me mad. I stopped going to school. My father got angry. He said "What is the matter with you?" but I didn't know and he hit me. My mother tried to stop him and then he left. He said we were all mad and he had to look after himself. I felt so ashamed. My mother took me to all sorts of people who said all sorts of weird things. They said somebody had put a curse on me. Then they said I was being called to become a healer. I don't believe all that stuff but I didn't know what was going on and then I wasn't sure of anything. My mother took me to the local clinic and the doctor there said she thought it was maybe this thing called schizophrenia and referred us to a specialist doctor at the hospital. I refused to go. I didn't want to called a mad person. I was not mad. I didn't want to be sick. I didn't want this to be happening. But I couldn't stop it. I began to notice strange things. It was odd and it made me anxious. It was as if I was getting signals but I did not know where this came from or what these signals meant. Things became blurred, they were no longer what they seemed to be. I could not understand it and then I began to think that people were playing tricks on me. Why should people be doing this to me? I had not hurt anybody. Why? It was so unfair. This got worse. I became afraid. I did not want to leave the house. Then one night I just lost control completely. I don't know what happened. Maybe I was possessed by the devil. I was just screaming and bashing my head against the wall so that there was blood everywhere. Maybe I was trying to kill something inside me. I don't know but it was bad and I was terrified. I ended up in hospital and that was also frightening. I thought the other people there were mad. They gave me some medicines and things got better and I was sent home. I didn't like taking the medication. I felt better and I didn't think I needed that stuff. Why should you take medicines if you are not sick? It made me think that maybe I was sick in some strange way that I didn't know and that made it worse. I did not believe that I would be sick again if I stopped the treatment. I refused to believe it. I am a young person. My life is ahead of me. I don't want to be sick. I am not mad. Maybe it was just the stress of the problems at school and my friends but I am over that now, I think. The social worker made an application for a disability grant because they said I had a mental illness and would not be able to work. That made me depressed but my mother said it would help because there was very little money and no support from my father. I had no friends now but the gangsters started coming around to the house. At first I thought they were quite cool. They made me think that I belonged but I suppose it was just the money from the grant that they wanted. They gave me drugs and that was also quite cool. It made me feel strong. It made me think I could do anything and that I wasn't sick in any way and that I didn't need the medicines. Then it all started going wrong again and it was worse and this terrible thing happened and now I am back in the hospital. I feel bad. I feel very guilty. I look at my mother and I see how disappointed she is and how tired and angry she is and I don't know what I can do to help her and my little sister. I feel like such a failure. Sometimes I think I would rather be dead. I don't know how I can go on like this".

37

Odd ideas, and very occasionally a strange beauty

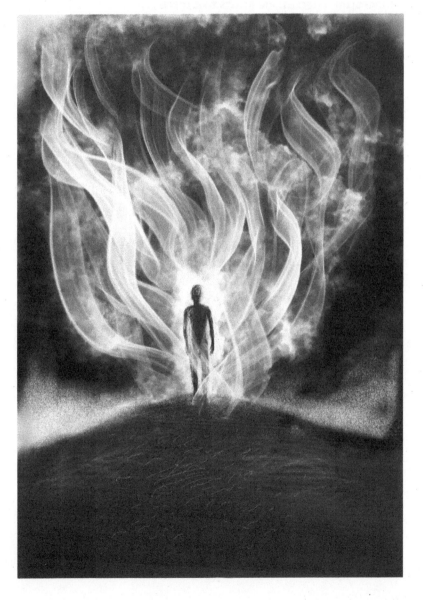

Reuben greets me affably. He could have been considered handsome but he was dishevelled and clearly paid no heed to his appearance. He shook my hand but the left hand was stuck down the front of his dirty trousers. After a few polite and formal exchanges I ask him why he is doing this. He laughs and says he is fine and there is nothing that I should worry about. He is nonchalant. I persist. He insists that there is no problem. I say that it is odd to put your hand down the front of your trousers, it is inappropriate. I hesitate but do not say that others will think he is crazy. He laughs again, and says, as if taking me into his confidence: "You see I have to. I must hold onto my penis all the time". "Why?", and this time I say, "people will think you have got a problem and you might scare them. What's going on?" Laughter again. "You must understand, I have to hold on because my mother has her hand rammed up my rectum. She is trying to rip off my penis". Then, as if to reassure me, he repeats: "it's okay. I'm alright. As long as I hold on tight she can't do it. I'm fine really". And then quite kindly: "Don't worry doc. There's nothing wrong with me. I can cope".

I ask for his permission to speak to his mother. She is a charming, immaculately dressed woman in her middle age. She is exhausted. She says this is a relatively good phase, because he is calm and he is polite to her. When things get bad she says he rages against her. He accuses her of trying to castrate him. His language is obscene and vituperative. He is violent. She fears for her life. She is resigned she tells me. She thinks that probably one day he will kill her.

Matricide is a rare event and when it does occur it is most often in this context. It is as if these young men living with schizophrenia find themselves in an intolerable trap. They cannot live without the mother and the mother is perceived as suffocating them, stifling them, castrating them, not allowing them to live and be free. The only, albeit psychotic solution to this problem is to either kill the mother or kill themselves. In this there is no strange beauty, only a relentless, enervating horror. She has lost her son but he is there, tormenting her, threatening her, and when she has gone who will look after him? Who other than a mother could bear this burden? The mothers seemed to most often bear the brunt of this. The fathers tend to withdraw or to flee, as do the siblings. Jan in a quite similar way was violent towards his mother. He had been an exceptionally bright young man but in late adolescence had become withdrawn. His academic performance declined and eventually to his parents' great distress he refused to go to school. The situation deteriorated steadily until it became clear that he was gravely ill. He assaulted his mother, accusing her of having sex with the gardener. Then in a rage he accused her of trying to have sex with himself. She was aghast. She could not understand what was happening. The family struggled until it seemed that something had to give. The father said: "I can't go on like this. It is either him or me". The mother felt she had no choice. She knew her son was sick but she did not know where to turn. The father left and so did the younger brother. When she brought Jan to see me she was trying to cope on her own and she was also exhausted.

Jan was unlike Reuben. He was distracted, perplexed and angry. He lacked the possibly protective nature of Reubens apparent calm. There is no stereotype of schizophrenia but Reuben did show some of its curiously characteristic features. The notion that schizophrenia constitutes a split personality is false. The split is in the integration of psychological states. There is a loss of congruence between the content of thinking and what might be considered the appropriate, corresponding emotion, and between the content of thinking and the corresponding behaviour. Reuben described what must have been an excruciating experience in the form of a somatic or bodily and persecutory delusion. The corresponding manifest emotion or affect was nevertheless for the most part a curiously bland indifference. Another feature he demonstrated was an extremely concrete way of thinking and acting. He was incapable of understanding that the experiences he described could have no basis in reality. That this could be construed as a delusion was beyond his capacity for abstraction. Furthermore there was a simple concrete solution to the problem. He just had to hold onto his penis. Then everything for the time being was going to be alright. This failure of an abstracting ability itself might seem an unhelpful abstraction in the attempt to make sense of the bewildering array of symptoms associated with the schizophrenia spectrum, and the corresponding havoc that ensues in the decline in functioning. A loss of the capacity for abstraction is part of a cluster of cognitive deficits loosely described as impairments of executive functioning. This is variously defined, but includes in addition to the problems of abstraction a difficulty in formulating goals and planning accordingly, of sequencing, problem solving and evaluating. It is quite possibly difficult to comprehend the devastating impact this has on young peoples' lives. Both Reuben and Jan had become helpless. Rendered unable to plan, to consider the future, to reflect and adapt, they were at sea, buffeted by randomness, at the mercy of circumstances they perceived to be either entirely out of their control or cruelly menacing.

The term executive function does little to convey the dramatic impact of its impairments. This may be more clearly comprehended in its effect on the mothers of these two patients. The capacity to function in a way that is dependent on intact executive functioning is at the core of what it might be to be considered personhood, to be able to act intentionally, to be self-reflective, to imagine. It is perhaps this loss that leads to the poignant refrain that I heard so often from the appalled mothers of sons living with schizophrenia: "Doctor please bring back my son".

This absence or loss is in stark contrast to the delusions and the hallucinations that are more characteristic of what are described as the "positive" features of schizophrenia. Positive and negative forms have different pathophysiological bases and tend to have different prognoses. The difference is such that the notion of schizophrenia as a clinical entity is questionable, and the term "schizophrenia spectrum disorder" is considered more appropriate. Positive and negative forms are furthermore not discrete, and may comingle.

I asked Xanta what he did during the day. He said, quite placidly, "nothing". I said he must surely do something, maybe wander about, occasionally prepare a meal, sleep and wake up. "No" he said, not emphatically, but blandly, unperturbed, "nothing, I do nothing".

"But surely you do not spend the entire day just staring at the wall?"

"Yes, that's what I do. I stare at the wall."

"Don't you get bored?"

He thought for a moment. Perhaps he sensed that in some way he had disappointed me and that I needed reassurance.

He said: "sometimes I get frightened. That's quite exciting."

Just a fear, no sense of even the slightest pleasure, no other emotion filled his empty days.

This strange flatness of emotion, this perplexing lack of responsiveness, an absence of being present can understandably be the most distressing aspect of the illness to family members. It can also not be interpreted as part of an illness, and this tends to happen in deprived households where overcrowding and a multitude of stresses result in the solitary, vacant young man in the corner simply being neglected, for weeks and for months until some dramatic event, a television set being destroyed for example, leads to a panicked call for help. This smashing of television sets is a curiously common occurrence, and as for Xanta, arises from the belief that characters in a drama are addressing one directly and in an abusive way. It represents an eruption of positive symptoms in the form of delusions from the otherwise empty and featureless terrain of schizophrenia.

The response of Hasim to his vivid delusions was less impassive than bemused. When I saw him in the outpatient department he told me that things had improved considerably. He was smiling, almost to himself, as if, with some distance that had developed between himself and his illness, he found the whole process quite fascinating. The briars patch he told me was slowly fading into background radiation. I asked him what the briars patch might be. He said it was a zone in his bedroom inhabited by a creature resembling a giant octopus. "When I'm schizophrenic this malevolent creature shoots out tentacles. These things jam into my mouth so that I cannot breathe". He laughed. He said:

"It's mad. It's terrible. It's just not cricket".

Laughter helps, sometimes. Nicolas told us that his goal in life was to set up an ice hockey team in Australia. We told him that we thought that was a rather crazy idea because Australia was a very hot country. He said that was not a problem. He would simply cast a spell on it to make it cold. He laughed. It was such a simple solution. Could we not understand? We asked him whether he could not rather cast a spell for rain as the province was encountering a severe drought at the time. He laughed again. That was not at all a concern for him. The ice rink in Australia was the big issue.

But more often there is no laughter. While the disjunction between the content of thinking and the associated emotion tone is suggestive of the diagnosis of schizophrenia, it is the ensuing behaviour that most often raises the alarm and leads to a hospital admission.

For Manto, and his family and his community the situation was dangerous. He had been admitted to the unit after trying to burn down his shack. This was his tenth attempt and considerable damage had been done. He lived in an informal settlement and neighbouring dwellings had been threatened. He had difficulty in trying to explain why he was doing this, and it was apparent that his psychosis was complicated by an intellectual impairment. He told us the voices told him to set fire to the shack. He had no control. He could not explain it further. His mother was angry and afraid. He was alone during the day because she had to leave for work early in the morning and she returned after nightfall. Gangsters moved into the house in her absence, exploiting the young man's handicap. They used drugs, stole whatever there was and ate all the food she left for him. They threatened to kill him if he complained or went to the police. He was trapped. The mother was despairing. She wondered, had her son tried to burn down the shack so that there would be nothing left for the gangsters to take. Was this his sort of solution? Her fears arose not only from her son's dangerous behaviour and from the gangsters but also from the neighbours. Fire is a constant source of anxiety in the informal settlements and she was terrified that the community would set upon her son when he returned from the hospital. She told us that they had threatened to kill him. His madness would cause a conflagration and be the end of them all. She begged us to keep him in hospital. It was the only safe place for him. We could not keep him, certainly not indefinitely. When the psychotic symptoms subsided we would have to discharge him. Out there nothing would have changed. The danger persisted. We all felt trapped in our different ways.

In such circumstances it seems that the alternative, more unperturbed responses to psychotic phenomena are preferable and provide at least a degree of protection. Stefan was pleasant but vague in his manner towards us. He was not distressed at all by the issues that had led to his admission. It was not a problem that his twin brother was not his brother, let alone his twin brother. He was "quite nice", this other person. He seemed to be quite caring. His mother was not his mother, but whoever she was she was also "quite nice". Although he did not seem to think that this was a problem his mother certainly did.

During the interview with Stefan I assume a posture of confusion. "I don't understand. I can't understand how you can refuse to accept that this woman who brought you into the world and who has cared for you all your life is not your mother". The disavowal is rigid. He gazes at me placidly, and asks, as if it is a matter of some debate: "Do you believe in parents?" I respond: "surely it is not a matter of belief. It is a biological fact of life. Children are born of parents". He is utterly unimpressed. It is simply a matter of belief, as is everything. He is imbued with a strange contentment, or maybe an indifference, as if all the world and everything that happens is not simply given but chosen, to be believed or not believed. This is possibly his way of regaining control. His impassivity makes him impervious to hurt as it does to the disappointment and dismay surrounding him.

That there should be any sort of strange beauty in these accounts might seem improbable if not preposterous. Any attempt to romanticize serious mental illness should be fiercely guarded against, and is more likely to do harm than good. It is ignorant and fails to register the gravity and the great distress of those living with schizophrenia and their families and their communities. Yet, while acknowledging this, I find it difficult not to see in these struggles to make sense of a confounding and often terrifying world a strange grace and a surprising sort of beauty. These stories do in a way represent determined often convoluted and bizarre but inventive strategies to survive, and to find some sort of solution, albeit psychotic, to the otherwise overwhelming problem of noise and meaninglessness.

38

Hearing voices, or listening

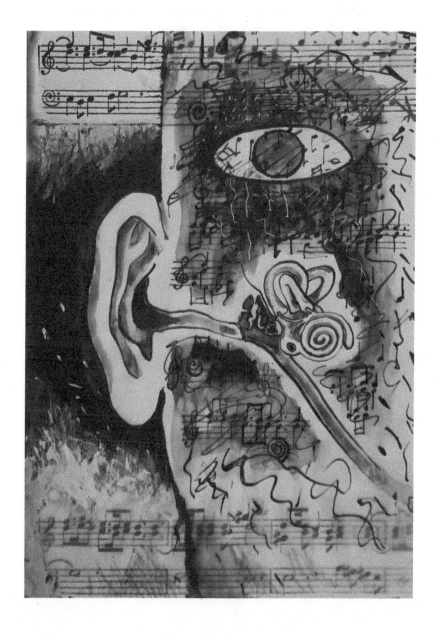

"When I'm sick the machine comes on...the voices are clearer...there is no barrier...I was too much into this thing to question it...it would drive me completely insane...it's a man's worst nightmare...this remote brain control...there's no escaping it. It is complex...how can I describe it...it's like snowing on TV...it's a sensation like that...it's the closest I can describe...it's not just what you visualize."

Marthinus, describing a psychotic episode from which he had recently recovered.

Hearing voices or auditory hallucinations are considered to be a core feature of psychosis or more specifically schizophrenia. Hearing voices does not indicate madness. We all in certain circumstances have the capacity to hear voices or noises of some nature that have no correspondence in the external world. This needs to be emphasized, as a misinterpretation of hallucinations has too often led to false diagnoses with baleful consequences. Voices or noises are perceived to arise in external space. The voice of God or the ancestors, or the voice of reason or conscience experienced internally are of course not hallucinations and thus not evidence of madness.

A further distinction which is not sufficiently emphasized in the academic literature is the distress associated with these phenomena. Marthinus, quoted above, describes his experience as the "worst nightmare". Hearing voices should not necessarily be distressing. One patient described being quite content, informing us that the voices he heard were enquiring whether they could befriend him on Facebook. The voices were companionable, and he saw no reason why they should be extinguished, and nor did we.

Clearly it is inadequate to consider that hearing voices is in itself in some way inherently pathological. For Marthinus the anguish seemed to arise more specifically from the belief that he was no longer in control. Any sense of autonomy was lost. There was no barrier between himself and the outside world. He had become engulfed by these external stimuli which, because they were beyond his control were understandably all the more intolerable. There was no escape.

Samuel regarded himself as being most fortunate to be alive and so did we. He had been found by his mother hanging from a clothing hook behind a bedroom door. She had heard a crashing sound presumably due to the weight of his body having dislodged the hook, and found him collapsed and blue in the face but alive. He had been behaving strangely for some days or weeks. He had become withdrawn and his appearance was ill-kempt. His mother had attributed this to adolescent problems, and this occurs frequently. It is a turbulent period. Perhaps he had been bullied at school, perhaps he had been rebuffed by a girlfriend, but whatever the reason what is familiar to any parent is the reluctance to divulge whatever might have caused the change in behaviour. Samuel was remarkably frank with us in the immediate aftermath of his attempted suicide. He said he did not want to die. He had had no intention of killing himself. He said he had everything to live for. The problem was the voices. This had started some weeks earlier, and initially was quite imperceptible, more an unfamiliar noise than any signal that he might be becoming ill. The voices had become gradually more intense, crystallizing into discernible words which then became derogatory and abusive. As he slowly crashed into psychosis he described the voices as incessant and increasingly commanding. He was told that he was worthless and deserved to die. He struggled to resist but the voices became too powerful. He lost control. His will, his fundamental instinct for survival was eroded. As for Marthinus it seemed to him then that he had no option other than to end his life. Sitting up in his hospital bed, fully recovered, in recounting these events he seemed bemused, as if this could not possibly have happened to himself, that in some mystifying way it must have been somebody else.

Describing these phenomena as auditory hallucinations seems inadequate. The aridly objective, notionally academic term gives no indication of the distress associated with the voices nor the behavioural consequences. These associated phenomena are closer to the core of what a patient might be experiencing and closer to what might be considered to be the priorities in terms of a therapeutic intervention. It was not the voices in themselves that prompted such anguish with disastrous consequences, but the disruption of something beyond, and something that might be considered innate and particularly human: a sense of self, of the privacy of the self, and a precarious notion of free will.

This chapter is ostensibly about hearing voices, but the argument is that it is not possible, and that it is a distortion to separate voices from the other intimately associated psychotic phenomena that afflict our patients. It does not happen that a person complains of hearing voices in isolation, and if this might happen on the rare occasion, it is unlikely that this would indicate the need for any form of intervention.

Marthinus described being "too much into this thing to question it". He shows insight into a loss of insight. The term psychosis is variously defined. It might be described as being characterized by delusions and hallucinations and thought disorders, or a common denominating feature might be articulated as a loss of insight. This is in itself problematic. Insight is a matter of degree, not an absolute, and requires qualification. For example, a registrar in presenting a patient to the consultant might say: "he shows some insight into the idea that he might be ill but has no insight into the need for treatment". It is a relative term. On whose authority insight or a lack thereof might be defined may be open to dispute. It might also be presumptuous to consider an absence of insight being limited to the mentally ill, as if those of us unburdened with such labels have a clear and unremitting insight into the vagaries of our thinking and behaviour, or are incapable of self-deception. Coupled to a lack of insight a defining characteristic of psychosis is that beliefs are held with conviction despite evidence to the contrary. Clinicians are wearisomely familiar with the indignant complaint: "What am I doing here? There is nothing wrong with me".

The same patient, Marthinus, described to me being bombarded with electric shocks from outer space. These bolts were intensely painful and were all the more distressing because he could not understand where they came from and why he was being persecuted in this way. He became increasingly agitated while telling me this. He said: "I know what you are thinking doctor. I know you think this is delusional, I know you think this is a relapse of the schizophrenia. But it's not. It's real. It's happening to me, and it's terrible". He was, as he said in retrospect too much into it, too engulfed by it to question whether or not it might be an expression of his illness. At the time however, he did show a degree of insight, being acutely aware of what I was thinking, prompting his indignant and pained response.

Again in this respect the term insight seems insufficient and requires elaboration in order to gain at least some idea of what a person might be experiencing. In these accounts patients have described being trapped. There is no escaping the predicament. There are no options. There is no freedom of will. There is no self to take action. What is described is not a hypothesis. It represents a brutal reality. It is irredeemably concrete. There are no other ways of seeing it. There are no metaphorical spaces.

What might be the source or the causes of these disturbing phenomena remains elusive. Functional scanning indicates that the hallucinations are self-generated. What a person is saying, without sound, appears to be perceived in external space. The wide range in the content of these phenomena has been described, with the possible common denominating factor being a loss of autonomy, or being in control, a loss of self with a degree at least of agency. Voices are most often in the third person, commenting on a person's thoughts or actions. "Look at what he is doing now: he has these bad thoughts now, he is bad", quite often ceaselessly, maddeningly intrusive, extending to commands: "He is so bad that he really should not be alive", and then: "Go on, do it".

Marthinus described the experience as "snowing" on a television screen. This seems an apt metaphor for an auditory perception. Snowing is the visual equivalent of noise. There is no signal, no meaningful pattern. The world makes no sense. There is no integrity, no continuity, no coherence, no means of making sense. This becomes insufferable. It is the "worst nightmare".

If in regard to the notion of a psychosis being by definition ununderstandable, what might be more understandable is the quite desperate struggle to make sense of the experience of noise, to mitigate it, to create a familiar pattern that might restore a sense of control and a degree of equanimity. It is also understandable that these strategies might derive from one's social or cultural context. In the middle class suburbs of the city a frequent complaint was that characters on television were talking to one personally, often in a code that was indecipherable but perceived as malicious. Young men from rural backgrounds described the voices as being those of displeased ancestors. However distressing these interpretations or beliefs might have been, they were less so than the noise and incoherence that possibly with some degree of intent they sought to dispel.

The biological basis for this perception of noise is uncertain. The neural correlates indicated by brain imaging might provide some clue. There is neural activity but a loss of signal. A useful metaphor might be provided by music. What is perceived as harmonious or beautiful or joyful is the expression of an extremely complex orchestrated process. A symphony for example consists of a wide range of instruments being played with great skill to a score and under the supervising coordination of a conductor. In the audience we do not attend to the component parts except perhaps when things go wrong. We celebrate or not the totality of it. We imagine we grasp the intent of the composer, enabled by the skill of the players and the conductor. All is harmonious. In the context of auditory perception all makes sense. The different parts fit more or less into the whole. But as this is a highly complex intricate process things can go wrong. The first violinist has omitted to take his medication for an attention deficit hyperactivity disorder. He rushes ahead hectically, ignoring the desperate attempts of the conductor to restrain him. The oboe player has fallen asleep. The percussionist, eager to impress the pretty second violinist overreaches himself on the kettle drum. The delicate balance is lost. The orchestra becomes disorganized. The music becomes a cacophony, mere noise.

Clearly in a biological context there are levels of explanation. A current, plausible model for psychosis is a dysconnectivity syndrome, or a dysregulation of the delicate and dynamic web of synaptic connections in the central nervous system, a disorganization of the orchestra. The underlying causes of this dysregulation are in turn indeterminate but probably concern the shifting and complex interactions of genetic and environmental factors. This is not discontinuous with what occurs in a healthy brain in the process of perception. On the basis of very limited sensory information and past experience we make inferences about what we might consider to be the most likely percept. The voice I hear and that speaks to me in a coherent and meaningful way is not a vibration of air molecules or the agitation of hair cells in the inner ear. The voice and the meaning I attach to its utterances is internally represented or constructed. It seems that this inferential process is what goes awry in psychotic states.

The way in which hallucinations and more generally psychoses are conceptualized has important implications for how these phenomena are managed. Within a strictly reductive biomedical model the hallucinations are symptoms of a pathological process. The content of the voices, and the person's experience and his or her response to these voices are without relevance. The implication is that that an appropriate treatment goal should be the elimination of the troublesome symptom. What the person might make of this is not clear, and is not taken into account. "It's just a symptom of the schizophrenia. It will go away with treatment". It is meaningless.

Alternatively, the symptom may be understood as an attempt by the patient to make sense of his or her experience. This might be cautious and idiosyncratic, but in all likelihood represents a striving for an explanation that is personally and culturally meaningful, and if so this needs to be acknowledged not necessarily suppressed. The decision to intervene requires careful consideration and should not be merely assumed. In this respect treatment in the form of the elimination of symptoms by pharmacological means may be experienced as a denial of one's tentative reality, and an interruption of a potentially therapeutic process. The symptom is considered as merely anomalous and invalid. This disregard might possibly be a factor in the widely prevalent and problematic non-adherence to treatment.

For the young man from the rural highlands hearing voices

might become listening to the ancestors. A pathological event is reconstrued as a culturally meaningful experience. It is validated. The young man is not ostracized. He is attuned. He is listening to the ancestors. This is of course contingent upon a particular set of cultural beliefs, but the implication in general is that it might be more helpful and useful to our patients for us to listen to what they are telling us, rather than simply suppressing the symptoms of psychosis. This is not an argument against pharmacological treatment but an attempt to redefine the principles and goals of treatment. A focus of attention beyond signs and symptoms, and an endeavour to attend to the experience and to the concerns of a person living with schizophrenia seems likely to be both more acceptable, less likely to do harm, and more probably beneficial. There is a world of difference between hearing and listening.

39

A family aghast

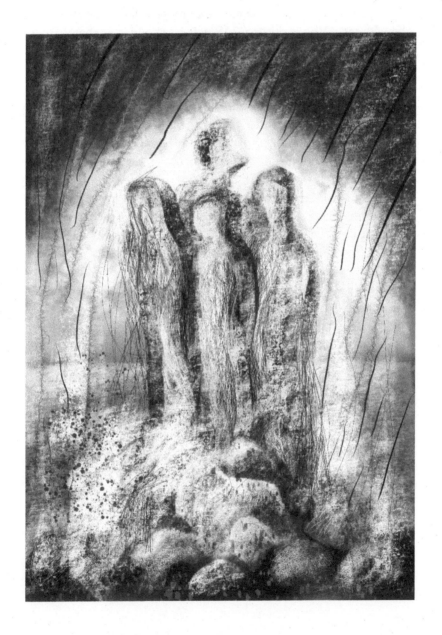

I have been fired by a patient. I have been told to go. He is angry and arrogant. He swaggers about the admission ward. He is a big shot. He is running the show. His name is Sayid. He fires all and sundry, including his fellow patients. He bellows: "You have to go. You are not up to it. I have to sort this mess out myself. All of you! Out! Now!" The staff are amused. The patients are bewildered. Who is this man? Why is he shouting at them? He is not one of the staff. He is a patient. Who does he think he is?

This is what usually happens when Sayid comes in. The bravado does not last long. Things break down fairly quickly and then Sayid becomes tearful and anxious and abject. It is poignant. The puffed up psychotic persona is perhaps something he imagines he should be, but it is unsustainable. He cannot be who he thinks he should be, or who he thinks his mother and his extended family wish him to be.

We have known each other for a long time. He is a pleasant intelligent young man who lives with an older brother and his parents in a fairly affluent suburb of the city. He has lived with schizophrenia from his middle teenage years. He has coped relatively well and has only required two or three admissions to hospital. He attends the out-patient clinic and usually manages to be quite cheerful and optimistic. His manner towards me is for the most part friendly and respectful. On these occasions it is unthinkable that in an altered state he might choose to fire me. He seems so well, so confident, so stable, with the support of such a caring and understanding family that nothing could possibly go wrong.

Probably in part because of his illness he did not achieve a matric pass. This does not seem to have deterred him unduly. He works for his father's building company and earns a small salary. He is clearly respected by his co-workers and he is loved by his family, and admired for the way he has not allowed himself to become downcast by his illness. They are a conservative and devout Muslim family. They have undertaken to inform themselves as fully as possible about this strange illness and they are supportive of Sayid, encouraging him to take his medication and to attend the out-patient clinics and to be hopeful. They maintain understandably the hope that maybe one day this might all pass, and he will marry and have children and perhaps take over his father's business.

Sayid has a close relationship with his older brother Mohammed. Generously, he has not allowed Mohammed's success to come between them. Mohammed did well at school, matriculated with a first class pass and started a degree course in engineering at the university. He was the pride of his family and of the community. Sayid shared in this pride and showed no sign of resentment at the greater attention inevitably shown to his older brother.

It was in the second year that Mohamed began to show the first signs of illness. He became withdrawn, he isolated himself from his friends and his academic performance began to suffer. The course convener expressed concern. The family were appalled. This could not be happening, not again, not to the pride and joy of their lives. They hesitated. Things got worse. Mohammed stopped attending classes. He locked himself in his room. He started shouting in the night, as if it seemed to his horrified family he was being terrorized by imagined assailants. The situation became intolerable.

I am not sure why the decision was made to seek help in the private sector. Maybe the family believed the treatment would be superior to that of the public sector. Maybe there was some wishful thought that if he was treated in a different system there would be a different outcome.

He was seen by one of my colleagues in private who is also of the Muslim faith. The referral was not discussed with me so I do not know what transpired but it seems possible that the family hoped that this psychiatrist would form a different opinion of the distressing course of events than my evaluation of his brother. It was not to be. A provisional diagnosis was made of schizophrenia. Medication was started. There was some degree of improvement and Mohammed returned with some hesitation to his classes.

Yet things could not be the same again. A confidence was lost. Everybody who was involved had become vigilant, anxious. What would happen? Would he be able to cope with the academic demands of his engineering course? Would it all be alright in the end? Would he please not follow the course of his younger brother. The family had coped with that as best they could, but also could not regard these events as anything but a sad and profound disappointment. How could they cope with having to go through this all over again, with their only other child, their hope for the future. Please let this not be happening. Please would it go away?

A tense and fraught time ensued. Mohammed did not seem to be quite himself. There was a distracted way about him. The family attributed this to the traumatic events of the recent past and chose to believe that it would take time to recover. Patience and their love and support and their prayers would bring him through this ordeal.

I do not know what prompted the family at that point to embark on a pilgrimage. I do know that this is required by the faith, and that neither Sayid or Mohammed had been on haj. I do not know whether in some way the family hoped that the holy rituals of the pilgrimage might accelerate and consolidate their troubled son's recovery. The family did not consult me, but there was no reason for me not to encourage the pilgrimage. When I saw Sayid before his departure he was full of excitement and anticipation.

The subsequent events are not clear and were reported to me by Sayid sometime later when he was still in a highly emotional and distraught state. Initially the pilgrimage had been thrilling. The family had felt swept along by the enormous crowds and the clamour and an overwhelming sense of a collective religious fervour. I am not sure if this was all too much for Mohammed. I am not sure if in an exulted religious state he chose to or merely omitted to take his medication. He became agitated and the family became anxious. The situation deteriorated rapidly. His increasingly disorganized behaviour could not in any way be interpreted possibly as a state of spiritual transportation. Increasingly fearful for his safety the family locked him in the hotel bedroom on the fifth floor of their luxury hotel. Left briefly unattended Mohammed found an open window in the bathroom and threw himself to his death. The family were aghast. Not only had they lost their beloved son in the holiest of places but many of the faith believe strongly that suicide is sinful. There was to be no consolation that their son would be on his way to heaven. He would more likely go to hell.

I could not address these issues with Sayid and his mother when I next saw them in the out-patient department. It did not seem appropriate and it was certainly not for me question an article of a faith that had sustained the family throughout their lives. On this occasion Sayid appeared to be putting on a brave front. He seemed to be determined to take on the role of his deceased older brother. His manner was almost nonchalant. He showed no signs of grief. His mother just stared ahead. She scarcely spoke. The father did not attend. The mother said his spirit was broken.

Six months later the father was murdered. It appeared to be one of those random brutal calamities that occur in the city. There had been an attempted robbery. The father had intervened to protect his property and in the ensuing struggle he had been stabbed to death.

In the conservative tradition of this bereft family Sayid is now the head of the household. When I next see him his manner is even more inappropriate than when I saw him following his brother's suicide. He is determined to show that he is strong, that he can cope. He is bluff. He is blandly aloof. His manner towards his grieving mother is cruelly abrupt. He appears to be impatient with her and oblivious to the tears running down her cheeks. He wants to show that he is the head of the family, that he is in charge. It is-sad and it is doomed. The mother, exhausted, shakes her head, nods, gestures as if to say it is all too predictable: he can't cope of course, it is all too much, he is becoming sick and she does not know what to do or where to turn.

The next time I see Sayid he has been admitted to our unit. He is indignant and enraged. He fires me and everybody else. Now he is on his own. There is no older brother. There is no father. He stalks about the ward, slowly becoming uneasy, fearful of his vulnerability.

It will be like this, time and time again. He will recover and he will make a great effort to cope. He tries to make a success of his father's business but he does not have the skills or the resources. The business fails. Mother and son have to leave the family home. It is too much. Things break down yet again and he is back with us, the king of the castle, the master of his tragic universe.

Sayid coped for some of the time, and at other times he could not cope and it seems possible that the psychosis was some sort of escape. He could madly be in charge at last. He could fire me, perhaps loathing the role I played in his life. He could for a while imagine that things were not as they were, and that he was magnificently in control. I cannot remember him formally reappointing me, but after a few days he would calm down and even show a degree of contrition. There was no more swagger, no more bravado. He was then just a very troubled and anxious young man in a painfully difficult situation.

Eventually and reluctantly on each of these occasions he accepts treatment. He gets better and he is discharged. Time will pass and then the mother will come back to the out-patient department, despondent, appearing to be worn down by the difficulties of her life. She does not have to explain very much. "It is all starting again. I can't manage". I cannot say it will be alright. I ask her to sign the necessary forms for an involuntary admission. We will go through the cycle again. He will get better again but the situation will not change. There would be no cure. There is no undoing of what has happened. There can be no enduring alleviation of the predicament of this most unfortunate family, and to presume otherwise is unhelpful and wrong.

40

Suicide and its aftermath

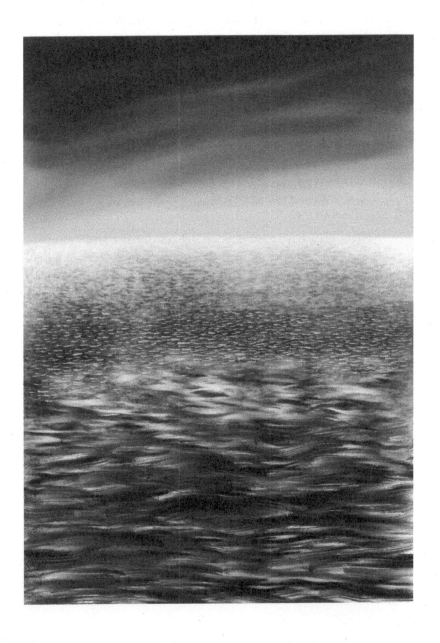

Suicide pervades to the core the clinical practice of psychiatry. The fear and the anxiety that attends every assessment made of risk, and the anger and the consternation that ensues following a self-inflicted death casts a long shadow. Suicide and its aftermath are devastating to all involved, and to the responsible clinicians it represents a sense of a profound failure. It haunts one for years, it undermines confidence, it carries with it a burden of self-reproach and helplessness. What could I have done to prevent this happening? We should have known. We should have picked up the signals. We should have been more cautious. Now it is too late.

I have known colleagues who have stopped practicing in the aftermath of suicide. The blame, however ill-founded it might be, the emotional turmoil and the anxiety that this might happen yet again weighs too heavily. My first night on call as a trainee psychiatrist compelled me to face these daunting and painful issues.

Night calls have always been difficult for me and I am sure for many of my colleagues. You are not able to withdraw, if only for a few hours, to reflect or to escape or to regain yourself. You are also alone. You are responsible. Anything can happen, and certainly in the early stages of training you have little reason to be confident that you will be able to cope with whatever crisis develops.

I had found the first few days at the beginning of my rotation predictably difficult. I was new to the hospital, there were unfamiliar routines and there were many members of staff with whom I needed to acquaint myself. There was also inevitably a degree of uncertainty as to whether this was the right choice for me. I was embarking on a four year training course in a speciality of which of course I could not know very much. This was in the UK and I was also needing to accustom myself to the often subtly different ways of thinking and doing things.

The first night call was I think on the fourth or fifth day of the beginning of this project and I was anxious. I think there might also have been some degree of resentment that I was not to be granted the respite of the short time I felt I needed just to cope with the demands of my new job. The first few hours were relatively quiet and I had just finished a routine ward round when I received a call from the head nurse. "You have to come to the admission ward, now!" he said, and there was a strain of urgency in this that intensified my feelings of apprehension. "What is it is?" I asked, only to be answered, "Just come" and again, "now!"

I arrived in the ward to find a cluster of nurses staring at the closed door of a lavatory. Nobody said anything. It was not immediately clear to me what I was supposed to do. It also seemed curious why a doctor was required to open the door, or why a closed door should constitute an emergency. Yet clearly the nurses gazing at the door were fearful. The silence was ominous. It seemed there was a great reluctance to open the door, in dread of something being confirmed that was deeply troubling to the nurses. The head nurse who had previously appeared to me as a man of great confidence and ability was now disconcertingly unsure of himself. He was fretful and indecisive. His staff turned to him. He turned to me. "Doctor, you do it. Please", he almost whispered, and it seemed to me for a moment absurdly as if he was asking me to do the honours. The group of observers stood back and I opened the door, knowing by then what was to confront us.

There is an appalling and confounding absence that surrounds a hanging body. We gazed upon our patient in horror. It is a vast stillness and a silence that extends beyond the lifeless body but binds us to it and shuts out the world. He was beyond us. He was dead but in the confusion of emotions that engulfed us all it was difficult not to imagine in that inert form a reproach, a now silenced howl of rage against a world that had forsaken him. He had gone, but I think for many of us he was then shouting at us. "Why did you not help me?"

I had admitted him hours earlier. He was a middle aged man who had been living alone on a farm some miles from the hospital. His brother had become concerned about his well-being. There was no history of mental illness but the brother had thought that he had become depressed following the end of his marriage in divorce some months earlier. The brother had suggested to him that he should seek help and he had agreed with some reluctance to attend the out-patient clinic. I had seen him on the afternoon of his admission.

His manner was cautious but he was pleasant, in a rather detached way towards me. I felt some sympathy from him, possibly owing to him seeing me as an inexperienced young doctor who could not possibly understand the darkness of the world that had come to envelop him.

His answers to my questions were vague and he gave an impression of being almost disinterested. He "might' be depressed, he thought. "It was a possibility", but "to be expected" in the circumstances. With regard to the possibility of suicide he was evasive. He shrugged his shoulders and after a moment shook his head, but this was without conviction. There was a weariness about him. He was scarcely attending to me. He was preoccupied and remote.

Living alone and with little support, being middle-aged and being depressed did put him at risk of suicide. When I tentatively suggested an admission he did not refuse but nor did he appear to welcome this proposal. He did not seem to care. I explained the procedures to him and he signed the necessary forms. I informed the nursing staff that the decision had been made to admit him, out of concern that he posed a risk of suicide, but I did not give an instruction that he should be under constant observation on a one to one basis. I did not think he posed that degree of risk. I was ignorant of the furious intent that suicide can demonstrate. I did not see him alive again, and it was not possible for me not to think that I was responsible, and that by issuing more specific instructions I could have prevented his death.

There follows the dreaded responsibility of the telephone call to inform the family. Nobody had told me how I should do this, but it seems improbable anyway that there might be a right way, and that it is not always going to be awful. I have undertaken this miserable task on a number of occasions, and it follows a curiously similar sequence. First the is confusion and bewilderment, then anger, then grief.

"No...no...there has to be a mistake...it is not true...please tell this is not true...this is not happening ...no!...but...but he was in the hospital...you admitted him because you were worried that he might do something...he was supposed to be safe in hospital...it can't be true...why did you allow this to happen...what sort of care is this...I don't believe this...tell me it is not true...I can't believe this...you tell me he is gone...that he is dead...that he hanged himself... no!.. please...please tell me there has been some sort of mistake...please not my brother, not my son, not my father...not somebody who meant the whole world to me...this person whom I cannot imagine living without...and now you have let him die...how could you?...How could you let this happen?"

Then there is the legal process, the court hearings, the apportioning of blame, the protracted bureaucratic process that inevitably ensues, and that might be imagined to attenuate the anger and grief but does not.

"What did I do that was wrong?, what did I miss, what could I have done to stop it?" are constant and quite possibly inevitable refrains that attend the aftermath of a suicide.

This becomes more acute or painful the closer it is to you. A colleague at work started to drift away from us. There was nothing dramatic. There was no apparent crisis. He just seemed to lose interest for the work that he was doing, and an enthusiasm in his professional behaviour to which we had become accustomed. There were a few minor mistakes or perhaps oversights, or lapses of judgement, but nothing that gave rise to a serious cause for concern. We suggested that he should maybe take some time off work. Perhaps there was a lot going on that we were unaware of and he should give himself time to sort things out.

He did not come to the clinic the next week and we chose to believe that he had heeded our advice and taken a few days off. His wife contacted our principal. He had been found in a remote area, some distance from his home. He was alive. Some children had found him in his car with a pipe leading from the exhaust to the interior. They had detached the pipe and opened the windows and he revived. He returned home. He returned to work. What had happened was impossible. It was inconceivable that this husband and father and successful and highly respected professional person should seek to kill himself. His desperate act was denied.

He disappeared the next week. Again he was found, this time in a different place, but again close to death with a pipe leading from the exhaust into the vehicle. It then became difficult or irresponsible to ignore the fact that there was a grave crisis, but for reasons that were unfathomable to me he was admitted to a surgical ward in a private hospital. I can only think that it was considered unacceptable that a colleague should be admitted to the acute unit of the public hospital where I worked as a consultant. I don't know whether it was thought of being somehow shameful. I don't know whether the situation was considered not sufficiently grave to consider such a radical intervention. I was not consulted or involved in any way in these decisions. So with all the respect owing to a colleague and specialist physician he was admitted to a private suite in a surgical ward with no restriction on his movement. He promptly went to a local pharmacy where he procured a wide range of sedatives and opiates which he prescribed for himself. He consumed the lot, climbed to the top of the building where the clinic was situated and threw himself to his death from the roof.

A turmoil of rage and grief and recriminations followed. How could this have been allowed to happen? All the signs had been there. What sort of nonsensical or wishful thinking was it that a doctor should be considered immune to desperation and to the risk of suicide? Why had his colleagues not seen what was going on, including a psychiatrist for god's sake? Why had we not done anything? Even in anguished retrospect I have no idea what drove my colleague to his suicide. It seems clear that he was determined, and it is not at all clear whether more decisive and restrictive measures would have saved him.

This fierce resolve is mysterious and can be deceptive. Perhaps it is within us all to refuse to believe that somebody, whether it is a patient or a friend or a family member has made a decision to end their lives. It appals us. It is unthinkable.

It is a curious and anomalous observation that in suicidal behaviour the most determined acts are not infrequently without apparent cause. Henri was a successful accountant, married with a nine year old daughter. He set off for work one morning without it seemed a care in the world. The office phoned his wife towards midday saying that he had not arrived at work. This was of concern as it was most uncharacteristic of him not to inform the office if for whatever reason he would not be coming in. His wife was mystified and went down to the garage of their home where she found her husband unconscious. He was lying in a pool of blood and in his hand was a knife with which he had slit his throat.

When I encountered him in the surgical ward he had fully regained consciousness but spoke with difficulty because of the pressure bandages around his neck. He was babbling. He seemed to be excited to be alive. At that time and on the many occasions afterwards when I spoke to both him and his wife he could provide no explanation for his actions. He said there were no problems in his life. He was happily married. He loved his daughter dearly. He enjoyed his work. He was utterly mystified as to why in such a violent manner he had attempted to end his seemingly most fortunate life.

Peter was employed by the university in an administrative capacity. He too was happily married with a young family and he too denied that there were any major problems in his life. The first time I met him he appeared to me as a character in a horror film. He was encased in plasters and splints. Pressure bandages enveloped his neck and forearms and his skull was protected by a helmet. He had first cut his throat. That was unsuccessful in ending his life but in great alarm he had been admitted to a private clinic. There he had managed to dive head first from the first floor into an atrium, fracturing his skull and his pelvis. After some days he had been allowed to leave the clinic for a few hours in the company of his wife. While her attention was momentarily diverted he had used a screwdriver to pierce the fibrous compartments of both forearms and sever his radial arteries. When he finally got to us, now as an involuntary admission, he was elated. He seemed delighted to be alive. He was fascinated by the curious behaviour of the other patients on the ward. He wanted to engage with them and do whatever he could to help them, but they shrank away from him in horror at his bizarre appearance.

He could not explain his behaviour. I do not doubt that he tried to make sense of what he had done to himself. He had come desperately close to killing himself, but for the years afterward when I saw him in the outpatient department he remained bewildered by his actions. At no point did he ever seem depressed. He went back to work and to his family and when I last saw him before he returned to private care he was cheerful, and seemed confident that there would be no recurrence of these unfathomable and violent events.

Suicide can be an understandable and rational act, but for the most part it is a source of profound distress to all, and confounds our deeply-held assumptions and beliefs in the value of life and the will to live.

41

HIV and madness

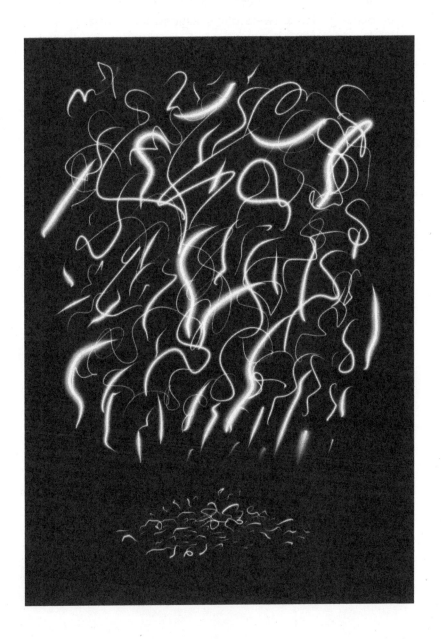

Maluti is adrift. He is vacant. He is elsewhere but I have no idea where that is. Dishevelled, he gazes at us with a disconcerting impassivity from his chair. He does not appear to be in distress. He is emaciated. He is not agitated. Anger about being where he is does not appear to account for his disengagement with his surroundings. He answers our questions, but with a delay, and slowly, without emotion. He is apathetic.

'Maluti, how are you coping? What's going on? How can we help you?' A long silence ensues. Can he hear us? Has he forgotten our questions? Is he beyond caring?

Then, quietly, with a degree of perplexity, almost to himself, he says, 'No, I am ... all right ... no problems ... yes ... it's all right.' And after a long pause, 'Thank you.'

There are a number of possibilities for us to consider and, as we so often preach to the students, it is unlikely that there is only one explanation. It is far more probable that there are a range of interacting factors that contribute to this rather enigmatic presentation.

Maluti has Aids. He has a low CD4 count. He also has tuberculosis. He also has schizophrenia. He also, possibly to cope with these problems, has a long history of alcohol abuse.

He has lived with HIV for over fifteen years. How he contracted the illness is again open to a range of possible factors. At that time, there was much controversy about what might cause of the illness, how it should be treated and, curiously, even whether it existed at all.

Garlic and the African potato were proposed as remedies by the Ministry of Health. In this context, it is quite possible that Maluti either ignored his symptoms or delayed treatment. The diagnosis of schizophrenia preceded the HIV. The self-neglect and the loss of any sense of self or control over his circumstances would certainly have rendered him vulnerable to infection. This would also have undermined his engagement with any treatment programme. Without support, it would perhaps have been expecting too much of him to adhere to the relatively complex treatment regimens of both schizophrenia and HIV. It therefore became grimly predictable that the HIV would develop into Aids and that, as a consequence of his impaired immunity, he would become afflicted with tuberculosis. Living alone, with little or no support from family or friends, it had then become even more improbable, or impossible, that he could have been expected to cope with living with HIV/Aids, schizophrenia and tuberculosis. It is not clear when alcohol became a problem, and that in itself is yet again a consequence of many likely factors.

He had moved many years previously from the Eastern Cape to the city in search of work. He had lost contact with his family and his community. The suspicions and social awkwardness of schizophrenia would have undermined the limited resources he had to seek support in a new and alien world. He had been unable to find regular work and was living in poverty in one of the many informal settlements that were developing on the peripheries of the city. In these dire circumstances, it is unsurprising that he should seek solace in alcohol. In the shebeens there was at least some semblance of a community and the illusory hope of putting aside, at least for a while, the hopelessness of his predicament. It is again quite understandable that, in these circumstances, he should seek comfort in sex – and that, given his isolation and his social unease, that this should have to be paid for. He had earned a small income from occasional, informal and unskilled work, and these pitiful amounts were spent on alcohol and prostitutes.

He had made some desultory attempts to attend the local clinics for his medication but this was for the HIV, not the schizophrenia. Even in his abject state he was fearful of being seen in the queue to receive psychiatric attention. The stigma of mental illness was greater than that of HIV/Aids. Predictably, he relapsed.

He had been brought to the emergency unit by the police, who had found him wandering in the traffic in the city centre. It did not seem to them that he was attempting to kill himself. He seemed confused and he was unable to give a clear account of himself. He was examined and the diagnoses of HIV/Aids and pulmonary tuberculosis were confirmed. Treatment was restarted.

Probably not knowing what to do with him, the medical staff referred him onward to our service.

This is often a source of rancour. The registrars perform a more or less ritual exchange. The psychiatrists will accuse the emergency physicians of dumping the patient. The medical team will say they are overwhelmed, they have done what they can, and they do not have the resources to assess and manage psychiatric disorders. The social workers usually join in the fray. This is time-consuming and enervating, and if a stalemate develops the consultant becomes involved. At this stage, there does not seem to be an option. Time is being wasted and goodwill is being undermined. I accept the transfer.

Maluti eventually finds himself in our ward, baffled, disoriented, stupefied by the sedative medications he has been given in the emergency unit.

Perhaps the most striking feature is his slowness. For this, there are many possible explanations. The most obvious is the sedative medication, given regularly in the emergency units for fear of the havoc that can be caused by a psychotic patient disrupting the emergency care of medically ill patients. In this circumstance, sedation does not seem likely. He is not drowsy. He is alert, but is not with us. Delirium is always a source of great anxiety. It can be life-threatening and, for Maluti, there are many possible causes, including the HIV, or the tuberculosis involving his brain, or both, or any other infective agent due to his compromised immune system.

The slowness could be explained by depression. There are many reasons for him to be depressed. People often do not say they are depressed. This tends to occur in the more severe forms of depression. If you are very depressed and consider your situation to be hopeless, what is the point of telling anybody that you are depressed? It seems very possible to us that this is what Maluti might be thinking and feeling. This sense of futility could in all likelihood be confounded by his being in a very unfamiliar environment, surrounded by inquisitive strangers speaking a language of which he has only the slightest grasp, asking inane questions like 'How are you?' and 'What is the matter?' – as if he knew, or could even begin to make sense of what had happened to him.

The slowness could be accounted for by the schizophrenia or by the medications that have been used to treat it. Delusions of persecution can induce a wariness that might be expressed in caution and slowness. The slowness might be a due to distraction owing to auditory hallucinations or intrusive commenting voices. Catatonia is a severe form of schizophrenia that can present with a dramatic slowness to the point of immobility and mutism. The negative forms of schizophrenia – the social withdrawal and emotional flatness and loss of volition often associated with cognitive problems, including impaired attention – are further possibilities that we need to consider. Antipsychotic medications can cause slowness in different ways, probably most commonly through sedation or by the curious parkinsonian side-effects induced by many of these agents, particularly when used at high doses.

Another possibility to account for Maluti's rather inscrutable presentation of being there and yet not being there is some form of dementia. We do not know his age, but he is probably in his forties, which would be early for the more common forms of dementia. Excessive consumption of alcohol is a not uncommon cause of dementia at this age. This is associated with a general lack of self-care, including inadequate nutrition – and, as happens so often in states of drunkenness, violence and repeated head injuries, all of which could be contributing to Maluti's slowness and possible dementia.

The most probable explanation is HIV/Aids. This has become one of the more common causes of dementia in younger people. A characteristic feature of this kind of dementia is slowness due to the damage caused by the virus to particular parts of the brain. Maluti's apathy could be explained by any one of these factors. It is more probable that some or all of these possible causative factors are interacting to produce what seems to be an intractable problem and a deeply sad and lonely predicament.

HIV can affect the brain in a number of ways. It can cause an encephalopathy or inflammation of the central nervous system that would usually present as a delirium, an altered state of consciousness. Through a suppression of the immune system, the virus may cause a wide range of secondary viral, fungal, parasitic and bacterial infections of the brain, including tuberculosis. It may cause a number of malignancies or rare cancers of the brain. It may cause dementias. Antiretroviral treatments may cause many psychological and neuropsychiatric problems. The associations of HIV and madness are complex and profuse.

There is another, non-biological and more figurative, way in which madness pertains to HIV. In the early part of this century, President Thabo Mbeki declares that the human immunodeficiency virus does not cause Aids. This is in defiant opposition to the scientific and medical consensus of the time. He is supported in this bizarre claim by the Minister of Health, Dr Manto Tshabalala-Msimang. 'Western medicine' is rejected. Aids activism represents a neocolonialist intervention, Mbeki declares. Tshabalala-Msimang commends as a cure *ubhejane*, garlic, lemon and beetroot. She becomes known as Dr Beetroot. As a result of the denialism of these two politicians, it is estimated in a report by Harvard University's School of Public Health that approximately 350 000 South Africans succumbed to preventable deaths.

My closest friend during my school and undergraduate years died of Aids. He was not in denial of his status. He had, perhaps, been in a quite mad denial of the consequences of the grave risks he took and in the apparent belief of his invulnerability. He excelled at everything he undertook. At school he was top of the class in most subjects. He captained the first teams in cricket and rugby and athletics. He occupied leadership positions and was held in high esteem by teachers and scholars. He continued to flourish at university. He was a star. He soared, it seemed, above us and beyond us.

His secret behaviour confounded me. He was a medical student. He knew all about HIV and Aids. He knew the danger of the risks he was taking with apparent abandon. He seemed compelled to test the limits, to fly as close as he could to the sun. I was unable to stop him. He laughed. Everything was a big adventure. His sexual exploits appeared to be all the more thrilling to him because he knew of the dangers. I think he was perhaps scornful of my concern and my caution. I found it increasingly difficult to be with him. What had at one time seemed almost heroically daring and creative now seemed wilfully destructive. We drifted apart. He flew on, further and further, more and more dangerously, until it became inevitable that he would burn and crash. When I last saw him shortly before his death he was weak and angry. Anger also confused my grief. It was such a terrible waste. He had been my best friend and I will never know what dark and mysterious forces led him to his early death.

There is, nevertheless, something in this story that is perhaps understandable and that is not confined to my friend's trajectory. In the sexual act, we abandon ourselves. We seek to lose ourselves. We are heedless of the consequences. Sex is dangerous. It requires taking risks. In relinquishing all control in a brief state of rapture, it is a moment of madness. It is outside reason and care and caution. The cruelty and sadness of it is that, in the moment of bliss and transcendence, there should fall the shadow of possible disease and destruction. In the Garden of Eden there will always be a snake, hissing and whispering in the leaves of the apple tree, driving us mad by burdening us with the preposterous notion that we might not be entirely in control of our lives, that innocence is transitory and paradise ephemeral.

Maluti is now beyond this madness. He is beyond caring and beyond seeking. He can be helped, to some extent. The tuberculosis can be treated. The schizophrenia can be managed and the HIV can be contained. He will be transferred to a home where his complex regime of medications can be supervised. He will receive a disability grant. It is unknowable whether, in the oblivion of his dementia, he might find some form of sanctuary.

42

Huntington's disease, syphilis and other tragedies of the damaged brain

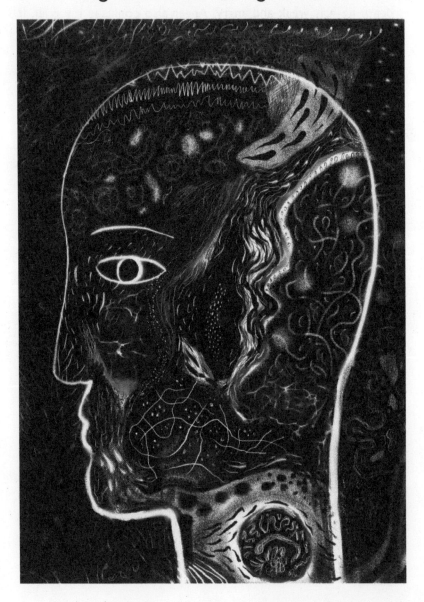

He is writhing about in a cot bed. He does not register us in any way. He makes curious distressing keening sounds. He beats his head against the side of the cot. He is wearing incontinence pads. His movements are purposeless. His eyes are vacant. He is my age. We were at school together. He was a champion tennis player.

The first indication had been a slight clumsiness. Nobody thought much of it at the time. He was in his early forties. Perhaps this was to be expected as we grow older. Perhaps it would pass. Then there were small, transitory lapses of attention. Perhaps this was due to stresses at work. Others mentioned similar problems. It was thought to be innocuous. It did not seem sinister. His wife described the movement and coordination problems becoming more marked and persistent. He became self-conscious about this. It seemed as if he might be drunk. His children then in early adolescence grew anxious and embarrassed. He had always paid scrupulous attention to his health. He had continued with the tennis and played competitively but now to his great dismay he was unable to perform what had been for him the most basic manoeuvres.

Alarm mounted. He appeared to have difficulty finding the appropriate words and his speech was at times slurred. At work his colleagues expressed a concern that decisions he made were at times ill-judged. This was affecting his performance and the business was beginning to suffer. They encouraged him to take leave. Initially he refused. He seemed to lack insight into the increasing gravity of the situation. Eventually there was no alternative. His colleagues insisted. As the movement and the cognitive problems persisted and seemed to worsen, it became apparent to the great distress of his family that it was increasingly unlikely that he would be able to return to work. Financial anxieties now compounded their fears. Then his father, a man in his late seventies began to show the same symptoms. It eventually became clear that both were afflicted by Huntington's disease. I think this must be one of the most cruel of all neurological disorders, and the reason for this is its genetics.

The tragedy that was engulfing this family was in some ways

unusual for Huntingtons. It is an inherited disorder. The transmission is autosomally dominant, indicating that the children of an affected person, regardless of gender, have a one in two chance of inheriting the illness. With regard to my school friend, and now my patient the diagnosis was perhaps delayed because there was no apparent family history of Huntingtons. It is recognized that symptoms may appear at earlier ages in succeeding generations, and it also seems probable that with increasing longevity a family history might become evident in an aging parent who would have otherwise died of another natural cause.

The son and daughter stood with their mother and myself at the end of their father's bed, observing in dismay his agitated figure, having to confront his inaccessibility, and their own threatened futures. Both were about to finish their schooling and both had plans to go to university. There had been no reason to doubt bright and happy and successful trajectories which is in the nature of their age, and now this was all thrown into a turmoil. They knew they had a one in two chance of inheriting this illness, and becoming like the demented father upon whom they now gazed in pity and horror. Not only were they having to contemplate the loss of their father but they were also facing the possible loss of their own futures. The mother held the hands of both her children. She was a source of immense strength and support for them. I am filled with a sense of wonder by the extraordinary resilience and the grace shown by this mother and grieving wife and by many others who cope in some mystifying and inspiring way with what seems to be a dreadful and unendurable situation.

It is possible to test whether one is carrying the Huntingtin gene but this raises a wide range of difficult issues, which are all the more complicated and agonizing for a young person. A positive test confers an inevitability. There will no longer be a tentative optimism allowed by a degree of uncertainty. My experience has been that for the most part the test is refused, and this is understandable. Why should a young person choose to close down hope, to live thereafter in a constant state of apprehension that any twitch or tremor might herald the onset of the disease, and an inevitable decline towards dementia and death? When a decision is made to be tested it is usually in the context of a young woman wanting to know whether she should start a family, and being determined not to pass the gene on to her children. It is a grave burden to bear.

The family of a colleague of mine was affected by this wretched illness. An older brother had died in a car accident, and it was suspected that he had begun to detect the early signs of the illness in himself and had chosen to end his life. My colleague's whole life had been in the shadow of Huntingtons. His ambition was to study medicine and specialize in neurology with the aim of finding a cure for the illness that had destroyed so many members of his family. For this reason he agreed to the test, arguing understandably that it would be futile to embark on such a long and arduous course if the symptoms of the illness were to make it impossible for him to realize his wishes. It was a very courageous thing to have done. The test was negative. He became a doctor. He has not discovered a cure for Huntingtons. At present it is not foreseeable.

Kobus is in good spirits. He greets the students cheerfully. He seems to enjoy the company of young people and he responds to their enquiries enthusiastically. I had asked the group to spend some time with him before the ward round. We reconvened five minutes later. I asked him whether he had met them before. He appeared to think this was rather a ridiculous question. Why should he have met them previously? He was nevertheless polite, and said, as if not wanting to offend: "No I don't think so. No I have never met these young people". They had spent about ten minutes with him. They were startled. In their conversation with him there was nothing at all to suggest that he had no short term memory. He was amicable. He was engaging. He had seemed to be well. Compared to the other patients on the ward they had seen he appeared to be intact. There did not seem to be anything the matter. The only slight problem was that he had been rather vague about the reasons for his admission, and this they probably registered only in retrospect.

This encapsulated phenomenon of short term memory loss is fascinating and disquieting. All other cognitive faculties remain intact. Kobus retained all his social skills. He spoke fluently and articulately. There appeared to be no damage and yet he was incapacitated. He was hospital-bound.

Kobus had spent the weekend as he had spent every weekend on the ward. He had alienated himself from his family and his friends. There was nobody willing to take him out of the hospital. Yet when we asked him how he had spent the weekend he embarked on a lengthy and delighted account of a hunting trip with friends. In the evening they had made a fire and cooked meat and yes, quite a lot of beer and spirits had been consumed, but it had been a most enjoyable occasion.

For a moment Kobus was at a loss as to how to account for the weekend. He had no idea at all. Confronted momentarily with a quite possibly terrifying sense of nothingness he retrieved long term memories. He had on many occasions in the past gone on hunting expeditions with his friends, and he had consumed excessive amounts of alcohol. This had caused the damage to the parts of his brain that make it possible for us to store short term memories. Kobus moved through life in the continuous moment of the present. Not knowing what he had been thinking or doing moments previously rendered him unable to function. There was no context. He had no story. The whole rambling edifice of a personal narrative had collapsed down to the vacancy of the immediate moment. He could make no sense of where he was and why he was there and what was going on around him because there was no past and there was no future. He could not move from point A to point B. He was trapped forever in the confined world of point A, the non-contingent present.

He was helpless but he used the other parts of his battered intelligence to hide this in confabulations. There was only a moment when his bewilderment showed, before he was able to fabricate a world that made some sense to him.

It is a mystery why alcohol should ruin these very small and specific parts of the brain, the mammillary bodies which form part of the diencephalon adjacent to the mid-brain. With continued use the damage spreads. Alcohol is one of the more common causes of dementia before the age of sixty five. Kobus was not demented. The damage and the deficit was localized. Had he continued his excesses he would have in all likelihood become demented, but he forgot who he was, he forgot the alcohol and what he had done to himself.

Dirk had also been profoundly affected by damage to a very specific part of his brain. I saw him regularly in one of the local community clinics. He had no problems with memory. He always greeted me pleasantly and by name. A familiar routine ensued. He was quite well thank you. He was living with a girl-friend and she was also doing well thank you. He was calm and composed and then quite suddenly he would burst into tears. The tears were profuse and appeared to be beyond his control. This embarrassed him greatly. In between the sobbing and scarcely audibly, he would say: "I am sorry Doctor. I am so sorry. I can't control it. I am not depressed. There is nothing wrong with me. It's just this crying. I can't stop it. It just comes over me suddenly. I can't stop it. My girl-friend gets angry with me. She doesn't believe me. She says there must be something wrong but there isn't". Then quite suddenly the tears abate. He composes himself and smiles at me. "I am fine, really. It's just this crying that I don't seem to control. It is completely unpredictable and it's embarrassing and annoying. People don't understand that it is because of the accident. They think there is something wrong with me. People don't cry for no reason".

Many years earlier Dirk had been involved in a motorbike accident. He had suffered a head injury and fractured his pelvis. After some months he appeared to have recovered completely from these injuries except for this one problem, an emotional incontinence that baffled and exasperated him. As a consequence of the closed head injury damage had been done to the inferior aspects of the frontal cortex. This highly evolved part of the brain mediates inhibition. His uncontrollable weeping was the expression of a disinhibition arising from the disruption of neurological circuits in this very specific part of the brain.

There is no other overt indication of damage and this

curiously causes much distress to those who are affected. There is no sign of a head injury. There is no paralysis nor any other dramatic feature to account for the changed behaviour. One has just lost control, or that is what people think, and that is shameful. There is one neurological signal of injury to this part of the brain and that is a loss of olfaction, or the capacity to smell due to damage to the olfactory nerve fibres that pass through the base of the skull into the nasal cavity. It is not overt but it is useful as an objective indication of damage to the brain. In a persisting dualistic way of thinking it is curious that patients may be reassured by being informed that their changed behaviour can be attributed to brain damage rather than psychological causes.

Disinhibition following a head injury has other repercussions that can cause further harm. Alcohol may be consumed to excess, leading to aggression and violence and an increased risk of another head injury being sustained. Sexual disinhibition may lead to unwanted pregnancies or sexually transmitted infections. In this respect HIV/AIDS is a particular cause for concern as the impulsivity resulting from a head injury would make the necessarily scrupulous adherence to treatment improbable.

These phenomena are consequences of fairly localized injuries to the brain. More diffuse injuries have more devastating effects, and this applies particularly to traumatic head injuries. The devastation is because these injuries are common and too often affect young people, ruining their and their families lives. It is every parents' nightmare to receive a call in the middle of the night to inform them of the accident. John or Sophie or Xolisi had been out celebrating their birthday with friends or their graduation or matric results and maybe somebody had been irresponsible and had had a few drinks before driving, or maybe it was somebody else's fault but in seconds everything falls appallingly apart. There will be no university, no family, no happiness, no future, no sadness even, except for others, just an enduring emptiness. Traumatic brain injuries are among the more common causes of dementia in young people.

Syphilis, and other sexually transmitted infections, especially HIV/AIDS are other causes of dementia. The two are associated.

Syphilis is on the rise for many reasons including HIV. Syphilitic lesions increase the risk of HIV transmission. HIV through impaired immunity accelerates the progression of syphilis from its primary stages to damage to the central nervous system. Another possible reason for the soaring rates of sexually transmitted diseases is that the sexual act is less fraught with anxieties. An oral contraceptive can prevent pregnancy. A pill can dramatically reduce the risk of HIV progression. Neither however will prevent infection as a result of unprotected sex.

Syphilis is difficult because the early signs can resolve spontaneously, without treatment, only to reappear in some unfortunate person years later, wreaking havoc in the brain.

I saw Jack for a few years in the out –patient clinic of the hospital before referring him to the local community clinic, when it became clear to me that there was nothing much more I could do for him. He had been treated for the neurosyphilis that had ruined him. He was demented but the progression had been halted. He was calm and appeared to be contented. He was vacant. There was no problem. He had no complaints. There was nothing wrong with him. he did not know why his family was making all this fuss. He was quite capable of looking after himself.

He was not, and it was to my great relief and that of the family that he agreed without complaint to being moved to a supervised home. The blandness, his passive acquiescence and apparent unconcern were part of the dementia but in this respect were to his advantage. He adapted in his way. He appears to be at peace in the world. He is not agitated. He is not in distress. He drifts on.

I have no idea what he is thinking but it is just possible that in some way his dementia might be protecting him from the pain of having lost his mind.

43

Why become a psychiatrist

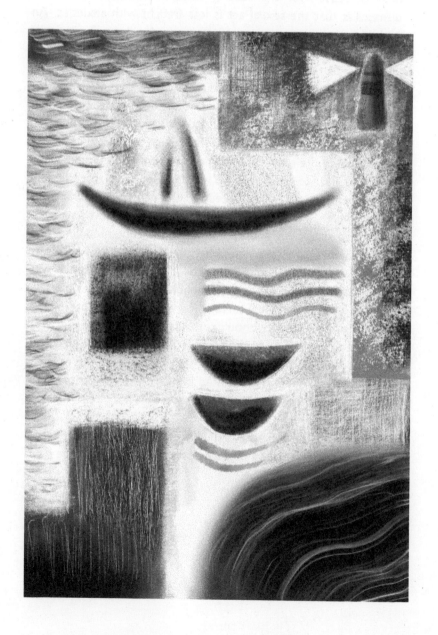

When I started my training to become a doctor I had no intention of becoming a psychiatrist. I did not consider it an option but nor did I have any plan to specialize in any other discipline. My goal at that early stage was simply to obtain a medical degree, I think in the rather romantic if not naïve belief that I would be doing something useful. I had spent three years doing a bachelor of arts degree, majoring in English literature and philosophy, and on graduating I wondered in a state of anxiety how I was going to make a living. I tried teaching. It was not a success. Without really knowing what I was letting myself in for I then embarked on a course of undergraduate training in medicine in South Africa and post graduate training in psychiatry in the UK that was to occupy ten years of my life.

The first years were difficult for me. It is possible that these very difficulties led to my choosing to specialize in psychiatry after I had completed my undergraduate studies. In the philosophy courses in particular I had been encouraged to think critically, to ask questions and to reflect. In the first years of my undergraduate degree in medicine this was certainly not encouraged. On the contrary these ways of thinking became a hindrance to the accumulation of large quantities of factual information. It is not helpful to question the basic principles of physics or chemistry or any other of the basic sciences we were required to absorb. The facts were out there and we somehow had to get all this stuff into our heads. In some unhappiness it seemed to me that what I needed to do was to turn myself into an empty vessel to receive as much information as possible. I am sure I had got it all wrong but at the time I felt I needed to become a passive recipient of knowledge, and to put aside the luxuries of critical thinking to which I had become accustomed in the faculty of arts. Somehow I muddled through, but I did worry whether or not I had made the right decision, and how I would cope as a doctor.

My first impressions of psychiatry were negative. This was in the fourth year of undergraduate training. By that stage I had become used to the rather convergent ways of thinking in clinical medicine and had developed a cautious respect for an evidence based scientific method. Psychiatry seemed vague. At the time a lingering belief in psychoanalysis still shaped the thinking of influential members of the department, and the lack of any evidence for what to a young medical student seemed bizarre propositions further alienated me. This was also at a time of a very different culture in medicine. Doctors and particularly specialists, not excepting psychiatrists, were aloof and condescending to all around them, including junior colleagues, nurses and especially patients.

The memory I have of one of my first encounters in psychiatry was a formal lecture on schizophrenia. I was one of about a hundred students gathered in a hall of steeply banked seats, facing an elderly and stern professor in a white coat. After a brief introduction to the subject he told us we were about to see our first psychiatric patient. This person had recently been admitted for the first time and the diagnosis was uncertain. We were to be privileged by observing the professor interviewing this patient and making a diagnosis which owing to his senior position was to be definitive. I recall a hush of excitement and apprehension among my fellow students. Psychiatry was unlike anything else we had encountered. It was deeply weird. Now we were going to see somebody that was quite possibly insane. Schizophrenia! I suppose we were all harbouring our own ignorant fantasies about what this might mean, informed probably for the most part by lurid and sensationalist depictions in film and fiction. We were told to be quiet and respectful. No questions were permitted.

A young woman was led into the lecture theatre by a nurse. She was not introduced to us and we were not introduced to her. Without preamble a few, it seemed rather random questions were asked. She answered hesitatingly. She seemed to be bewildered. I do not remember her being asked what she thought the problem might be. The questions were more of a "Do you hear voices?" nature, requiring an affirmative or negative response. There was no enquiry as to how she was coping with what must have been for her an ordeal. Eventually the professor grimly nodded his head and she was led away. We all knew what this meant. The dreaded diagnosis had been made. The learned professor had pronounced her mad. She was a "schizophrenic". She had been haughtily dismissed. She was condemned. I remember this event vividly and with some shame. We should have demanded to know how he came to what seemed to us a peremptory diagnosis that we knew would have devastating consequences. We were cowed. We were just medical students. What did we know?

The next morning we gathered in a smaller group in one of the hospital wards. On this occasion the psychiatrist was a fairly young woman. She was sympathetic and kind and rather nervous. She told us she was going to introduce us to a woman in the manic phase of a bipolar mood disorder. We waited for what seemed a long time. Maybe this patient was bravely refusing the degrading exhibition that had taken place on the previous day. Then there was a commotion and a very fierce woman hurtled into our midst. She glared at us, her hands on her hips and shouted "I want to fuck"... surveying the group of students cowering away from her, imperiously jabbing a finger at me, "you", she yelled. My colleagues were sniggering. I was deeply embarrassed. The woman was led away, bellowing, furious and indignant, down the long corridors back to her ward. It was not a propitious introduction to psychiatry.

Perhaps in retrospect one of the more troubling aspects of the earlier charade was the application of a rigid and restrictive biomedical model to the practice of psychiatry. In this respect a number of specific questions are asked and signs are elicited to make a diagnosis according to rigorous or operationally defined criteria. A crushing chest pain with shortness of breath and the pain radiating down the left arm, and specific electrocardiogram changes and blood samples showing raised enzymes indicating heart damage will lead to a diagnosis of a heart attack or a myocardial infarction.

The fear associated with this, the dreaded anticipation of death is an irrelevance. Delusions and hallucinations might suggest a diagnosis of schizophrenia. The content of these phenomena, the belief that your mind is controlled by a machine, or the voice telling you that you are worthless and deserve to die, according to this restrictive model are of no consequence. This is clearly inadequate.

You go to see a doctor because you have lost a lot of weight and you have noticed specks of blood in your sputum. This is a very skilled and efficient young specialist, well versed in the conventions of the biomedical model, and confident in the advances it has represented in his speciality. The necessary questions are asked, the examination is performed and the appropriate investigations are ordered. When this process is completed he calls you to say that you have lung cancer and will probably be dead within the next six months. This would be absurd. It is offensive and grotesquely insensitive, but in a limited sense this young doctor has done what is required of him. He might argue that it is not his job to ask what support is available to you, how you will cope with this news, or what your fears might be. That is for a psychologist or a priest. It is not his job to be nice or kind he says. His duty is to make the correct diagnosis and recommend the most effective treatment.

It should not be like this. Obtaining a fuller history, understanding the context, developing some idea of a person's strengths and weaknesses, enquiring about what symptoms might mean to the person and what hopes and fears there are is not being merely nice, it is surely being a better and more effective doctor. In the first scenario it seems very likely that you will be angry and disbelieving, and either deny the diagnosis or turn to somebody else who you might be better able to trust. The second approach is more likely to be useful and helpful. It is also more acceptable and more respectful. You do not see yourself as an object, as a cancer. You are a subject with a history and a future, belonging to a family and a community. You hold a set of beliefs that are important to what sense you make of this diagnosis and how you will cope with it. Being a patient should not be degrading. You cannot be irrelevant to your diagnosis.

The terms "biomedical" and "biopsychosocial" represent, loosely, more an approach rather than a model, and should not be considered as opposites. It is not one thing or another but rather a matter of degree. It would be simplistic in the extreme to consider that a biopsychosocial approach is appropriate to psychiatry and a biomedical approach more appropriate to general medicine or surgery. Of course it will not be helpful to embark on a lengthy history in a medical emergency. Nor does one want to be asked how one feels about having a heart attack. One wants the problem to be solved as quickly and as effectively as possible. A question as to how one might be coping with a recent diagnosis of a terminal cancer is however appropriate. Not making such an enquiry, and not asking about available support and plans for the immediate future is negligent. Meanings are not outside science or clinical medicine. A fractured wrist in a young and ambitious concert pianist will have a different meaning to him or her than a fractured wrist in an elderly woman suffering from dementia. As clinicians we are obliged to attend to this.

Luthando is referred to me with a probable diagnosis of schizophrenia. I could use a checklist approach to identify particular symptoms according to some arbitrary diagnostic manual, confirm the diagnosis, prescribe an anti-psychotic medication and then call for the next patient. This would be ridiculously insufficient. I need to know Luthando's background. I need to know his family history and I need to have an understanding of the genetics of schizophrenia. I need to know this because Luthando's mother is going to ask me if he can have children and what the risks are of them developing schizophrenia. I need to have a medical knowledge in order to be sure that the symptoms might not be due to a general medical condition. I need to know what the family's beliefs are regarding psychosis. I need to know whether they have consulted a traditional healer because I need to have some indication as to whether or not they will accept the diagnosis and what it means to them because this will determine to a great extent his adherence to a treatment programme. I need to know, among much else, about Luthando's resources, the friends he might have and the support available to him. I need to have an understanding of neurophysiology and neuropharmacology in order to prescribe the appropriate medication, and to deal with the possible side-effects. I need to have an ethical sense to decide how to manage the possibility of

Luthando refusing treatment and I have an obligation in the domain of public health to raise awareness, for example, of the association of cannabis use and schizophrenia, the nature of mental illness and the harm done by stigma and exclusion. I don't think that these lines of enquiry are specific to psychiatry but I do think the integration of such a wide range of perspectives, from basic neuroscience to psychology to some understanding or awareness of socio-economic, political and cultural contexts and ethics and religion is probably more fundamental to psychiatry than to other medical specialties.

Given these concerns that one or another approach should not be restricted to a particular discipline, a broadly defined integrated biological and psychosocial approach is or should be intrinsic to psychiatry, and that is what makes psychiatry deeply intriguing. It is inevitably intimate and intense, and to me profound because one is dealing with the disruption of the very faculties that make us who we are.

In many ways it is a personal issue, and one's choice of a speciality a matter of interest and values rather than aptitude. Broken bones are very different from broken minds. I can understand my orthopaedic surgery colleagues' disinterest in psychiatry. Fractured minds are not readily fixable. Psychiatry is messy, but not in a physical way. These perceptions are distorted to my exasperation by the misapprehension amongst my colleagues outside the field of psychiatry that severe mental illnesses cannot be effectively treated. The medical profession is not immune to the need of the "other", and curiously the discipline of psychiatry is itself often elided with this disregarding epithet. Madness is "other". Psychiatry and psychiatrists are also in some other domain.

I am very fortunate and happy to be there. It has been for me a domain of wonder and intellectual fascination.

44

Meaning and madness

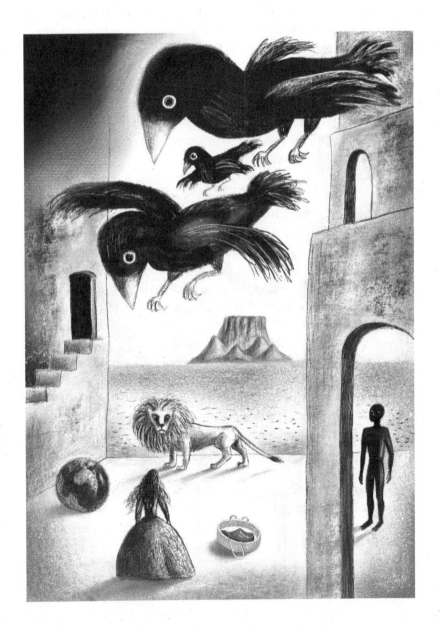

At the Monday morning feedback meeting I am informed by the nursing staff that there are three Mandelas on the ward. They are behaving in a courteous, dignified way towards each other. There is no dispute as to who the true Mandela might be. They appear to respect the choice that each has made to be an eminent and revered figure. There has never been a Jacob Zuma on our ward. The ex-president is currently facing charges of corruption. He is not a popular figure in our refracted world. Some time ago a very large and fierce black man from the DRC was admitted to the high care unit insisting he was Helen Zille, a recent premier of the province. This was curious because Helen Zille is a middle-aged white woman. It is also surprising that a recent immigrant from central Africa a should have known who the premier is, and that he should have chosen to be her.

Choice is not generally a consideration in psychoses. You don't choose to be psychotic. It is inconceivable. A common theme in psychotic disorders is that one is helpless. Things happen to you over which you have no control. These things are usually bad, and it is unimaginable that such adverse experiences should be willingly sought. I do not think a psychosis is chosen but I do think it is possible that at some level there is a degree of agency in regard to the content of delusions. The choice to be a Mandela, for example, rather than a Zuma I believe is not random. It is not without meaning. These are two political figures who symbolize very different philosophies and moralities. The one features on our ward and the other does not. There are at any one time an array of doctors teachers healers and others who might be considered to have in common a wish to make the world a better place. I think our patients want the world to be safer and kinder, and in their strange and deluded ways they believe that by being who they are they can possibly help themselves. Being a doctor, however mad, puts you in a position to help others and yourself, and that in itself brings hope.

I struggle to recall any patient in our system who believed he was evil, or was in any way at ease with this perception of himself. A young man was admitted to the high care because he was considered to be a high risk of harming himself. He had come to believe that he had killed his family. This caused him great anguish and he insisted that the only way this calamity could end would be for him to be killed in turn. However deeply mired our patients were in their private psychotic worlds, for the most part a discernible theme was evident in their aspiring to help themselves and others, and perhaps to do good. This man believed that he had something that was terribly wrong and he wanted justice to be done, even though that might require his own death.

Thabo was brought to the hospital by the police. He had presented himself at the Houses of Parliament earlier in the day and declared to the bemused security officers that he had come to take over the government which in his mind was corrupt and incompetent. It is not clear why this should lead the conclusion that he was mentally ill, but he was referred to our unit to be assessed. He was not an angry man. He was not violent in any way. Overthrowing the government for him was more of a duty than a self-righteous insurrection. We did not think he was dangerous and he was moved to an open ward. I found him sitting at the fence looking at the birds on the river. He said: "Our time will come. We have to be patient. My army of birds are awaiting my command. Then we will take over the government. My birds are ready. Our time will come". He was calm. He was at peace with himself. He had a plan and he believed it was a just plan. The birds drifted unperturbed in the shallow waters of the river.

At a biological level the experience of psychosis might be imagined as noise. A complex array of interacting factors contribute to this final pathway of disintegration. These might include a number of genetic variants, none of which are sufficient in isolation to precipitate the illness, epigenetic factors and adverse events in early and late childhood. A common precipitating insult in our practice is the abuse of substances, usually cannabis or methamphetamines. These toxic processes appear to disrupt the very precise and complex interplay of neurotransmitters and receptors in the central nervous system, leading to a disorganization of the synchrony of neuronal networks and the experience of madness or mere noise. The delicately embroidered elegantly folded fabrics of the mind are torn apart. The musical notes are scrambled. The complex interaction of forces, the foundations and the buttresses and supporting walls can no longer withstand the storm and the whole apparatus comes crashing down.

In this state all is noise and chaos and devoid of meaning. It is difficult to imagine, our lives are so much made up of light and sound and thoughts and feelings that form meaningful patterns and which help us to make sense of our lives and may grant us pleasure. The patient experiencing a psychotic episode is robbed of these harmonies. We cannot know the mind of another, and certainly not the mind of a psychotic another, but we can imagine that such noise, such a dissolution of meaning would be intolerable. In this context it becomes understandable that a person in such a state should urgently seek to find or construct meanings, and in this process to employ themes that are culturally or spiritually familiar, albeit in very often deeply strange ways given the disorder of mind.

The formation of a delusion might therefore represent the emergence of a struggle for restoration, an attempted reframing of a terrifying and meaningless event into something that might just begin to make sense and restore a degree of control. If this might be so, we need to think very carefully about the ways in which we intervene. The focus of attention would then shift from simply eliminating or suppressing the symptoms of psychosis to reducing the significance or the control these symptoms have over a persons' life and the associated distress.

One critical step in this process is to reimagine the symptom not merely as a sign of a pathological process but an endeavour to find meaning and regain control. This would entail acknowledging rather than dismissing these often bewildering symptoms. I have no idea why this man from the DRC should come to believe that he is the white female premier of the province. I have more of an understanding why the others have become Mandela, but they do share in some way an aspiration of being in power and holding authority. In this respect these delusions can be imagined as strategies to cope with otherwise unbearable feelings of helplessness and hopelessness.

"I need the drones for my mining projects…I will be opening up a number of silicon mines in Brazil…it's no problem…the land is there for the taking…you just take out the silicon and you wash it…it is no problem…"

In a country where ownership of land is a vexed and politically fraught issue this is a pleasant if not facile solution. On the other side of a vast ocean there is land that is simply for the taking. It also contains great riches. It is a fleetingly sustaining fantasy that finds concrete but temporary form in a delusion that is harmless.

Marius and Joan are sitting on a bench in the shade of a pine tree, holding each other's hands in a contented intimacy. They are gazing at the birds on the river. There is a curiously serene and dignified demeanour about them, a stillness that is unusual in psychotic states. She is the Queen of England and he is her rather bewildered Prince. She is the authority and she bears herself with regal grace. Marius is shambolic in appearance and does not seem to be inclined to make much effort in being royal. He just goes along with it, I think for Joan's benefit.

She does not bother too much with this lack of enthusiasm on his part. I think she is grateful for the companionship. They look after each other in their own way. They glide along in their gentle madness with dignity. They are allowed to be who they choose to be. Nobody says to them: 'You are not the queen. You are not a prince. You are just mad old people". They are not mocked. They are treated with some deference. There seems to be a shared belief that nothing is to be gained by taking away their delusions of nobility. It would be merely cruel, and there would be nothing to put in its place.

Simon was admitted after he had assaulted his mother. He worked in an embassy and had come to believe that listening devices had been installed in his office. This belief gradually increased in intensity and shifted to his home. He became convinced that his movements in all the rooms of the house he shared with is mother were being observed, and then that not only his movements but his thoughts were being monitored by some sinister and unknown organization. I think he was trying to explain to his mother that, owing to the nature of his psychotic illness his precarious sense of his self as being private had broken down, and that this understandably angered and frightened him. His poor mother became agitated and intolerant. She had been through this too many times before. She told us she no longer had the patience to listen to his crazy ravings. She said she was exhausted by his recurrent breakdowns and no longer had the reserves to attempt to understand what he was going through.

She told him he was ill and that he needed to be in hospital. Her dismissal of what to him was a terrifying reality had maddened him. It was this refusal to acknowledge his ordeal he said, rather than the invasion of his privacy, that had tipped the balance. In a fury of exasperation he had assaulted her and now he was ashamed of what he had done. If only she had been able to believe him or at least hear him he believed this would not have happened. His mother said she could not understand what he was saying to her. She no longer was willing to try to understand. It was meaningless. It was just this terrible illness and why could he not accept it?

This loss of hope and meaning is also described by those in severe states of depression. Moletsi said to me after he recovered, because in the midst of his illness he was mute: "There was no colour, no light and shade. There was no value to anything. There was nothing to give me direction or purpose. There was no meaning to anything. That was perhaps the worst of it, the loss of meaning, and with it hope".

Whether it is through god or the ancestors or whether it arises from our own needs there is within us all, whether or not we suffer from some form of mental illness, a need to find meaning in our lives, however meaningless that might be in some other implacable order of things.

Epilogue

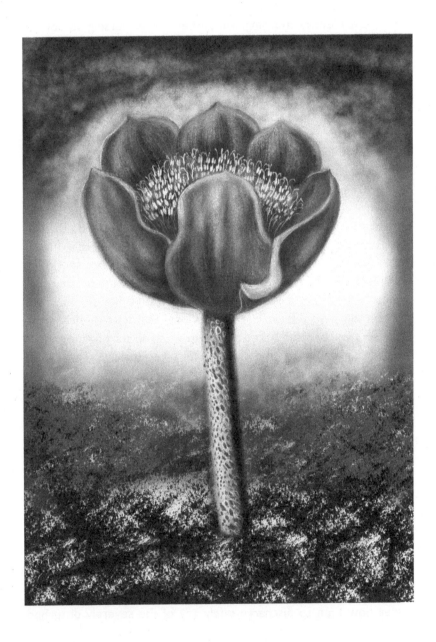

Hope is ephemeral. Hope is elusive. It is fragile. It is without reason. It is something to which we resort when there is no hope.

I am not sure how I would have coped in the hospital for as long as I did without hope.

On Monday morning, we gather in the nursing station to discuss the new admissions. There have been ten over the weekend. Sibusiso is back, having been discharged only six weeks ago. He was well when he left. Then, according to his mother, he stopped the medication after about two weeks and started to use methamphetamines. Despondency descends upon us. What are we doing? What are we hoping to achieve? It seems we are just patching things up. The nursing staff are demoralised. They say they are understaffed and the female members say they don't feel safe at night. All complain that they can't do their jobs properly because they have to fill in too many forms. The social worker is disgruntled. She says she has more important things to do than fill in application forms for disability grants. The occupational therapist says she cannot possibly provide an adequate service as she is on her own covering two wards. She says the nursing staff must help her but they say they cannot because they are occupied with their own duties. The occupational therapist says then the patients will become bored and frustrated and start fighting and it will just make things all the more difficult to manage. There is an awkward and sullen silence.

I receive a call from the bed manager. She is very considerate but there is a plea in the voice. 'Please,' she says, 'there are thirty-five patients now on the waiting list. I am under a lot of pressure. Is there anything you could possibly do?' She is politely asking me to discharge as many patients as soon as possible to create space for at least some of these thirty-five patients. They are being accommodated in the emergency units of hospitals and clinics in the greater urban area. If they need admission to our unit, I know they are causing havoc. They will be harassing the nurses and disrupting emergency procedures and making everybody very angry with psychiatric patients.

'I will do what I can,' I say to the bed manager, having little idea how I am to discharge safely any of the severely disturbed young men currently in our wards.

The clinical psychologist weighs in with an angry contribution. She is disabled and the hospital management has not yet been able to organise the necessary assistance for her. She is extraordinarily determined and resilient, but she says she does not think she will be able to attend these meetings for much longer. There is more silence. Gloom envelops us. I am the nominal leader of this group. I know I need to do something to stop this unhappy mood,-but what that might be is not apparent. Nobody told us at any stage of our training that maintaining morale would be an important part of our responsibilities.

A weary defeatism now looms in the confines of the nursing station. The patients peer anxiously through the partition, as if sensing our predicament. We are on the verge of being confounded by the futility of it all. I become a little bit desperate on occasions like this and absurdly bring cakes to the meetings, as if that could make things better.

I need to instil hope, if not in the expectation that things will get better then at least in that what we are doing, however inadequate, might just be helpful, to some degree, in some way. It is what we need to think, or believe, in order to cope and not become downcast.

Hope is a form of seeking. We seek food and sex and shelter to survive. We need hope to survive.

Frequently, I don't know how families cope. I don't know how Sibusiso's mother manages after he has been admitted yet again, for the same predictable and exasperating reasons. He gets well. He promises to take his medication. He promises to attend the local clinic. He promises not to use the drugs. 'Don't worry,' he laughs, wanting to reassure us, 'I have learnt my lesson. You are not going to see me again in this hospital. Never again! I need to get on with my life.' He has said this, again and again, and now his mother sits in our interview room, gazing balefully at us, angry and disconsolate.

'Why don't you doctors keep him? You know what is going to happen. You know he will come back. He is clever. He knows what to say so that you will release him.' We have been through this before. She knows that we have no option other than to discharge her son. Another oppressive silence ensues. She seems reluctant to leave. 'Tell me, Doctor, is this a lifelong illness? Is this going to go on until I die and then what will happen to him? The people in the community say that there is no cure for this and that he will never get better. Is there any hope?'

'Yes, of course there is. We don't know what the future holds for Sibusiso. Anything is possible. There is always hope.'

Uncertainty is difficult to live with, but it does provide a space for hope, and certainty in this circumstance would be false. 'It is true that there is no cure but that goes for many illnesses, such as heart disease or diabetes, and people learn to live with these problems,' I say. But diabetes is not like schizophrenia. It does not change the way you are. It does not cause you to scream at imagined voices or turn violently against your mother in the belief that she has become a witch.

It is necessary and respectful to be honest, but honesty does not need to foreclose on hope. We need to find some creative balance between acceptance that is not resignation and a hopefulness that is not hopeless. Our patients and their families guide us.

Sibusiso will leave with his mother. They will go back across the river. She will not give up hope. This is what happens in the great majority of such circumstances. There is a profound and inspiring dignity and strength in the resilience that these mothers show. It is mostly the mothers. Perhaps they will have to put some things aside. There will need to be a re-evaluation of priorities and a reconsideration of what is most important in life. It is probable that Sibusiso will not become the man she had once dreamed he might be, but she tells us that will not stop her loving him. He is her son and he will always be her son and she refuses to give up hope.

I don't think Sibusiso has the intention of deceiving us. I do not doubt that he wants to be well and get on with his life. I don't think he has given up hope. He cannot afford to. I hope he will find a direction in his life, and some meaning that will give him purpose, however strange and different that might be. Hope is not fragile or desperate. Hopefully it will provide him with the strength he will need, and we all need.

Beyond hopelessness and reason and madness there is only hope.

Acknowledgements

I want to acknowledge and thank the following who in many different ways have contributed to the development of the ideas expressed in this book, for which in the end I must hold sole responsibility:

Tony Morphet, Ingrid de Kock, Nigel Penn, Sean Kaliski, Sue Hawkridge, John Parker, Penny Busetto, Judy Gathercole, Berit Maxwell, Johan Liebenberg, Lara Foot, Steve Reid, Leslie Swartz, and all my colleagues in the Department of Psychiatry and Mental Health in the Health Sciences Faculty of the University of Cape Town.

I wish to acknowledge and express my gratitude and admiration for the nursing staff and all other staff working at Valkenberg Hospital in Cape Town, who worked with impressive care and dedication and skill in very often difficult circumstances.

I wish to acknowledge and thank Michelle Emerson for her thoughtful and very skilled design of this new publication for The Conrad Press.

I am thankful to Jeremy Boraine of Jonathan Ball Publishers for encouraging me to embark on this project and to Caren van Houwelingen for her supervision of the process and to Angela Voges for her careful attention to the arduous process of editing the text, and especially for her engagement with the themes I have sought to articulate.

I will always be in gratitude to my family Fiona, Anna and Clara who have brought light and beauty into my life and who have throughout continued to sustain and inspire me.

I am in wonder at the illustrations for the text created by Fiona, which vividly and mysteriously express what reaches beyond words.

I wish to acknowledge with great respect my patients and their families with whom I have worked for so many, to me fortunate years, who have prompted me to write this book and to whom it is dedicated.

Sean Baumann

Data Collection Research Methods in Applied Linguistics

Data Collection Research Methods in Applied Linguistics

Heath Rose, Jim McKinley and Jessica Briggs Baffoe-Djan

BLOOMSBURY ACADEMIC
LONDON • NEW YORK • OXFORD • NEW DELHI • SYDNEY

BLOOMSBURY ACADEMIC
Bloomsbury Publishing plc
50 Bedford Square, London, WC1B 3DP, UK
1385 Broadway, New York, NY 10018, USA

BLOOMSBURY, BLOOMSBURY ACADEMIC and the Diana logo
are trademarks of Bloomsbury Publishing Plc

First published in Great Britain 2020

Cover design: Toby Way
Cover image © DavidGoh/Getty Images

A catalogue record for this book is available from the British Library.

A catalog record for this book is available from the Library of Congress.

ISBN: HB: 978-1-3500-2583-7
          PB: 978-1-3500-2584-4
          ePDF: 978-1-3500-2586-8
          eBook: 978-1-3500-2585-1

Series: Research Methods in Linguistics

Typeset by Integra Software Services Pvt. Ltd.
Printed and bound in Great Britain

To find out more about our authors and books visit www.bloomsbury.com
and sign up for our newsletters.

Contents

List of Illustrations

Figure

Tables

Preface

For research in applied linguistics, the successful elicitation and collection of data is a key challenge to obtaining reliable and valid results in a research project. In our review of research books available in our field, we noticed that many textbooks tend to focus on research designs with far less attention paid to the important step of obtaining data. For example, textbooks tend to provide detailed accounts of experimental designs in second language research, but little advice on the tools used within these designs to collect data from participants. Likewise, research methods textbooks might give comprehensive overviews of field research or ethnographic research but little guidance on how to obtain good data when in the field, whether it be via observations, interviews or field notes. Much applied linguistics research is conducted in the field, and therefore, researchers often face innumerable challenges and obstacles in collecting good data. Our book aims to provide guidance in this area by squarely focusing on the things researchers do to obtain data in their research projects.

We have also observed a tendency in research methods books to conflate data collection methods with approaches to research design, which our book aims to remedy. For example, questionnaires (a data collection method) are often discussed interchangeably with survey research (a research design), even though some questionnaires are used for purposes other than 'to survey' and survey methods can utilize more than just questionnaires to collect their data. In some books data elicitation tasks and tests (data collection methods) are listed alongside elements of methodology such as experimental studies (a research design). While we acknowledge that certain data collection techniques often accompany certain research designs, we feel there is a need to uncouple these two dimensions of research to encourage more freedom and creativity in applied linguistics research. Because, in fact, multiple data collection research methods can be (and are) used within a variety of research designs.

One book which does not conflate research design with data collection methods is Brian Paltridge and Aek Phakiti's edited collection, *Research Methods in Applied Linguistics*, published by Bloomsbury Academic. This book consists of thirty-one chapters on various research methods, and research areas, but intentionally does not touch on data collection research methods. Paltridge and Phakiti (2015), therefore, provide a clean overview of designs, within which a multitude of data collection methods can be used by the reader. For this reason, we believe that our book acts as a suitable companion text to this volume by adding this missing dimension to research in applied linguistics research methods. The commendable decision of these editors to not conflate data collection with research designs and topics is one of the reasons why we approached Bloomsbury to publish our textbook, as, together, these two textbooks offer a comprehensive overview of research methods in applied linguistics.

When data collection is discussed in methodology textbooks, there tends to be an overemphasis on interviews and questionnaires as the main qualitative and qualitative methods to collect data in our field. This sends a highly constrained message to novice researchers in terms of the repertoire of techniques available to them as researchers to collect their data. To expand this realm, our book explores frequently used data collection techniques, including, but not limited to, interviews, focus groups, field notes, observations, stimulated recall tasks, corpus building questionnaires, and tests/measures. It also introduces techniques that are widely used in other social science disciplines and are only beginning to make inroads into the mainstream of applied linguistics research, including the use of journals and focus groups.

While the methods outlined in this book will be of interest to all researchers, our target readership consists predominantly of postgraduate students of applied linguistics and language education research (including TESOL), who are being introduced to research methods for the first time. Our aim is to provide a book that will complement the traditional formats of research methods training in postgraduate settings, which are generally organized around abstract notions of design: case studies, ethnographies, surveys, experiments, action research or narrative inquiry. Alternatively, we present research methods in terms of the tangible actions that researchers take to collect data. This perspective should be of primary relevance to novice researchers, who are often highly concerned about obtaining usable data for their projects. Thus, we hope the book will become an essential resource for all applied linguistics researchers and will be used as a valuable textbook for research methods courses worldwide.

Each chapter in this book focuses on one area of data collection, outlining key concepts associated with the method, discussing ways to increase the reliability and validity of data collected, as well as covering the procedures needed for good data collection. Each chapter also showcases several real examples of published research projects where the method was used to collect data. It does this to provide tangible examples to the reader so that they can better understand how these techniques are put into action by experienced researchers. In many cases, we draw on our own published studies – not because we believe they are better than others available but because we have a more intimate understanding of the processes behind the scenes in the data collection phase of the research.

The introductory chapter provides an overview of research methods and data collection. This is intended to act as an abridged version of the content provided in most research methods book by providing an examination of common research designs such as experiments, surveys, case studies, ethnographic research and action research. This information is then used as a platform to discuss how research designs can incorporate multiple data collection techniques and how these techniques are not bounded by particular research methods. This chapter will lay the foundation for a focus on data collection as its own dimension of research methodology.

The next four chapters in the book focus on data collection research methods used to collect data directly from participants. Chapter 2, on data elicitation tasks, provides an overview of the variety of tasks used by researchers to collect data on various language learning processes. Chapter 3 then explores retrospective and introspective tasks as a further way to directly monitor unseen processes of acquisition of language use and language using/learning behaviours. Key challenges explored include issues such as time between the task and data collection, the provision of suitable stimuli, external factors affecting task completion, issues surrounding think-aloud tasks and issues surrounding self-report measures on cognitive processes. Chapter 4 looks at validated tests and measures and explores issues surrounding the construction of valid and reliable measures, as well as issues surrounding the adaptation and use of measures constructed by other researchers for similar research purposes. Chapter 5 looks at observations, contextualizing the data collection research method in a wide array of applied linguistics contexts. Types of observation frameworks are outlined, including time-sampling and event-sampling designs.

The next four chapters explore indirect methods to collect data from participants who self-report on the constructs being investigated. Chapter 6 provides an overview of interviews and interview types and problematizes the way interviews are currently used in much applied linguistics research.

Next, Chapter 7 outlines the use of diaries, journals and logs, differentiating the varied use of this data collection technique by drawing on robust work in the field of psychology. Following this, questionnaires are explored in Chapter 8. While this is a common topic covered in many research methods books – and one of the few data collection instruments that is given emphasis alongside research designs – it is a popular one in our field, and deserving of a chapter in itself. Chapter 9 explores issues surrounding focus groups and outlines the major differences between interviews and focus groups in order to problematize the unreliable way they have been applied to much research in our field thus far.

The next two chapters focus on methods that collect discourse (written and spoken) which are then subjected to various methods of data analysis in our field. Chapter 10 explores the use of documents in research, in that researchers collect these secondary sources upon which to conduct primary research. This chapter explores the use of archive documents (such as newspapers), policy documents, textbooks, online communications (such as websites, blogs and social media comments), but also research documents themselves in the form of systematic reviews. Issues surrounding the identification and selection of documents are discussed in terms of making informed choices to enhance the reliability and validity of data collected. Chapter 11 outlines the collection of discourse in order to build corpora for linguistic analysis, which is a huge area in applied linguistics research. This chapter mostly centres on the issues and procedures surrounding the recording of spoken discourse in real-world settings, although the collection of written discourse is also addressed. While other methods aim to collect data with a specific research question in mind, data for corpora are collected to build a resource that other researchers may draw upon in answering a range of future research questions.

The final chapter concludes our volume and explores macro-perspectives of issues associated with good data collection. It discusses triangulating data collection and offers advice on the realities of data collection, which is inevitably a messy process. It also explores core issues rising to prominence in our field such as a need for replication research and research transparency, which involves making available data collection instruments for researchers use in their projects.

Heath Rose
Jim McKinley
Jessica Briggs Baffoe-Djan

1

An Introduction to Research Methods

Pre-reading activities

Think

Before reading this chapter, make two lists of all the research designs (e.g. experiments, case studies) and data collection methods (e.g. interviews, questionnaires) that you can think of. Consider the differences between a research design and a data collection method.

Discuss

In small groups, or as a class, compile your lists into a master list. Then attempt to further organize these terms into categories based on similarities and differences. Then discuss the following: (1) How difficult is it to organize methods/designs according to a qualitative and quantitative dichotomy? (2) Is there a better way to categorize these methods and designs?

Imagine

Imagine you are conducting a study of second language acquisition during a study abroad programme. Your participants are based in Turkey and are doing a 6-month study abroad in Ireland. You are interested in discovering the language proficiency gains in English in terms of reading, writing, speaking and listening proficiency, plus knowledge gains in vocabulary. Furthermore, you want to understand if learner motivation affects gains. Design a study to research this topic. What data collection instruments might be useful?

Introduction: Why study research methods?

An understanding of research methods is essential for all applied linguistics postgraduate students, novice researchers, as well as practising language teachers. A knowledge of research methods can help students to develop a critical eye when reading research. Research methods training is essential for postgraduate researchers embarking on research for the first time or entering into unfamiliar research domains. An understanding of research methods can also heighten novice researchers' awareness of the repertoire of approaches to research design, data collection and data analysis available to them. An understanding of research methods is also essential for language teachers, who are increasingly encouraged to undertake practitioner-based evaluations of their teaching practices and curriculum innovations. While the aim of such research may not be formal publishing, knowledge of research methods can help inform teachers of the various ways to collect data within educational contexts. Research methods can make classroom-based inquiry more robust, thus giving the findings from such research more clout in terms of impact on practice. Finally, a good grounding in research methods can help people to be more discerning consumers of research in general.

Key terms

In this book, we make an important distinction between research design and data collection methods. While both are part of research methodology, a *research design* refers to the methodological structure of a study, which informs the research approach. Popular research designs include, but are not limited to, surveys, case studies, experiments, action research, field research, corpus research and ethnographies. *Data collection* refers to the actual methods used to gather data for analysis. Popular data collection research methods include, but are not limited to, questionnaires, interviews, focus groups, tests, language elicitation tasks, corpora and observations. Research designs do not dictate how data are collected but rather provide the framework and philosophy within which a researcher collects the data. For example, survey research, which involves the widespread examination of the prevalence of a particular construct within a population, is often paired with questionnaires as a data collection method but could equally make use of data collection techniques such as document analysis, depending on its appropriateness to the topic. Field research, which involves a researcher exploring in-context phenomena, could make use of a combination of data collection methods such as interviews, observations and questionnaires.

Book structure

While the focus of this book is on data collection in applied linguistics research, this opening chapter provides an overview of research designs in order to establish the methodological foundation upon which to discuss the collection of data. Many research methods books tend to focus on design as methodology, neglecting the procedures of collecting the actual data. To fill this gap, the focus of our book is on exploring research methods through the lens of data collection to provide a practical perspective of applied linguistics research. Of course, research designs are important in providing methodological structure to data collection; thus, we first focus on common research designs in this introductory chapter. For a fuller overview of methodology from a research design perspective, readers should consult the resource, *Research Methods in Applied Linguistics* (Paltridge & Phakiti, 2015).

Popular research designs

In this section, we explore research designs that are prevalent in applied linguistics research. Rather than present these designs in the abstract, we do so via an illustrative example of a hypothetical study. This hypothetical study centres around a language education researcher who wants to conduct research into the effects of a new language learning software called Software X on students' learning.

Experimental and quasi-experimental research

Experiments are considered the gold standard of showing causation in research methodology. Indeed, the rigour of experimental designs is often used as a benchmark to evaluate the validity and reliability of other methods.

A true experiment attempts to isolate cause and effect of a 'thing' being manipulated (referred to as the *independent variable*) and the effects of that manipulation on the 'thing' being measured (referred to as the dependent variable). A true experiment aims to measure effect by trying to eliminate alternative explanations of observed relationships between variables. In our software example, the independent variable would be Software X and the dependent variable would be language learning development. It is important to understand that in the social sciences it may be impossible to capture the true dependent variable, which in our case is language development. So a proxy of that variable is needed (such as a language proficiency test), which needs to be appropriately justified as a valid measure of the dependent variable. In intervention studies, an experiment usually embodies a pre-test/post-test design, where the dependent variable is measured before and after the intervention. If time is considered to play an important role, a delayed post-test might also be used to ascertain whether the effects are short term or more sustained.

Essential features of true experiments require: (1) random allocation of participants to experimental conditions and (2) full experimenter control over the independent variables and other *external variables*. Control groups are often used in experimental research to compare the results of a group receiving the experimental condition (in our case Software X) to a group that does not receive it. To avoid confounding variables or factors, the only way to claim that an observed change is due to the independent variable (e.g. Software X) is to make that variable the *only* difference between the experimental groups. External variables in the software example could be anything external to the software that could affect language learning gains, such as participants' aptitude, existing differences in language proficiency, language learning history, motivation, age, teachers and so on. Thus, true experiments often require laboratory-like conditions.

Not only are true experiments difficult to carry out in social science research, they can be seen as problematic in that they may not authentically capture the effects of the independent variable in real-life settings, where external variables are a real part of participants' everyday lives. To remove these variables could also be seen to reduce the ecological validity of a study. Ecological validity refers to the extent at which the control a researcher exerts over a study still remains representative of the real world. Moreover, in educational research, a researcher may not be able to randomly assign participants to groups and may need to settle for roughly matched classes. In these cases, researchers can choose to adopt a quasi-experimental design.

Quasi-experiments are not required to meet the two conditions of a true experiment (random assignment and full experimenter control) but rather try to get as close to them as possible. In quasi-experimental research the control group is often referred to as a comparison group due to ethical issues arising from a design which requires this group to receive no treatment at all. In our software example, rather than receiving no language instruction at all, the comparison group might continue learning the language via the existing methods of teaching. In some quasi-experiments no comparison group is used, especially when it is neither feasible nor ethical to have one. However, researchers must be aware of the limitations of such a design when attributing observed changes to the intervention.

'Before' measures are also a way for researchers to gain control over their experimental condition. For example, a researcher might collect data on students' aptitude, motivation, previous learning experiences and current language knowledge to see whether these initial differences might explain differences between the two groups. In our software example, good before measures would tell a researcher whether the two groups (those that received Software X and those that did not) were comparable in the first place. Good before measures could lead to statistical analysis to measure how much of the difference could be predicted by other variables (e.g. motivation or aptitude) and how much by the software.

If external variables are thought to create too much 'noise' in the data, a researcher could decide to adopt a same-subject design, where the same 'subjects' (people) receive all treatments (e.g. Software X and the regular teaching method). The advantage of a *same-subject design* is that individual differences of participants are the same for each treatment. The disadvantage of same-subject designs is the risk that each treatment may be affected by the subjects' previous experience. That is, the experience of earlier experimental condition (e.g. using the software) could affect the outcome on later encountered conditions (e.g. studying in the usual manner). If treatments can affect or 'leak into' each other in terms of impacting the dependent variable, this is not a good design to use. If same-subject designs are used with multiple interventions or treatments, it is good practice to switch the order of the treatments for some participants (if possible) to counter such effects. Readers who are interested in knowing more about experimental designs in applied linguistics research are encouraged to consult Gass (2015) or Phakiti (2014) for a good overview.

Experimental research can also take the form of other types of design, where variables are manipulated by the researcher to understand their relationships and effects. These types of experiments are explored further in relation to the various tasks and tests used by a researcher to elicit language in order to measure the effect of a manipulation.

Field research

While experiments aim to control for external variables in the study of a construct, *field research*, sometimes referred to as naturalistic research, aims to embrace these variables as an important part of the phenomena under investigation.

> The social and educational world is a messy place, full of contradictions, richness, complexity, connectedness, conjunctions and disjunctions. It is multilayered, and not easily susceptible to the atomization process inherent in much numerical research. It has to be studied in total rather than in fragments if a true understanding is to be reached. (Cohen, Manion & Morrison, 2018: 288)

Naturalistic research, therefore, aims to research the world in its natural setting – thus, embracing the world's 'messy' nature. Field research is an approach to conducting research in the 'real world' and is not an exclusive category of research with strict parameters in itself. As a result, field research can include other approaches to research, such as case studies or ethnographies (discussed later in this chapter).

Field research is sometimes considered the opposing design to classical experimental research, and indeed many elements of field research are positioned as ideologically opposite. While experiments try to control for variables, seeing them as contaminating the design, field research embraces them, seeing them as central to understanding the context under investigation. In our example of researching Software X, field research would be less interested in measuring the effects of the software in terms of language gains measured by proficiency tests (although this could be part of the data it collects) but would be more interested in entering classrooms where the software is being used to understand how teachers and learners are engaging with it to gain a rich understanding of how it is being implemented and received. Field research usually requires flexible uses of multiple data collection methods such as (in our software example) interviews with teachers and students, observations of its use, curriculum documents related to its implementation or the collection of test scores in the observed classes.

Because field research requires direct engagement of the researcher with the research setting, the nature of the researcher's role is an important consideration. This role can generally be placed into five categories on an insider–outsider continuum:

1 Complete participant (e.g. enrolled in the class as an actual student)
2 Participant (e.g. acting in the role of a participant during research)
3 Observer as participant (e.g. working alongside participants during research)
4 Observer (e.g. sitting in the corner of a room, taking notes)
5 Detached observer (e.g. video- or audio-recording the classroom)

The positionality of the researcher during fieldwork has implications for the study design and also how the data should be interpreted later. If a researcher presence is likely to impact the activities being observed, the researcher should try to be as detached as possible. If the events being observed require the researcher to take an active role, then a participant role may be more appropriate. Researcher roles during observation are discussed further in Chapter 7.

Case study research

A case study research design involves the in-depth and contextualized study of the 'particularity and complexity of a single case' (Stake, 1995: xi) or multiple cases. In social science research, cases are primarily people, but in applied linguistics a case can also be positioned as a class, a curriculum, an institution, a speech community, a piece of text or a collection of text types.

Case study research, with its in-depth examination of a single case (or small number of cases), generally falls into three case types:

1 An *intriguing case*, where the peculiarities of the case are the primary focus of research.
2 A *typical case*, where the event is the primary focus, and the case is of secondary importance.
3 A *multiple case*, where the event is the primary focus and multiple perspectives are required to capture variability.

In our Software X example, an intriguing case could include a class where the software was reported to work extremely well; thus, a researcher might be interested in understanding how the software was implemented in this class to understand why it was so successful. Results could then be used to inform future implementation in other contexts. A typical case would be less interested in the peculiarities of the case itself but would rather explore how 'typical' students engage with the software. Multiple case studies increase the scope of a study's findings by exploring multiple perspectives of how students engaged with the software (if students are positioned as cases) or how multiple classes integrated the software (if classes are positioned as cases). In multiple case studies a variety of non-probability sampling techniques can be used. While there is no magic number of how many cases constitute a multiple case study, ideally researchers limit the number of cases to less than twelve in order to deal with the richness of each case appropriately (Miles & Huberman, 1994).

There are a number of advantages to case study research. Results are easily understood by a wide audience, as they are strong in reality and easily relatable. They catch unique features lost in large-scale data collection designs, and these features might be key to understanding the situation. They are also flexible in design and thus are adept at embracing unanticipated events and uncontrolled variables. Case studies also have a number of disadvantages. Their highly contextualized research design means that findings are not generalizable to other situations, unless the reader sees an application. Findings may be highly subjective and selective due to inability to 'cross-check' findings with a target population. They are also prone to problems of observer bias and researcher inference.

To increase the reliability of case study designs, studies need to show a 'chain of evidence' so that an external researcher can track and check each step of the study (Yin, 2009: 41). Detailed descriptions of the methods and analysis also increase the trustworthiness of a researcher's interpretations and thus increase the transparency of the design. As a rule of thumb, the procedures, instrument, context and results need to be written with a 'thick description' (Macpherson et al., 2000: 56) that would enable a replicated study to take place. Readers who are interested in reading more about case study research designs are encouraged to consult the work of Robert Yin (e.g. Yin, 2018), who is one of the world's authorities on case study research. In terms of resources specific to the discipline of applied linguistics research, further detail can be found in Casanave (2015).

Action research

Action research refers to a type of research conducted by practitioners in their own classrooms to trial innovations in teaching practice to improve learning or solve problems. Action research increased in popularity in language teaching research throughout the 1990s. According to Kemmis and McTaggart (1988), who were the early advocates and formulators of action research:

> A distinctive feature of action research is that those affected by planned changes have the primary responsibility for deciding on the course of critically informed action which seem likely to lead to improvement, and for evaluating the results of strategies tried out in practice. Action research is a group activity. (Kemmis & McTaggart, 1988: 6)

However, action research is more than just practitioner research and follows a strict methodological framework.

Action research is conducted in carefully planned cycles of planning, implementation, observation and reflection for further planning. It is usually depicted by cycles of research. In our software example, a teacher might first plan to use the software in class in a manner they see fit (e.g. to see whether it encourages out-of-class autonomous learning), and then they would try to implement the software and observe the effect of the software (e.g. via automatic user logs of software use and progress, and weekly questionnaires with students). The teacher would then analyse and reflect on these data to inform future plans to improve use of the software. For example, if students were not using the software as much as hypothesized, the teacher might tweak activities to incentivize its use. This then leads to the second cycle of action research, where the amended format is then implemented, observed and reflected upon.

Action research carries with it a number of advantages. It is ideal for problem-solving in real situations and is perhaps one of the few approaches that are strong for evaluating the impact of teaching methods, curriculum innovation and policy implementation. As the design sees the researcher's 'insider' status as a strength rather than a limitation, it is an ideal method for practitioner-researchers. Similar to case study research (as in essence the researcher's own classroom is like a single case), a disadvantage of the design is that it is highly contextualized, meaning that findings are not generalizable to other situations.

Reliability of findings can also be an issue as, unlike quasi-experiments, it is difficult to eliminate factors external to the interventions that may have influenced the result. As action research is usually driven by a teacher's desire to initiate change, and often tests innovations teachers believe might work, it is difficult for some researchers to maintain unbiased objectivity in their interpretations of the data. Action research is inherently messy as the teacher and students are participants in the research in real-life settings where numerous factors interplay with the innovations being trailed. However, messiness need not be interpreted as a lack of rigour, as Cook (2009: 290) argues:

> If an indicator of our successful work as action researchers is the integration of the development of practice with the construction of research knowledge, then we must provide honest accounts of that process and incorporate mess as an integral part of a rigorous approach.

Thus, like case study research, a thick and honest description of the processes of action research is needed to enhance exactitude of the results. Rich in reality, action research's embracement of the social world's messiness should be seen as a strength of the design, rather than a weakness. To understand more about action research designs within the field of applied linguistics, good overviews can be found in Borg (2015) and Banegas and Consoli (2020).

Ethnographic research

Ethnographic research positions the participants (and its communities and cultures) as the primary focus of investigation. Ethnographies can entail both descriptive and analytical explanations of participants' behaviours, values, beliefs and practices. As ethnographies involve the study of people within their natural contexts, there is understandable overlap between ethnographic designs and field research designs, except it is the person rather than the context that is being researched.

There is also a natural overlap with case study design, except with subtle differences. In our software example, an ethnographic study would include the study of participants' behaviours, beliefs and practices surrounding the introduction of the new software into their learning environment. Rather than measuring the impact of the software on learning within a case context, an ethnographic study would be more interested in the impact of the software on the learners themselves.

A subcategory of ethnography, which is gaining in popularity in applied linguistics research, is autoethnography. Autoethnographies 'draw together features of autobiography and ethnography' (Paltridge, 2014: 100), and the research design allows the researcher to report on their own lived experiences in relation to the phenomenon being studied. For example, an autoethnography might include a researcher reporting on their experiences learning a language (see Casanave, 2012), or in our software example, using Software X as a teacher or learner.

When presented as a 'joint autoethnography', two or more authors can discuss shared lived experiences to create new meaning by offering different perspectives. This type of autoethnography is also referred to as a *duoethnography*, which is the study of 'how two or more individuals give similar and different meanings to a common phenomenon' (Norris, 2017: 2). Examples of joint autoethnographies include Adamson and Muller's (2018) self-exploration of their academic identities of teacher-researchers and Rose and Montakantiwong's (2018) lived experiences of teaching English as an international language in Japan and Thailand. Outside applied linguistics, autoethnographies are flexible in the methods they use to present data, often including such fictional-style writing as poetry and prose (Ellis & Bochner, 2000); within applied linguistics, they tend to be more conservative following traditional methods of qualitative data presentation according to emergent themes.

A further subtype of ethnography is *critical ethnography*. Critical ethnography takes a subversive worldview by challenging the beliefs and practices observed within ethnographic research with the aim to explore what these beliefs and practices *could* or *should* be (see Thomas, 1993). Critical ethnography is often linked to theories from other disciplines in the humanities and social sciences such as queer theory, race theory or feminist theory to explore power relationships among the people being studied (Cohen, Manion & Morrison, 2018). In applied linguistics, critical ethnography is often conducted via *critical discourse analysis*, which explores the power relationship between people or communities of people represented in the language used by and about them.

Survey research

Survey research involves the widespread exploration of a topic within a target population. Survey research generally aims for representativeness in its findings and also to cross-sectionally explore differences in segments of the population according to key variables. Census data are the ultimate example of survey research, where huge financial and human resources are placed in mapping the population of a country with an attempt at collecting data from a near-total sample of people within the target population.

In research, surveys try to be as representative as possible of the population being studied and aim to collect a large enough sample to reduce the margin of error. If large numbers of respondents cannot be obtained, researchers ideally apply a probability-based sampling technique to gather data from participants in the target population to minimize bias in the data. For an overview of survey research in applied linguistics, see Wagner (2015).

Corpus and document research

Corpus and *document research* involve the analysis of language and content within a collection of texts (written, spoken or multimodal). The design phase of the method typically involves the assemblage of a suitable body of texts. When a large number of texts are collected and compiled via a systematic method, the result is usually referred to as a corpus. Corpora are intended to be representative of language used in a particular genre and are generally used to analyse language. When texts are collected for the purpose of analysing content (rather than analysing linguistic features in *text analysis*), this is usually referred to as document research. There are many subcategories of document research including policy research in the case of the collection of language-related policy and planning documentation, or textbook analysis in the case of materials evaluation.

The data collection phase of document or corpus research typically involves the extraction of suitable materials for analysis. In the case of document research, this may involve extracting relevant elements from the larger sample for qualitative analysis (discussed further in Chapter 10). In the case of corpus research, this could include tagging the corpus for its linguistic features for further analysis (discussed further in Chapter 11).

Data collection research methods

Unlike the research methods outlined above, which inform the design and structure of a study, data collection research methods refer to the ways in which data are collected within such designs. Some research designs lend themselves to certain data collection research methods – for example, experimental designs often collect data via tests; survey designs often collect data via questionnaires, and ethnographic designs are likely to include interviews. In reality, however, data collection methods can be used within almost any design, creating multiple possible combinations for a creative, innovative researcher seeking to provide original contributions to knowledge in the field. For example, an ethnographic research design might involve collecting data from participants via tests and questionnaires, or a survey might collect data via oral interviews. As an example, the landmark *Kinsey Reports* (Kinsey, Pomeroy & Martin, 1948, 1953), which were large-scale surveys of human sexual behaviour in the United States, collected data from in-depth, face-to-face interviews with 5,300 males and 5,940 females, respectively.

Data collection methods available to social science researchers are so numerous it is impossible to cover all of them in a single volume; thus, this book aims to cover the most commonly used methods within applied linguistics research, plus others which are increasing in popular use in the field. These include:

- interviews, which are useful to capture the experiences, thoughts and behaviours as reported directly by the participants themselves (covered in Chapter 6);
- focus groups, which are useful to capture group consensus of target populations on surrounding issues under investigation (covered in Chapter 9);
- questionnaires, which are useful for collecting data from large populations (covered in Chapter 8);
- diaries, journals and logs for capturing life as it is lived by participants when the researcher is not present (covered in Chapter 7);
- observations, which provide first-hand collection of events and contexts being investigated (covered in Chapter 4);
- introspective and retrospective tasks (including stimulated recall and think-aloud protocols), which can provide insight into participants' thoughts and behaviours (covered in Chapter 3);
- tests and validated measures, which aim to provide objective measures of a construct (covered in Chapter 5);
- document data collection, which includes a range of techniques to collect data from written documents as varied as graffiti, students' essays or language-related policy (covered in Chapter 10);
- corpus analysis, which includes the collection of written and/or spoken data into large banks of texts for linguistic analysis (covered in Chapter 11);
- language elicitation tasks, which involve any activity designed to have students produce language or indicators of language processing for the purpose of analysis (covered in Chapter 2).

Qualitative, quantitative and mixed methods designs

Qualitative versus quantitative research

Perhaps the most oft-discussed dimension of social research is the qualitative and quantitative divide; however, this divide is not as distinct as some research methodologists indicate. Creswell (1994: 1–2) sees the divide as a methodological one, describing quantitative research as 'an inquiry into a social or human problem, based on testing a theory composed of variables, measured with numbers, and analyzed with statistical procedures' and qualitative research as 'an inquiry process of understanding a social or human problem, based on building a complex, holistic picture, formed with words, reporting detailed views of informants, and conducted in a natural setting'. Such descriptions seem to suggest that experimental designs, with their testing of theories composed of variables, are part of the quantitative research paradigm, and naturalistic field research, with its holistic examination of real-world settings, is part of the qualitative research paradigm.

However, the simplistic nature of this distinction soon rings untrue for research designs that collect data in the form of words in experimental research and in the form of numbers during naturalistic field research. It further rings untrue for data analysis techniques that perform complex statistical analysis of data in the form of words (which is true for many corpus linguistic studies) or qualitative analysis of data in the form of numbers, such as the profiling of data to reveal participant case profiles as is the case in Latent Case Analysis and Latent Profile Analysis. If we return to the *Kinsey Reports* examples mentioned above, the reports consist mostly of statistical analysis of key demographic variables within the population, despite a data set that was originally composed of interviews. In such cases, it seems more useful to adopt Bryman's (2016) position that quantitative and qualitative methods are approaches to data analysis, rather than divisions of research design or data collection. Within this view, the *Kinsey Reports*, while qualitative in data collection (interview based), are examples of quantitative research because of their approach to the analysis of the data.

If we accept all of the varying views of the divide between qualitative and quantitative research, there are three levels of the qualitative–quantitative dimension in research and eight possible combinations (although some are more feasible than others).

Mixed methods research

Mixed methods designs blur the lines between qualitative and quantitative research. Onwuegbuzie and Leech (2005) have argued that historically social science researchers have focused on the differences between the two categories, rather than the similarities, concluding that all graduate students need to be open to both types of research to develop as pragmatic researchers (i.e. those who have the methodological knowledge to combine methods to answer any given research question). Mixed methods research, however, involves more than just piecing together a 'quantitative' design (e.g. surveys) and a 'qualitative' data collection method (e.g. interviews). As Table 1.1 shows, the mixing of methods can occur at any stage of research: from epistemological stance of the research design, data collection or data analysis (Johnson, Onwuegbuzie & Turner, 2007). In this book we explore mixed methods research from a data collection perspective.

Mixed methods designs at the data collection stage often take two forms: those that apply complementary methods concurrently (e.g. QUAN + QUAL) and those that apply complementary designs sequentially (e.g. QUAN → QUAL). For example, in a QUAL + QUAN study exploring vocabulary gains during study abroad, a researcher might concurrently give participants a writing task (for qualitative analysis of productive vocabulary) as well as a vocabulary test (to quantitatively measure vocabulary knowledge). For other studies, a researcher might decide to adopt a sequential mixed methods design, where one phase of research leads into the next. For example, a QUAL → QUAN study on language attitudes might conduct focus groups with learners to generate qualitative data, which are then used to create items on an attitudinal questionnaire to be used in a second stage of research.

Table 1.1 Levels of qualitative and quantitative research

Level	Qualitative	Quantitative
Research design	Building a complex, holistic picture of the research construct (e.g. case studies, naturalistic field research)	Theory-testing, composed of variables related to the research construct (e.g. experiments, surveys)
Data collection	Consisting of words	Consisting of numbers
Data analysis	Analysis of content, themes and language (e.g. qualitative text analysis, conversation analysis)	Statistical analysis of numbers (e.g. analysis of variance, correlation, regression)

Hashemi and Babaii (2013) have noted that in applied linguistics research, concurrent designs for the purposes of data triangulation are most prevalent. They also argue that few studies in applied linguistics have achieved high degrees of integration of mixed methods approaches.

In some mixed methods research, one type of research might be prioritized over the other. In this chapter, we represent this design via use of upper- and lower case letters – a technique used elsewhere (e.g. Creswell & Plano Clark, 2011) to indicate one method is subordinate to another. For example, in a QUAN + qual mixed methods survey, a researcher might deploy a questionnaire with a large sample of participants, accompanied by an interview with a much smaller subset of the respondents to add depth to their data (N.B. even though interviews occur after the questionnaire, this is not a sequential design because the questionnaire data are not used to inform the design of the interviews). In a QUAL + quan in-depth case study of foreign language learning anxiety, a researcher might concurrently collect data from participants via learner journals and a questionnaire, prioritizing the journal data due to it being more suited to the case study approach.

Example case studies in applied linguistics

This section showcases a range of studies that utilize a variety of research methods to provide real-world examples of research designs in practice. In this table, we have highlighted some of our own studies, as these are research designs with which we are most intimately familiar – a practice we continue throughout the book when available. These studies are outlined in Table 1.2.

Briggs' (2015) study of 261 learners of English explored the relationship between out-of-class language contact and vocabulary gain in a study abroad context. Briggs collected data via a vocabulary test at the beginning and end of the study abroad period in addition to a language contact questionnaire towards the middle of their stay. Although this study appears to be quasi-experimental in its collection of data at two time points, the study adopts a survey design. Like most survey designs, it aims to generalize its findings to the wider study abroad experiences of students. Also, like most survey designs, it aims to cross-

Table 1.2 Examples of various methods in applied linguistics research

Study	Topic	Participants/Data source	Research design	Approach	Data collection methods
Briggs (2015)	Vocabulary gain during study abroad	Adult, mixed-L1 study abroad learners of English (n = 241)	Survey (with some quasi-experimental elements)	QUAN + QUAN	Two questionnaires at two time points
McKinley (2017a)	Writer identity in argumentative EFL writing	Students (n = 16) and teachers (n = 4) in a university in Japan	Field research with ethnographic elements	QUAL (Qual) + QUAL	Interviews (based on observations); text analysis
Rose (2013)	Mnemonic strategies for learning written Japanese	University-aged learners of Japanese (n = 12)	Case study	QUAL (Qual) + Quan	Interviews (embedded with stimulated recall); questionnaire
Galloway and Rose (2014, 2018)	Teaching Global Englishes to language students	University-aged English language learners in Japan (n = 108)	Action research	(QUAL + QUAL) → QUAL	Interviews, learner journals, written reflections
McKinley and Rose (2018)	Native speaker bias in academic journal author guidelines	Journal guideline documents (n = 210)	Document research	QUAL (quan)	Content analysis (with embedded corpus analysis)

sectionally explore variables within the data such as the study abroad location and the length of stay, even though it also contains a longitudinal element to measure vocabulary gain.

Galloway and Rose (2014, 2018) showcase two cycles of an action research project which aimed to raise awareness of Global Englishes within English language classes at a Japanese university. They collected data via listening journals and interviews, as well as written reflections after a presentation task. Together these studies demonstrate the flexibility of an action research design, as well as an openness to collect different types of data to measure the effects of a classroom intervention. A further cycle of this project, which involved a debate activity, is reported in Rose and Galloway (2017).

McKinley (2017a) investigated the construction of writer identity in English academic writing by Japanese university students in Japan. This study is a typical example of field research as the researcher had to work within the context of his study over a year-long period to collect students' written texts and curricula documents and conduct monthly student and teacher interviews and classroom observations. A total of sixteen students and their four teachers participated in the study, and the contextualized approach allowed in-depth analysis of how learners' identities were shaped by their learning experiences. As the learners were foregrounded in much of the data presentation, this study could also be considered to adopt an ethnographic design.

McKinley and Rose (2018) is an example of a study which uses documents as a source of research. Their study involved the analysis of academic journals' author guidelines to explore bias towards native forms of English, thereby prejudicing nonnative writers. In total 210 guidelines were collected, and qualitative text analysis (see Kuckartz, 2014) was conducted to categorize the guidelines according to their rigidity or flexibility towards nonstandard forms of English. Embedded within this design was a small quantitative element to the study, where corpus tools were applied to examine keywords within the guidelines.

Rose (2013) is an example of a case study consisting of twelve learners of Japanese at universities in Japan. The study explored the mnemonic strategies deployed by learners to memorize Japanese written characters called *kanji*. The main data collection instrument was interviews, which had a stimulated recall component embedded within them. Data were also collected via questionnaires, but data were used only as stimulus for discussion, rather than for statistical analysis, and this aspect of study is represented in lower case letters (quan) in Table 1.2.

Implications for researchers

Choosing a research design

While research methods tend to be presented to novice researchers as neatly packaged designs that can be applied to any suitable research topic, they are in fact flexible in nature. For example, ethnographic field research can also be a case study, in the example of exploring the experiences of a select number of participants in the field. Surveys can also be document research in the example of a survey of language requirements set out in admissions policies in universities in a particular region. As designs are malleable, they should be considered a framework within which to position all methodological decisions made when constructing a study. A creative researcher can adapt certain elements of a design if a logical argument can be made to do so.

Research designs are also fallible even when perfectly implemented. As Rose and McKinley (2017: 3) have noted, 'There are innumerable ways in which a research design faces obstacles in the research process, no matter how carefully a project was planned.' An important takeaway from this introductory chapter is to understand that a research design is only an idealized blueprint; it informs a researcher's approach to data collection, rather than dictating it.

Choosing a research approach

It is important that novice researchers are not caught in the crossfire of the qualitative and quantitative 'paradigm wars' (Gage, 1989) and understand that the divide is a lot more complicated than it first appears. Indeed, in this chapter we have only scratched the surface of the various combinations of mixed methods designs. Hashemi and Babaii's (2013) investigation of mixed methods designs in 205 applied linguistics articles revealed an array of complicated designs, such as those represented as follows:

- QUAL → QUAN + (QUAN → QUAL)
- (QUAL + QUAN) → (QUAN + QUAL)
- (QUAN + QUAL) → QUAL

In Table 1.2 we have also attempted to capture the complexities of our own research studies in terms of their integration of methods to answer a research question.

We concur with Onwuegbuzie and Leech (2005) that postgraduate researchers need to understand the benefits of both quantitative, qualitative and mixed methods designs to make informed decisions of the best possible approach to answer their own questions. Based on this knowledge, researchers then need to choose methodology according to the 'right reasons', such as that the chosen design yields the most appropriate data for the research questions. The 'wrong reasons' for choosing a design include the following:

- Choosing a quantitative design because they are worried that qualitative research is not as highly valued by examiners, reviewers or their peers (this is simply not the case)
- Choosing a qualitative design because they fear statistical analysis (quantitative data analysis can be no less time-consuming and difficult than qualitative analysis)
- Choosing a qualitative design because they are worried that a quantitative design might end up with a null result (a finding of no significance is still an important finding in itself)
- Choosing a mixed methods design because they believe it is the only way to achieve data triangulation (triangulation is easily achieved in QUAN + QUAN or QUAL + QUAL designs)

In short, for the creative researcher, there are vast opportunities to integrate a variety of data collection methods within a research design, so long as the design logically fits the research questions of the study, and researchers are able to cogently communicate their rationale for adopting the design.

Choosing a data collection research method: The purpose of this book

This opening chapter has focused on the fundamentals of research design, as too do other research methods books written for applied linguistics (e.g. Dörnyei, 2007; Paltridge & Phakiti, 2015). For research in applied linguistics, the successful elicitation and collection of data is a key challenge to obtaining reliable and valid data for analysis. As much applied linguistics research is conducted in the field, researchers can often face extra obstacles in collecting good data. The remainder of this book, therefore, turns to the topic of data collection in its exploration of frequently used data collection research methods.

Each subsequent chapter focuses on one area of data collection, outlining key concepts, procedures and practical concerns for good data elicitation. Each chapter also showcases a handful of model research projects where the data collection techniques have been used to collect data in a successfully completed study. In our experience as doctoral and masters research supervisors, we find that data *collection* research methods tend to be more tangible to novice researchers, rather than the abstractness of research designs and approaches. Thus, in organizing the remainder of our book around the methods to collect the data, we hope to provide the reader with a more perceptible roadmap to conducting research successfully in applied linguistics.

Post-reading activities

Reflect
Reflect on the three levels where qualitative and quantitative approaches can be delineated within a research project (Table 1.1). Thinking of the Software X example, where you want to conduct a study exploring the effects of a new language software on language learning in a Year 8 French classroom, think of ways that a mixed methods approach could be achieved at each level.

Expand
Locate one published study that is in your area of research interest. As was done in Table 1.2, provide a summary of the study topic, participants, design, approach and data collection methods. Provide an evaluation of how the study adhered to (or deviated from) *typical* descriptions of the study design in methodological literature. To conduct this evaluation, you may need to refer to the descriptions and further readings outlined in the section 'Popular research designs'.

Apply
Return to the hypothetical study in the pre-reading activity of this chapter. Drawing on the concepts in this study, as well as on additional research related to the topic of language gain, motivation and study abroad, map out a suitable design for a study.

Resources for further reading

Paltridge, B., & Phakiti, A. (2015). *Research methods in applied linguistics.* London: Bloomsbury.

This book is a comprehensive resource of research methods in applied linguistics. It consists of thirty-one chapters on various research methods and research areas. The book is broken into two parts. The first part outlines research designs including experimental research, narrative inquiry, case study research and action research. The second part of the book outlines broad subfields of applied linguistics research including writing, language learner strategies, speaking, motivation and teacher beliefs. Each chapter follows a similar structure of embedding a real example of applied linguistics research within the chapter to act as a case study for the research method or research area. Unlike many other research methods books, this publication does not conflate methods with data collection. For this reason, we believe that the Paltridge and Phakiti edited volume is the best supplement to this book for a full coverage of research design and data collection methods. Together, these volumes offer a comprehensive overview of research in applied linguistics.

Dörnyei, Z. (2007). *Research methods in applied linguistics.* Oxford University Press.

This book is a highly accessible text on the topic of research methods in applied linguistics, covering the basics of research methodology. As an introductory text, it provides an excellent overview of common research designs; however, this coverage does not extend to providing extensive examples or explanations of data collection instruments, which are relegated to just two of its chapters. Dörnyei's book is probably one of the best starting points for novice researchers who are embarking on their very first research project.

2

Data Elicitation Tasks

Pre-reading activities

Think
Before reading this chapter, think about your answers to the following questions: How might researchers and/or teachers probe how language knowledge is processed and stored in learners' minds? How might we find out what learners can do with their linguistic knowledge?

Discuss
In small groups, or as a class, discuss the following: (1) For what reason might researchers devise specific tasks to elicit data from learners, rather than observing them using the language in naturalistic conditions? (2) What does production data tell us about learners' competence in a language? What does it not tell us? (3) To what extent might the methods we use to elicit language production (i.e. learners' speaking or writing) affect the data yielded by them?

Imagine
Imagine you are designing a longitudinal study that aims to investigate the development of pragmalinguistic competence – specifically, mitigation of requests (e.g. 'I was wondering if I might chair today's meeting?') – among L2-English economic migrants to the UK. You would like to measure development in your sample's ability to mitigate workplace requests over their first 3 months in UK-based employment. Devise a data collection plan to collect these kinds of data and pay attention to the following questions: How many data collection tools might you need in order to be confident that your data are a comprehensive portrayal of your participants'

workplace request mitigation competence? To what extent might features of your data collection methodology influence the type and quality of data you collect? How time-consuming (for you and/or your participants) might your data collection methodology be? Can you think of any other methodological issues that might arise?

Introduction

Elicitation of linguistic knowledge forms the basis of much of the data collection methodology in second language research today. In the early literature, scholars tended more towards naturalistic observation of their participants: for example, in the case of child second language learning, studies often comprised longitudinal case study observation of children playing with their parents or the researchers (e.g. Paradis & Genesee, 1996; Swain & Wesche, 1973), and some adult-focused studies similarly focused on purely naturally occurring production data (e.g. Poplack, Wheeler & Westwood, 1989). However, as time has passed, scholars have tended to introduce more control to the elicitation of their participants' second language. Notwithstanding the labour-intensive nature of transcribing multiple observation sessions, this is primarily because in naturalistic data it is common for some linguistic structures or functions to appear infrequently (if at all) and such under representation cannot confidently be interpreted. Likewise, naturalistic data do not easily facilitate concrete judgements about participants' comprehension and/or processing of language.

In response to the limitations of naturalistic data collection research methods, data elicitation tasks have been widely employed in second language research. Such tasks provide the researcher greater control over what is elicited from their participants, thereby reducing some of the ambiguity of naturalistic data as outlined above. Some elicitation tasks resemble naturalistic settings in that the level of researcher control is relatively low and the tasks are highly contextualized (e.g. role plays); whereas others are very highly controlled, experimental in nature and wholly decontextualized (e.g. semantic categorization tasks). Therefore, data elicitation tasks encompass a broad spectrum of data collection methods and techniques and, concordantly, yield a very wide spectrum of data types – from long transcriptions of meaning-based spoken L2 production to response times measured by the millisecond. Considered together, however, good use of data elicitation tasks in applied linguistics research allows the researcher to draw inferences about language knowledge, ability, storage and/or processing beyond the task environment and in a focused, comparatively time-efficient manner; bad use of elicitation tasks can yield little data and/or data with lamentable ecological validity (i.e. correspondence to the real world).

In this chapter we focus on language production tasks and experimental elicitation tasks as two of the primary ways in which applied linguists can probe participants' knowledge, storage and processing of language. Each of these task types is outlined and discussed below, followed by a discussion of the procedures and practicalities inherent in their use in empirical research.

Language production tasks

A wide range of language production tasks have been developed by applied linguists interested in researching specific aspects of language knowledge and ability. Comprehensive lists of language production tasks can be found in Doughty and Long (2000) and Chaudron (2003): here we focus on four of the most common in the applied linguistics literature, described below in order from the most highly controlled and decontextualized to the least controlled and most contextualized.

Discourse completion

Discourse completion tasks (DCTs) present respondents with a situation and/ or prompt to which they respond in oral, written or cloze form. DCTs have most commonly been used in second language research to probe learners' *pragmatic competence*, particularly as regards specific *speech acts* such as requesting, complaining or apologizing (e.g. Schauer & Adolphs, 2006). DCTs are useful data collection tools because they allow the researcher to manipulate not only language but also highly specific features in the situation or prompt relating to power relations, social distance or imposition (Brown & Levinson, 1987). For example, focusing on the speech act of requesting, a DCT can be modified to reveal whether a change in power dynamic between interlocutors (e.g. student → student vs. student → professor) leads to changes in how the speech act is formulated. One drawback to this level of control is that DCTs limit the respondent's capability to demonstrate the full range of his/her pragmatic competence.

DCT data can be coded by speech act strategy (e.g. Cohen, 2010) in terms of five key criteria: (1) the ability to use the correct speech act, (2) the typicality of the expressions used, (3) the appropriateness of the amount of speech or amount of information provided, (4) the level of formality and (5) the level of politeness (Cohen, 2004). One of the key criticisms of DCTs relates to the huge variation in their design (Sweeney & Zhu Hua, 2016), which makes it difficult to compare studies' findings at the macro level. One good resource for DCT design is Hudson, Detmer and Brown (1995), who recommend that situations and prompts should be as authentic and unambiguous as possible.

Role play

A staple of communicative second language classrooms the world over, *role plays* are another useful task for eliciting data on pragmalinguistic competence among L2 learners. Role plays constitute an interactive (usually dyadic) task in which interlocutors are assigned a role and tasked with interacting on a given topic within a defined situation. Dyads may comprise participant–participant or participant–researcher pairs. Role plays have been found to yield similar data to DCTs in terms of the speech act strategies employed (e.g. Sasaki, 1998); however, role plays produce a greater amount of data and enable the participant to display a broad range of interactional pragmatic competence, including topic management and turn-taking (Kormos, 1999). Similar to the design of DCTs, roles and situations in role play tasks should be clearly defined and correspond to real-world discourse.

Storytelling

Storytelling is an incredibly useful means of eliciting production data from a sample. Preselected stories can be presented to participants in picture form, for example Lennon's (1990) use of the International Picture Stories (Timms & Eccott, 1972) to study the indicators of perceived fluency. With *video stimuli*, participants may either retell the story after watching (e.g. Towell, Hawkins and Bazergui's (1996) use of the cartoon 'Balablok' to explore longitudinal development on temporal measures of fluency) or simultaneously narrate while watching for a more 'on-line' elicitation, such as Gass et al.'s (1999) use of vignettes from 'Mr. Bean'. Alternatively, *story stems* may be presented to participants orally or in written form, and the respondent tasked with completing the story (in oral or written form) (e.g. Philp, 2003). The primary benefit of using story(re)telling as a data elicitation task is that the researcher knows and has control over the sequence of events in the story, thus enabling relatively straightforward comparison of data across participants. However, the longer the stimulus, the more likely it is that certain events will be omitted from participants' retelling, and – regardless of the stimulus length – wide variation in token count (i.e. the number of words produced by different individuals) should be expected.

Oral proficiency interviews

The *oral proficiency interview* (OPI) is a standardized measure of L2 speaking ability usually comprising of a 20–30-minute guided conversation between test-taker and examiner that is designed to elicit oral proficiency. OPIs usually elicit both monologic and dialogic speech and commonly follow a three-part format that includes picture description, sustained speech and conversation. The predominant US-based OPI is the American Council of Teachers of Foreign Languages OPI. UK-derived equivalents include the speaking components of the Cambridge ESOL examinations (including IELTS). In some cases, *simulated OPIs* are employed, wherein the examiner is replaced by computer-based prompts and the test-taker delivers his/her task responses to a microphone.

OPIs are a widely used task to elicit spoken production data in the applied linguistics literature: for example, in a study of the relationship between phonological memory and learners' oral production, O'Brien et al. (2006) administered an OPI to adult L1-English learners of L2-Spanish at the beginning and end of an academic semester, between which the sample was either taking Spanish classes at a US university or was studying abroad in Spain. The data were analysed to yield measures of productive vocabulary, narrative ability, accuracy, fifteen elements of inflectional morphology (e.g. affixation, vowel change) and use of subordinate and coordinate clauses. As stated by Chaudron (2003), because OPIs combine the use of a number of commonly employed oral data production tasks, they themselves can be considered a legitimate data collection research method. However, criticisms of OPIs arise in relation to the power imbalance between examiner and examinee (possibly resulting in suboptimal oral performance) and the extent to which the reliability of the method depends on the consistency and conduct of the examiner (e.g. Bachman, 1990; Lazaraton, 1996).

There are a number of advantages to using language production tasks in research. The obvious main advantage, relative to collecting naturally occurring data, is that the researcher can manipulate the task such that certain productions are elicited. More relevant data can be collected from a larger number of participants in a given data collection period. Second, given that production task instructions and materials can be presented to participants in the L1 or in non-linguistic format (e.g. pictures, cartoons, videos), many language production tasks can be used with respondents of any L2 proficiency level, thereby making them a useful means of comparing participants grouped by proficiency on task performance. Concordantly, if a researcher is focusing on a population of language users at a particular proficiency level, production tasks can be devised to target the specific developmental stage of the sample by eliciting a target feature that they are in the process of acquiring. Furthermore, because the task is designed to elicit specific linguistic features and the scope of the language production is controlled, production task data are comparatively straightforward to transcribe and analyse (but see 'Procedures and practicalities' below for issues of reliability in transcription and coding protocols). Finally, language production task data, depending on the extent of authenticity and contextualization of the task, can be a window into real-world ability in a given situation or genre.

In terms of drawbacks, one key issue with using language production tasks is that even in the most carefully designed task, participants may avoid using the target linguistic feature or indeed producing much language at all, leaving the researcher with a paucity of data with which to attempt to address their study's research questions. This is a particular danger when eliciting production data from populations of younger learners, for whom adjustments should be made where possible in order to simplify cognitive or motor task demands and to promote task engagement. Furthermore, individual and group differences such as culture, personality or foreign language anxiety may mean that some respondents do not conform to task demands or respond to the task in a predictable way.

Experimental elicitation tasks

Experimental elicitation tasks are necessarily more controlled and decontextualized than language production tasks because they seek to isolate perception or processing phenomena at the micro level. Here we discuss three elicitation tasks that are commonly used in the applied linguistics literature to scrutinize the processing of lexical and grammatical input.

Lexical decision

Lexical decision tasks (LDTs) are a type of yes/no identification task that are used in psycholinguistic research as a means of probing how lexical items are organized and processed in the mind (i.e. for research into the mental lexicon), thereby providing key insights into how language is learned and stored. LDTs require respondents to quickly decide whether a target string of letters on a computer screen is a real word or a *pseudoword* (sometimes termed *nonsense words, non-words* or '*nonce*' words). Different types of LDTs have been categorized in different ways. For example, Jones and Estes (2012) distinguish three types:

1 *Continuous LDTs*, whereby two lexical strings are presented simultaneously and the participant responds to each string separately.
2 *Standard LDTs*, in which two strings are presented consecutively (i.e. the first string is presented and then removed before the second string is presented) and the participant responds only to the second string, denoting that the first string functions as a *prime* and the second string is the *target* word.
3 *Double LDTs*, whereby two strings are presented simultaneously and the participant makes one single response to them both.

LDTs can further be categorized by the means with which the lexical strings are presented to the respondent: aurally, visually or both (Jiang, 2012).

LDT data are commonly analysed for *response times* (also termed *reaction times* or *response latency*) and *error rate*, meaning that they yield information on the speed and accuracy with which respondents can identify real and pseudowords. One early example of the use of LDTs is that of Meyer and Schvaneveldt (1971), who developed a double LDT in which pairs of words that were either (1) real + real-related (e.g. 'DOCTOR' 'NURSE'), (2) real + real-unrelated (e.g. 'DOCTOR' 'TREE'), or (3) real + pseudoword (e.g. 'DOCTOR' 'PLAME') were presented to respondents in the form of photographs on a projector (this before the widespread prevalence of computers). Participants were tasked with pressing one button on a response panel if both words were real words and another button if either word in the pair was not real. They found that response times to related pairs of words are faster than to unrelated pairs, suggesting that when a real word is read, it activates other, related words in the lexicon.

Semantic categorization

Another type of yes/no lexical identification task is the *semantic categorization task* (also termed *semantic judgement task*). The dependent variable in semantic categorization tasks, as in LDTs, is usually response time and error rate, and they similarly make use of prime-target word pairs. In semantic categorization tasks the respondent must decide whether each target word belongs to a predetermined semantic category (e.g. 'pets'). In a standard (i.e. consecutive) LCT, target words (e.g. 'CAT') may be preceded by a semantically related L2 prime (e.g. 'DOG' 'CAT') or a semantically unrelated prime (e.g. 'TREE' 'CAT'), or the prime might be the L1 translation equivalent of the target word (e.g. 'GATO' 'CAT') or a semantically unrelated L1 word (e.g. 'ÁRBOL' 'CAT'). Target words that belong to the semantic category (e.g. CAT = pet) are termed *exemplar targets*, whereas target words that do not (e.g. TREE ≠ pet) are *non-exemplar targets*.

Grammaticality judgement

Experimental tasks are not limited to lexical classification but can further probe grammatical sensitivity. *Grammaticality judgement tasks* do just that: sentences are presented to the respondent, who judges whether they are grammatical or not (in some cases participants are instead/also tasked with identifying, correcting and/or explaining ungrammatical forms). Grammaticality judgement tasks can be timed or untimed with timed versions providing less opportunity for learners to use explicit knowledge when making their determination (e.g. Ellis, 2009; Loewen, 2009) and yielding response time (RT) data in addition to response accuracy and error rate measures. Stimuli can be delivered aurally or visually (i.e. in writing) and usually focus on a single target feature (Plonsky et al., 2019). For a detailed discussion of judgement tasks in SLA research, see Spinner and Gass (2019).

There are many advantages to using experimental elicitation tasks as a data collection method. First, they are generally straightforward to administer, being programmed onto a computer system (e.g. laptops, tablets and smartphones) in advance. Likewise, experimental tasks are (usually) simple for the respondent to complete, requiring merely the pressing of one or two keys on a keyboard or response panel or the production of a single word (but see, e.g., Declerck and Kormos (2012) below for the increased complexity of the dual-task paradigm). Allied to the more mechanical administration of experimental tasks, scoring experiments is also straightforward: responses to trials are either correct or incorrect and response times are a unitary count in milliseconds.

There are also some drawbacks to using experimental measures such as LDTs, semantic categorization tasks and grammaticality judgement tasks. For example, the artificiality of such a controlled task type means that unless the phenomenon under investigation has a clear link to the real world, the findings will lack ecological validity (i.e. they will mean very little beyond the confines of your study). Furthermore, where tasks are 'on-line' (i.e. administered under pressure of time and therefore designed to tap into more unconscious or automatic responses to linguistic stimuli), the data they yield are inevitably affected by the necessity of using motor movement to indicate a response (i.e. response times necessarily encompass the time it takes to press a response key).

Key concepts

In this section, we explore concepts fundamental to the use of data elicitation tasks as data collection methods. These concepts inform the design and theory underpinning the development and use of data elicitation tasks.

Language production tasks

Some scholars have postulated specific principles to apply in the design of language production tasks. Loschky and Bley-Vroman (1993) suggest that a particular language feature can be incorporated into a task – and thus be elicited by the task – via three key considerations:

1 *Task naturalness*, whereby the task could feasibly be completed without use of the language feature, but the language feature can reasonably be expected to occur frequently and naturally during task completion. For example, it is possible to complete a map-reading direction giving task without using the imperative ('Please take the second right'/'You

should go straight on'), but it is highly likely that the task will elicit imperative use ('Go straight on'/'Turn left').

2 *Task utility*, whereby once more the task could feasibly be completed without use of the target feature but using the target feature will make the task easier to complete and will promote task success. For example, it is possible to complete a picture description task without using prepositions ('There is a woman'/'There is a horse'/'The horse has a ribbon') but easier to successfully complete the task with their use ('On the left there is a woman on a horse that has a ribbon in its tail').

3 *Task essentialness*, whereby the task cannot be completed successfully without use of the target feature, and thus the target feature is the essence of the task. For example, a story completion task in which a learner reads the first part of a story and then must ask questions to find out how it ends cannot be completed without the use of question forms, and therefore question formation is essential to the task.

Unless a researcher is absolutely certain (based on ample previous studies' findings and/or their own extensive piloting) that naturalness and/or utility will elicit the target feature in sufficient quantity and with sufficient range, it is recommended that the task essentialness principle is applied in production task design. Key to applying all of these principles is the proficiency of the sample: the participants' stage of development should be taken into account such that the task corresponds to a target feature that participants are in the process of acquiring. Conversely, if a researcher approaches their study from the perspective of foregrounding the target feature, the participants' proficiency level needs to correspond.

More broadly, Philp (2016) argues for a three-way balance in data production task design, between

1 *authenticity* (i.e. eliciting the target feature in an authentic context – thus enhancing ecological validity),

2 *creativity* (i.e. promoting inventive use of language) and

3 *engagement* (i.e. presenting a linguistic and cognitive challenge to the participant).

She posits that authenticity and creativity concern the quality of the elicitation, whereas engagement concerns motivating participants to the task.

Experimental elicitation tasks

Here we discuss a range of concepts related to the development of experimental elicitation tasks. While this is by no means a comprehensive treatment of the issues, which could fill a volume in and of itself, we highlight some of the key considerations for researchers in the experimental paradigm.

Modality

Modality of task delivery is a key consideration in experimental task development because the manner in which the stimulus is presented to the respondent is likely to affect the speed and accuracy with which they respond to it. For example, Murphy (1997) compared modality of stimulus presentation (aural vs. visual) in grammaticality judgement tasks among L1 and L2 users of French and English to find that all participants – particularly L2 users – were slower and less accurate in the aural condition. Researchers may wish to mirror the input modality of the data collection methods used in studies that foreground their own experiments as a means of facilitating comparison between findings.

Stimuli

Selecting words as stimuli for LDTs and semantic categorization tasks is a complex issue because words can vary in a number of different ways (e.g. frequency, abstractness, syntactic category, length, number of syllables). When selecting words, it is crucial that the only systematic (i.e. non-random) differences between their characteristics are those that are of specific interest to the experiment (e.g. semantically (un)related, (non) cognate). Word frequency is of particular importance to take account of because the use of low-frequency stimuli in experimental tasks creates noise in the data. Research suggests that low-frequency words engender low response consistency and slower response times; that is, respondents are inclined to respond differently to the same low-frequency target word in different trials (Diependaele, Brysbaert & Neri, 2012). Similarly, the more real-like the pseudowords in a task, such as one-letter transpositions (e.g. 'GRAET') or pseudohomophones (e.g. 'TREET'), and the more that pseudowords resemble high-frequency real words in particular, the longer the response latency in reaction to both pseudowords and real words in that task (Lupker & Pexman, 2010). Thus, the selection of real words and pseudowords in a task can have a significant effect on the results. It is also important for stimuli to be randomly dispersed throughout a task as far as possible so that any latent presentation order effects are mitigated.

Fillers

A *filler* is a task item that is excluded from the main data analysis yet included in the task to distract the respondent from developing a subliminal understanding of the distribution of the stimuli in an experiment such that they might alter their behaviour based on that understanding (i.e. display *bias*). For example, if the target feature of a study is the passive voice and the study uses grammaticality judgement tasks as a data collection method, then filler items may include ungrammatical uses of other structures, such as the past progressive and/or grammatical use of other structures. It is important to include as large a number of fillers in an experiment as possible (keeping *participant fatigue* in mind) and to ensure they are interspersed throughout the task as randomly as possible (while also ensuring that randomization has not produced large blocks of stimulus trials without any fillers).

Counterbalancing

Counterbalancing is a technique applied in experiential research to mitigate *order effects*. For example, if an experiment is designed to compare participants' performance on semantic categorization task trials in their L1 and L2, a *counterbalanced design* would involve half of the sample completing the first half of the task in the L1 and the second half of the task in the L2, and the other half of the sample completing the first half of the trials in the L2 and the second half in the L1. By doing this, when the sample data as a whole are analysed, the researcher can be confident that any effects of language have not been confounded by presentation order.

Priming

Priming describes the phenomenon that exposure to one stimulus affects the processing of a later stimulus. *Positive priming* improves processing of the target stimulus and improves the response time as with semantically related primes (e.g. the prime 'DOG' leads to faster processing of 'CAT'), whereas *negative priming* interferes with target item processing (e.g. the prime 'TREE' interferes with the processing of 'CAT'). Prime-target pairs can be presented in the same modality, or primes can be aurally presented with targets visually presented or vice versa (i.e. *cross-modal priming*). *Masked priming* refers to the presentation of a prime which is either forward masked (i.e. preceded by a series of symbols, such as '######'), backward masked (i.e. followed by a series of symbols) or both. The prime is displayed for a very short amount of time (typically around 50 milliseconds) and this, coupled with the masking, makes the prime almost imperceptible to the respondent. The masked priming paradigm is important because it offers a window into priming effects where respondents are not consciously aware of the prime–target relationship.

Procedures and practicalities

In this section, we look at the specific processes involved in using data elicitation tasks in applied linguistics research. Common challenges to and issues inherent in collecting and analysing elicitation task data are outlined, and strategies for overcoming these challenges are suggested.

Time commitments for production tasks

Language production tasks such as OPIs and storytelling may carry a significant burden of organization and time as regards data collection because often only one participant can be recorded at a time. This has a knock-on effect in terms of sample size, which is an unavoidable trade-off which should be a consideration at the study design phase and certainly prior to planning data analysis. Likewise, transcription of spoken data is incredibly time-consuming: if researchers intend on transcribing audio data personally, sufficient time for this should be factored into the research timeline from the outset.

Administration of production tasks

It is imperative that administration of the chosen data collection tools is as consistent as possible across participants so that data are reliable: the data collection protocol should be the same for every recording session, even down to the interaction between the researcher and their participants before and after completion of the task. Researchers should plan in advance some comprehension questions that they can ask to each respondent to check that they have clearly understood the task instructions and know exactly what to do (particularly if any written instructions are not presented in the participant's L1). Researchers should try to administer tasks in a quiet place so that respondents are not distracted by any environmental disturbances and so that the quality of the audio recording is protected.

Data preparation and analysis for production tasks

Unless the audio/video recordings themselves constitute a dataset, production data must be transcribed prior to analysis, and this process involves a series of decisions about what to include in the transcript. There is no single 'correct' way to transcribe L2 data because the decisions a researcher takes will depend on the chosen theoretical lens and research aims and these will vary from study to study. Mackey and Gass (2016: 113–116) provide a useful discussion of L2 production data transcription, including an overview of commonly used transcription conventions.

It is challenging to condense advice on analysis of all types of production task data given the huge variation between the available tasks and the types of data they yield: certainly, how a researcher analyses their data will depend very much on the research questions they are asking. One traditional approach to analysing production task data is to determine the percentage of target-like utterances/productions, non-target-like utterances/productions and omissions in light of the total number of obligatory contexts (in this case, it is not advisable to analyse only subsections of the dataset). Furthermore, non-target-like utterances/productions can be coded by error type (for detailed discussions of error analysis/classification, see, e.g., Corder, 1974; Dulay & Burt, 1974; Lott, 1983; Richards, 1971). However, if the construct of interest is, for example, spoken fluency or pragmatic competence, a researcher is likely to adopt specific coding procedures that go beyond identification and classification of non-target-like forms. We recommend reviewing a range of studies that have investigated the same or highly similar constructs to that which a study is focusing on. We further recommend aggregating, possibly in tabular format, information about the analytic approaches applied in those studies, including any relevant comments about the strengths and drawbacks of each approach. Doing so will enable clear comparisons and evaluations of analytic options and help researchers to decide on the most appropriate, valid and reliable method for their research.

Software for experimental elicitation tasks

There are a number of software packages on which psycholinguistic experiments can be developed and administered for researchers without knowledge of programming languages: some are licensed at a price (e.g. SuperLab, E-Prime, Presentation), whereas others are free to download but may only be compatible with certain operating systems (e.g. DMDX, PsyScope). The graphical user interface on most of these tools is easy to use, especially with the help of manuals for use that are openly available online.

Stimuli for experimental elicitation tasks

There are a number of web-based word generators that will generate words and pseudowords for use in psycholinguistic experiments. These include the English Lexicon Project (http://elexicon.wustl.edu/), Macquarie University's Non-Word Database (http://www.cogsci.mq.edu.au/research/resources/nwdb/nwdb.html) and the Orthographic Wordform Database (http://www.neuro.mcw.edu/mcword/). Such generators offer the researcher a range of parameters to apply (e.g. length, number of syllables) and generate large lists which can be copied or pasted from the web browser or mailed directly to the researcher. Most web-based generators apply to English words only; others deal with multiple languages (e.g. http://globalwordnet.org/wordnets-in-the-world/). It is recommended that researchers check that pseudowords are not brand names (e.g. via http://www.kunst-worte.de/markennamen/) and do not have a meaning in current usage (e.g. via http://www.urbandictionary.com/). There are likewise databases of picture stimuli (e.g. http://crl.ucsd.edu/experiments/ipnp/; http://csea.phhp.ufl.edu/media/iapsmessage.html; http://wiki.cnbc.cmu.edu/TarrLab), and if a researcher is working with populations of young language learners, the CHILDES database enables extraction of word frequency specific to children (http://childfreq.sumsar.net/).

Data analysis for experimental elicitation tasks

Experimental data are commonly analysed with regard to the response time of correct trials. Therefore, the first step in data analysis is to establish the percentage of accuracy in each condition. To do this, trials in which the respondent either failed to identify a target or failed to make any response should be identified. An internal consistency coefficient, such as Cronbach's alpha, should be estimated and reported for task scores (see Chapter 4 for a discussion of interpreting reliability estimates). Next, response time data should be screened for extreme values and outliers: these can be adjusted to a certain number of standard deviations beyond the mean (usually around 2.5 SDs), replaced with the item mean (Lachaud & Renault, 2011) or otherwise eliminated from the dataset. Due to the motor constraints of pressing a response key, response time data are commonly non-normally distributed with a positive skew: if so, log transformation can be performed prior to analysis. The specific parametric analyses used will depend on the number of factors in the task: typically employed in the literature are t-tests, ANOVA and regression models.

Improving reliability and validity

Now that we have explored the practicalities of using data elicitation tasks, our attention turns to factors which may threaten reliability and validity of the information yielded by tasks during data collection. It should be noted that an important means of ameliorating threats to validity and reliability in any study is piloting of the instruments and procedure: as stated by Derrick (2016: 146), piloting '[ensures] that the instructions and tasks are clear, that the instrument has good reliability, and that test tasks are measuring the intended construct or ability'.

Language production tasks

A major threat to the reliability and validity of language production tasks as a data collection method is the notion that the linguistic forms produced in a language production task are a function of the task itself as opposed to the linguistic knowledge or competence of the respondent (see, e.g., the work of McDonough (2006) on syntactic priming). For this reason, it is common for researchers to utilize multiple data elicitation measures in a single study such that they can *triangulate* findings across data collection tools (discussed in Chapter 12) and are thereby better able to confidently tease out data which represent the participant's underlying competence (see as an example Galante and Thompson, 2017) below. Validity can also be achieved via *convergence* of a study's findings on the findings of other studies that have used similar techniques to investigate the same phenomenon. If multiple uses of a data collection methodology across similar studies point to the same fundamental conclusions, then there is an argument for the validity of the chosen approach.

Even where multiple production tasks are employed in a single study, it is pertinent to keep in mind that productive language knowledge is usually preceded by receptive knowledge (e.g. Keenan & MacWhinney, 1987). Thus, production task data cannot reliably be said to be comprehensively representative of an L2 user's entire linguistic knowledge. Accordingly, any claims made in the discussion of the findings should acknowledge this.

Experimental elicitation tasks

As regards the validity and reliability of experimental elicitation tasks, it is imperative that experimental settings and protocols, such as those in which an LDT is administered, are comparable across participants. For example, practice sessions and interaction between researcher and participant should ideally be identical every time data are collected so that contextual variation is not a factor affecting the participants' responses at an individual level. It is also imperative that the participants in the study know the real words that are included as stimuli in the trials: if they do not, the response times will not reflect the type of processing the task is intended to measure.

Another key consideration regarding response times is that they are notoriously subject to a range of factors that have nothing at all to do with stimulus processing speed. For example, participants may, due to environmental distraction or lapses in concentration, accidentally press a key. Where there are two keys from which to choose (as in yes/no identification tasks), participants may press the wrong key even where they have correctly identified the target. Furthermore, right-handed participants' left-hand responses may be slower than their right-handed responses (with the opposite true for left-handed participants). One alternative to the two-key yes/no format that goes some way to reducing such variability is the *go/no go format* in which there is only one key to press: the respondent must press the key when they identify a real word and do nothing when they identify a pseudoword. Another option is to employ voice-activated triggers (whereby the participant responds orally), yet factors such as background noise and coughs/sneezes threaten reliability in this method.

To reduce variability in experimental elicitation task data, it is recommended that participants receive extensive practice trials prior to the experimental task and that large numbers of trials are included in the experimental blocks, as in Fitzpatrick and Izura (2011). *Buffer trials* (i.e. trials that look like experimental trials to the participant but are excluded from the data analysis) can be included at the start of each experimental block so that by the time the true experimental trials begin, the participant has acclimatized to the task. Furthermore, if large numbers of trials are administered in one session, participants should be given a break between blocks of trials to combat fatigue.

Case studies of data elicitation tasks in applied linguistics research

Table 2.1 comprises summaries of a number of applied linguistics studies that have utilized data elicitation tasks for their data collection methodologies. From this selection, we choose two to showcase in more detail.

Galante and Thomson (2017) and Nassaji (2017) are included here because both studies employed multiple language production tasks. In the case of Galante and Thomson (2017), these were all oral tasks because their variable of interest was oral L2 proficiency. Two of the tasks were picture narrations, one was a video narration, one a monologue without pictures and one a role play. The researchers used multiple task types 'to ensure some tasks did not favor one group over another' (2017: 125), which is logical seeing as their intervention was drama based and therefore more closely related to some task types (e.g. role play) than others. Similarly, Nassaji's justification for using multiple language production tasks was to negate any effect on the findings of the tasks themselves, and he selected his tasks to elicit different types of knowledge of the target feature. He administered (1) an

Table 2.1 Examples of data elicitation tasks in applied linguistics research

Researchers	Topic	Participants	Research design	Data collection method
Azaz and Frank (2017)	The influence of perceptual salience on acquisition of the construct state in Arabic	L1-English learners of Arabic at a US university grouped by proficiency (n = 55)	Cross-sectional; pre-testing; ANOVA	Oral proficiency interview; written sentence completion task with picture prompts
Galante and Thomson (2017)	The effects of drama-based L2-English pedagogy on oral skills	Adolescent Brazilian learners of English in São Paolo (n = 24)	Intervention with experimental and control groups; pre- and post-tests; ANOVAs	First-person picture narration; third-person picture narration; video narration; role play; monologic speech sample
Grey et al. (2015)	The roles of study abroad experience and cognitive capacity in L2 lexical and grammatical development	L1-English advanced learners of L2-Spanish in Spain (n = 26)	Longitudinal; pre- and post-tests; t-tests and correlation analyses	Working memory tests; grammaticality judgement task; lexical decision task
Kim and Taguchi (2015)	The relationship between task complexity and L2 pragmatic competence development	Korean junior high school learners of English (n = 73)	Intervention with experimental and control groups; pre-, post- and delayed post-tests; non-parametric analyses	Discourse completion task

Continued

Researchers	Topic	Participants	Research design	Data collection method
Nassaji (2017)	The effect of L2 grammar learning of extensive and intensive recasts	Adult ESL learners of various L1 backgrounds in Canada (*n* = 48)		Oral picture description task; written grammaticality judgement task; written storytelling task
Shiu, Yalçın and Spada (2018)	The influence of task features on L2 learners' grammaticality judgement performance	Taiwanese EFL university students (*n* = 120)	Cross-sectional; correlation; repeated-measures ANOVAs	Four grammaticality judgement tasks
Wolter and Yamashita (2015)	The influence of L1 collocation patterns on the processing of L2 collocations	L1-English university students in the US (*n* = 27) and L1-Japanese university students in Japan (*n* = 50)	Cross-sectional; mixed modelling	Double lexical decision task

oral picture description task (to elicit oral implicit knowledge of L2-English articles since the task required spontaneous production in meaning-focused activity), (2) a picture-prompted written storytelling task (to elicit written implicit and explicit knowledge) and (3) an untimed written grammaticality judgement task (to elicit explicit knowledge of articles).

Kim and Taguchi (2015) and Azaz and Frank (2017) both utilized discourse completion tasks as data collection tools but in different ways and to investigate very different linguistic features. Kim and Taguchi (2015) administered a fifteen-item DCT which tested knowledge of request expressions in discourse situations comprising differing levels of power and distance between interlocutors and of imposition of requests. Each item situation was described in the L1 (to ensure understanding), and slightly modified wording was used in the test at each time point to negate any practice effect. Azaz and Frank (2017) developed a sentence completion task to test the role of salience in the acquisition sequence of the 'construct state' in L2-Arabic – a grammatical marker of the first noun of a genitive construction (e.g. 'the queen of Sheba') used to indicate possession of the first noun by the second noun. The task was accompanied by picture prompts and was designed to elicit the target structure while participants were engaged in a meaning-focused activity (describing the pictures). The order of the pictures was counterbalanced because, as Arabic is a right-to-left script, it was hypothesized that the participants may strategically but wrongly assume that the right-hand picture should appear first in the nominal construction.

Turning now to studies that have employed experimental elicitation tasks, we look at the use of grammaticality judgement tasks in Shiu, Yalçın and Spada (2018), the use of LDTs in Wolter and Yamashita (2015) and the combination of both of these task types in Grey et al. (2015). Shiu, Yalçın and Spada (2018) explored the effects of different grammaticality judgement task features on the grammaticality judgements of Taiwanese EFL students. They devised four computer-based grammaticality judgement tasks to measure combinations of timed vs. untimed and aural vs. written tasks. The timed tests (aural before written so as to reduce any practice effect) were administered on the same day with a 30-minute break in between; the untimed tests were administered 1 week later (to decrease any memory effect).

Wolter and Yamashita (2015) used an LDT to investigate whether acceptability judgements pertaining to L2 collocational patterns are influenced by collocational patterns in the L1 among Japanese speakers of L2-English. The researchers developed a double LDT designed to test the hypothesis that L1 collocational links are 'copied and pasted' in the mental lexicon to corresponding L2 lemmas and therefore that response times to L2 word pairs which constitute acceptable collocations in Japanese but not English will be faster.

Grey et al. (2015) employed a grammaticality judgement task and an LDT to measure the effects of short-term study abroad on the development of lexical and grammatical L2 knowledge of L2 learners of Spanish. The grammaticality judgement task targeted word order, noun–adjective number agreement and noun–adjective gender agreement; the LDT tested accuracy and speed of recognition of real and pseudo Spanish nouns.

We choose now to showcase two studies to highlight the use of the two types of data elicitation tasks under focus (language production tasks and experimental elicitation tasks) with each study offering insight into the employment of these types of tasks.

Galante and Thomson (2017): A study using multiple language production tasks

The first illustrative study is that of Galante and Thomson (2017), who employed a pre-test and post-test design to investigate the effects of a 4-month-long drama-based English language programme on spoken fluency, comprehensibility and accentedness among Brazilian adolescents in São Paolo. Participants were assigned either to the experimental drama-based condition or received traditional EFL pedagogy (communicative language teaching) during the 4-month period. Pre and post the intervention period, the researchers administered five language elicitation tasks to the sample, all of which were audio-recorded: (1) a first-person picture narration, (2) a third-person picture narration, (3) a video narration, (4) a role play and (5) a monologue. A sample of thirty untrained L1-English users was recruited to rate excerpts from the speech sample recordings: each rater listened to 240 speech samples (24 speakers' excerpts from two time points on five different tasks) and rated each speech sample on fluency, comprehensibility and accent using a nine-point scale. From the rating data, a mean score for each sub-construct (fluency, comprehensibility, accentedness) at each time point was calculated. These variables were then employed in mixed-between-within analyses of variance, taking task (five levels) and time (two levels) as within-subjects variables, and group (two levels) as the between-subjects variable.

Of particular interest in Galante and Thomson (2017) is the differences by task type in their raters' scores: contrary to previous research that followed a similar data collection methodology (i.e. Derwing et al., 2004), Galante and Thomson (2017) found that picture description tasks yielded higher ratings than monologues and role play tasks, with first-person picture description showing particularly strong ratings as regards accentedness and comprehensibility. The researchers explain this finding by drawing a somewhat tenuous link between first-person description and the role of an actor. Another possible explanation is that the task itself facilitated better spoken proficiency among the sample as a function of its specific linguistic and content demands. Whether or not this is the case, Galante and Thomson's (2017) findings serve to underscore the importance of a multi-instrument data collection approach when using data production tasks: if performance might vary by task type, using multiple task types is the most valid and holistic approach.

Grey et al. (2015): Lexical decision and grammaticality judgement in a study abroad context

A second illustrative study is Grey et al. (2015). This study is methodologically novel because it uses highly controlled experimental tasks in a field of study (literally administered 'in the field') where they have not commonly been applied (study abroad) to investigate nuances in L2 development over a short period of time. Their grammaticality judgement task was interesting in that it focused on three target features, all of which were areas of key difference between the L1 (English) and L2 (Spanish) of their population (word order, noun–adjective number agreement and noun–adjective gender agreement). Their visual LDT focused on Spanish nouns: real-word stimuli were non-cognates, known to the sample (they appeared in the sample's Spanish textbooks), normed for frequency (using an online Spanish corpus) and an equal balance of abstract and concrete nouns. Pseudowords were one-letter transpositions of the real-word stimuli that maintained orthographic and phonological acceptability (e.g. ventana → ventapa). The tests were administered in situ in weeks 1 and 5 of the sojourn, a methodological move made possible by remote electronic administration that overcame some of the confounding variables inherent in testing participants after a sojourn has ended (e.g. post-study abroad L2 exposure).

Through the employment of experimental elicitation tasks, Grey et al. (2015) were able to isolate nuanced linguistic development that would likely not have been identified in their study had they adopted a less controlled data collection methodology, such as via the use of data production tasks: while accuracy of responses to real Spanish words in the LDT did not significantly change over the 5-week study abroad period, there was a significant decrease in latency scores, suggesting that automaticity of lexical knowledge (i.e. the ease with which the mental lexicon is accessed) had undergone development. The grammaticality judgement task data revealed that accuracy on two of the three target features significantly improved, but response times did not change on any of the targets considered separately from one another, although overall there was a significant effect on latency. The scholars suggest that this lack of significant effect on individual target feature latency was a function of the test itself: in total their grammaticality judgement task had thirty ungrammatical items with ten for each target feature, and they posit that this low item count may have limited power at the analysis stage such that latency effects on individual target features were obscured. This study therefore highlights the complexity of testing multiple target features in a single grammaticality judgement task and the importance of considering at the point of instrument development the likely subdivisions of data at the analysis stage such that sufficient numbers of items for each target feature are included.

Implications for researchers

A recurrent theme throughout this chapter has been the relationship between task control and ecological validity, which is the extent to which the control a researcher exerts over a task diminishes the real-world relevance of the data. The specific data elicitation tasks discussed in the chapter vary wildly when considered by level of researcher control, but is it the case that the greater the level of control, the lower the ecological validity? For example, is the relatively less controlled OPI more ecologically valid than the very highly controlled LDT? Since control over how data are elicited has a direct relationship to *internal validity* (in simple terms, how well the research is done and avoids the influence of possible confounding variables), is it possible to maintain a healthy balance between internal and ecological validity when using data elicitation tasks?

There are some notorious examples of social science research in which the quest for ecological validity has led to a disastrous lack of control on many levels. Think, for example, of the infamous Stanford Prison Experiment. However, we believe that a workable balance can be struck at both the macro level (i.e. converging evidence across studies) and micro level (i.e. in one particular study) if careful equal consideration is given to internal and ecological validity from the outset of the study design process. For example, it may be the case that the research questions being asked require the use of highly controlled experimental elicitation tasks which arguably bear little relation to what language users do in real life. If so, ecological validity can be achieved via other means, such as sampling a range of categories of language users, administering experiments in real-world settings (as in Grey et al., 2015), and/or using multiple measures and triangulating the data they yield. On a broader level, when discussing data elicitation task findings, we recommend situating observations beyond the specific methodological paradigm of the study to take account of evidence that illuminates the phenomenon of interest from a broad range of perspectives.

Post-reading activities

Reflect
This chapter has suggested that there is a trade-off between using data elicitation tasks and ecological validity. Do you think that in the case of some of the data elicitation tasks discussed in this chapter, that trade-off is too large? In other words, are there task types that you deem too inauthentic? How might ecological validity with regard to these task types be improved?

Expand
Individually or in small groups, choose one of the studies in Table 2.1 to read and critique. After reading, consider and discuss: (1) What was the data elicitation task able to tell us about the variable of interest? What was it unable to tell us? (2) Were there any aspects of the methodology which could have been improved in design or implementation? (3) Did the researchers consider the ecological validity of their data collection methodology? If so, how? If not, how might they have done so?

Apply
Design a cross-sectional study that aims to determine whether L2 lexical and grammatical sensitivity is influenced by the cognate status of the L1 (i.e. whether or not the L1 is a cognate language to the L2, such as with Spanish and English). You are particularly interested in establishing whether there is an effect of L1 cognate status on recognition of L2 non-cognate language features (words, grammatical structures). Plan a methodological approach that would collect this type of data and pay particular attention to the following decisions: What task modality would you adopt, and why? How and where would you administer your tasks? How would you ensure reliability and validity of the data?

Resources for further reading

Chaudron, C. (2003). Data collections methods in SLA research. In C. J. Doughty & M. H. Long (Eds.), *The handbook of second language acquisition* (pp. 762–828). Oxford: Blackwell.

Craig Chaudron's chapter on data collection in SLA research is a clear and accessible overview of a range of data collection research methods with excellent sections on language production tasks and experimental methods such as the lexical decision task. Particularly useful is the categorization of data elicitation tasks on a continuum from naturalistic to experimental, and the detailed discussion of the advantages and disadvantages of each category of task that is discussed.

Doughty, C., & Long, M. H. (2000). Eliciting second language speech data. In L. Menn and N. Bernstein Ratner (Eds.), *Methods for studying language production* (pp. 149–177). Mahwah, NJ: Lawrence Erlbaum Associates.

This chapter draws links between methodologies used to elicit speech data from L1 language users with those designed to elicit L2 use, highlighting the key differences between L1 and L2 populations and discussing the implications of these for data collection methodology. The chapter then focuses on three research domains that speak to describing and understanding L2 production (developmental linguistic profiling, descriptive linguistic profiling, documenting the role of L2 production in acquisition) and discusses the strengths and limitations of each with reference to specific studies.

3

Introspective and Retrospective Protocols

Pre-reading activities

Think

In applied linguistics, introspective protocols involve participants voicing their thoughts or explaining their behaviours while simultaneously carrying out a language-related task. Retrospective protocols involve participants voicing their thoughts or explaining their behaviours after completing a task. What are the strengths and limitations of each data collection method?

Discuss

Thinking of the range of topics covered by applied linguistics research, what types of language-related tasks would be better suited to introspection, and what kinds of tasks would be better suited to retrospection?

Imagine

Imagine you are conducting a study into the writing processes that learners engage in when completing the IELTS written exam. You want to understand how students monitor and make corrections to their own language while writing within this exam condition. You decide to employ a retrospective protocol because the act of voicing thoughts while writing will disrupt the natural writing process. Accordingly, you decide to interview students after they have finished the writing task. What would you do as a researcher to ensure that the data yielded is as reliable as possible?

Introduction

Introspective and retrospective protocols have a long tradition in second language research. Introspective protocols involve tasks that require participants to look inward at their own behaviours, thoughts and beliefs and communicate these actions and processes to the researcher. Retrospective protocols are a type of introspection and require participants to look inward regarding a recently completed past activity. Depending on the topic being researched, introspection or retrospection might be deemed more appropriate.

Larsen-Freeman and Long (1991: 15) claim introspection is the 'ultimate qualitative study' in second language research, 'in which with guidance from the researcher, learners examine their own behaviour for insights into SLA.' Some SLA researchers question the validity of these insights due to learners not being able to accurately report the subconscious processes taking place within their own learning. Other researchers, however, argue that alternative methods such as observation cannot provide access to learners' conscious thought processes. We concur with both camps, seeing introspection as both powerful and limited depending on how it is implemented and depending on the task being researched.

In this chapter, we argue that introspection remains a useful data collection research method in applied linguistics, particularly for research pertaining to second language learning processes. However, due to the effects of memory deterioration and researcher bias on introspective data, certain precautions need to be taken in order to alleviate threats to validity. This is especially true of retrospective designs, when time has passed between the event being researched and data collection. For these reasons, versions of introspective and retrospective protocols have been developed to minimize negative effects: think aloud, retrospective think-aloud and stimulated recall. The most widely used introspective technique in applied linguistics is the think-aloud protocol, which aims to capture introspection simultaneously while the task is being carried out by the participant. By collecting data at the same time as the event being studied, the protocol eliminates memory decay, thus enhancing the accuracy of the data collected. Other protocols such as retrospective think-aloud protocols and stimulated recall protocols aim to combat memory deterioration in other ways.

This chapter aims to navigate novice researchers through the various decisions that need to be made in order to develop the most appropriate protocol for introspection and retrospection in applied linguistics research. We first cover basic protocols and their subtypes before diving deeper into ways a researcher can improve the reliability and validity of data collected via such protocols. We will also discuss how advances in technology have enhanced introspective and retrospective research designs by allowing the researcher to better capture and present stimuli for memory prompts or to collect supplementary data via eye-tracking software or keystroke logging software.

Key concepts

In this section, we explore three basic types of introspection: think-aloud protocols, retrospective think-aloud protocols and stimulated recall protocols before touching on some associated methods of eye-tracking and keystroke-logging.

Think-aloud protocols

A think-aloud protocol involves a participant voicing their thoughts or explaining their behaviours during the task being researched. Think alouds have been used widely in second language acquisition studies which aim to understand the thoughts of learners during language learning processes. Gu (2014: 74) notes that although there have been numerous methodological concerns raised regarding the disruptive nature of thinking aloud on the phenomenon being researched, 'it is now widely agreed that various versions of thinking aloud are the most direct and therefore best tools available in examining the on-going processes and intentions as and when learning happens'. He argues that recent additional methods of collecting data on learning processes (such as eye-tracking, discussed later) have shown think-aloud protocols to be quite robust and accurate in their collection of data.

Think-aloud protocols are particularly useful in writing research, where evidence has shown that verbalization of thought processes has little impact on students' writing in controlled conditions (Yang, Hu & Zhang, 2014). However, some scholars note that think-aloud protocols do not provide a complete picture of the complexities of thinking processes (see Hyland, 2016).

Retrospective think-aloud protocols

Retrospective think-aloud protocols are a less commonly used version of introspection and require interviewing a participant immediately after the event being researched. Retrospective think-aloud protocols are usually suited to tasks where the act of thinking aloud is seen to change participants' primary cognitive processes or is disruptive to the observed action (e.g. during a speaking task). The protocol is usually manifested as a retrospective interview and aims to collect data on participants' thoughts and behaviours while they are still fresh in the memory of the participant. This protocol is different from general interviews (discussed in Chapter 2) in that general interviews broadly capture participant experiences and thoughts, whereas retrospective think-aloud protocols aim to capture data surrounding an associated task given to the participants. To combat memory deterioration, retrospective think-aloud protocols are best conducted immediately after the event being studied.

Stimulated recall protocol

Stimulated recall is a type of introspection which aims to gather data after the event being studied using stimuli to help improve the accuracy of a participant's recollections. In second language research, 'learners are asked to introspect while viewing or hearing a stimulus to prompt their recollections' (Mackey & Gass, 2005: 366). Stimulated recall protocols require the use of a tangible prompt, such as a visual or audio cue, to encourage participants to retrieve and verbalize their thoughts at the time of the event (Mackey & Gass, 2016: 87).

Stimulated recall has potential problems related to issues of mistaken memory and retrieval, ill-timing and poor instructions. To combat these issues, Mackey and Gass (2005) make four suggestions to carefully structure stimulated recalls:

1 Data should be collected as soon as possible after the event that is the focus of the recall.
2 The stimulus should be as strong as possible to activate memory structures.
3 The participants should be minimally trained; that is, they should be able to carry out the procedure but should not be cued into any aspects that are extra or unnecessary knowledge.
4 The researcher should take care to not lead or interfere with the recall process.

These suggestions should be considered when conducting the stimulated recall for any study.

Procedures and practicalities

In this section, we draw on the hypothetical IELTS writing research project presented in the opening activity of this chapter to provide an illustration of how each protocol can be used to collect data on an applied linguistics topic. Our hypothetical study aims to investigate the writing processes that learners engage in when completing the IELTS written exam, focusing particularly on how students monitor their language and make corrections while writing within an exam context.

Think-aloud practicalities

In our hypothetical IELTS study, a think-aloud protocol would involve capturing thoughts and processes while the participants are simultaneously taking a mock IELTS exam. Think-aloud protocols work best when a researcher is present, rather than asking a participant to think aloud independently. To minimize researcher bias, the researcher should prompt the participants to voice their thoughts aloud without leading them. This will ensure that the participant is able to focus on the concepts of interest to the researcher while the minimizing impact of the researcher on the event being studied.

In our IELTS study, a researcher might sit with a participant while he or she completes the IELTS task. Periodically, the researcher might ask the participant to voice what they are thinking in terms of monitoring their own writing and what they are doing when observed to engage in editing. For example, when a participant appears to be engaged in proofreading or correcting their work, the researcher could gently ask them to explain what they are doing.

Retrospective think-aloud practicalities

There are many reasons why a researcher would opt to conduct a retrospective think-aloud protocol for our IELTS study, instead of a simultaneous design.

A researcher might deem the process of thinking aloud to be too disruptive to the writing process, thereby destroying the very thing being researched. Likewise, a researcher might decide that a mock IELTS task does not adequately capture the pressure and anxiety associated with participants writing in a high-stakes examination context. For either reason, a researcher might decide to interview participants immediately after they take a mock or real-life IELTS examination.

In our IELTS study, the researcher would aim to sit down with the participant immediately after they complete the IELTS written test. They would get the participant to talk the researcher through the processes they used to monitor their writing and to edit their work during the task. As recall of these processes may be difficult, it would be wise if, prior to going into the writing task, the participants were mildly privy to the focus of the think aloud. This awareness would make them more cognizant of their thoughts and behaviours during the task. It may be useful in some retrospective think-aloud studies for participants to make notes of their thoughts and behaviours during a task to later discuss with the researcher, but only if this is not seen to disrupt the activities being researched. Other researchers opt to bring some artefacts of the event to the retrospective think-aloud interviews to aid discussion (Azaz, 2017). In our hypothetical study the researcher could ask the student to bring a copy of the exam prompt and their written notes.

Stimulated recall protocols

Retrospective think-aloud protocols are susceptible to memory deterioration when participants cannot accurately remember all of their thoughts and behaviours after a completed event. In such cases a stimulated recall protocol might be deemed a more appropriate means to gather introspective data. A stimulated recall protocol for our IELTS study would involve the use of stimulus from the writing task to jog participants' memories during the retrospective think-aloud task. Useful stimuli for the IELTS writing task might involve a screen recording taken throughout the writing task (in the case of an IELTS internet-based test) or a video recording of the participants' hands and paper (in the case of a paper-based test) to capture the writing process. This video would then be played back to the participant during the retrospective think-aloud interview to provide a strong stimulus for participants to recall their actions and their thoughts during the writing process. The researcher could either sit with the participants and go through the entire writing process in real time (thus getting the participant to think aloud alongside the stimulus) or preselect segments of the stimulus where the participant appears to be heavily engaged in corrections or monitoring.

Sanchez and Grimshaw (2020) state that advancements in technology have facilitated improvements in video recording for stimulated recall, including split-screen video recordings to capture multiple perspectives. Jackson and Cho (2018: 35) state that viewing multiple perspectives together such as a student view and a contextual view 'may serve as stronger stimuli for the reminder of events and prompt participants' recall through the provision of situational and contextual support'. Other advancements such as wearable technology to capture the participants' point of view during interactions offer further opportunities for stimulated recall.

Table 3.1 An example stimulated recall procedure

Setting up

1. The researcher will ensure good recording of stimulus in the form of split screen video capture that includes the work being written and edited and the participant engaging with it.
2. The researcher will confirm a meeting time with each participant within 48 hours of the task completion. The researcher should organize a quiet room for the stimulated recall interview.
3. Before the interview, the researcher will watch the recording and select the most active moments where the participant is observed to engage in monitoring and correcting their writing (e.g. proofreading and editing).

During the stimulated recall

1. The researcher explains ethical issues and how recording of the stimulated recall interview will be used.
2. The researcher explains the protocol.
3. The researcher initiates recall by providing contextual clues: 'We are going to watch some segments from your IELTS writing task. Do you remember what the topic of the writing task was? Do you remember where you were sitting and how you were feeling when you started the task?'
4. The researcher plays the first segment of stimulus without stopping: 'I am going to play the segment once, and I just want you to listen and recall the lecture.'
5. The researcher probes learner on their listening processes: 'What were you doing?'; 'How were you checking or correcting your work?'
6. The researcher plays the segment a second time and gives the student ability to pause the recording to explain their behaviour: 'We are going to play back the same segment, and feel free to stop the recording at any time to tell me anything you were thinking or doing. You can stop to tell me anything you remember.'
7. Repeat protocol for two other strong stimuli.

If some time has passed between the event and the stimulated recall task, it is good practice to provide participants with sufficient contextual information so that the reliability of their remembered experience will be enhanced. During stimulated recall, steps should be taken to ensure that participants do not make inferences that go beyond the task. The researcher should ensure this by only asking direct questions specifically about the stimulus via broad open-ended questions. An example of a stimulated recall procedure for our IELTS study is shown in Table 3.1.

Analysis

Analysis of think-aloud data requires careful consideration as the outside researcher is required to interpret an insider perspective. Gu (2014: 75) states, 'Rarely can we find in standard research methodology books as to how think-aloud data can be coded and analysed. Most published research using think-aloud protocols have not presented the nitty-gritty details of coding and analysis, not to mention problems therein.' We concur with Gu and extend this observation to other types of introspection and retrospection. That being said, Mackey and Gass (2016) have laid a solid foundation for analysis of stimulated recall methodology in second language research.

How introspective data from think-aloud and stimulated recall protocols are analysed depends entirely on the purpose of the research. If the purpose of introspection is to look for meaningful patterns in learning processes, then counting and quantifying of the data is a necessary step. Introspection, while qualitative in data collection, is often quantitative in terms of data analysis. If the purpose of the research is to understand the complex nuances of learning in dynamic contexts, then qualitative analysis might be deemed more appropriate. As Chapter 1 has outlined, mixed methods approaches can examine data from multiple perspectives, particularly when mixing occurs at the data analysis stage. It may be possible, given adequate participant numbers, to explore data both quantitatively in terms of frequency and qualitatively in terms of exploring complexities.

A further consideration during data analysis involves how researchers code the data to ensure they are not imposing etic coding frameworks upon emic data (Gu, 2014). Introspective data analysis is at its core emic data (i.e. data from inside the participants and his or her social context). However, researcher interpretation during data coding causes this data to become etic (i.e. interpretations derived by the researcher from outside the participant and his or her social group). Data analysis is essentially two steps removed from the event being researched, which can be problematic in terms of accuracy: the analysed data is the researchers' interpretation of the participant's interpretation of the actual thing being studied.

As the data themselves are participants' own voiced interpretations of actions and thoughts, it is important then that researcher does not force his or her own interpretations on the data during coding. Gu (2014: 80) states:

> Researcher coding of think-aloud data is always an etic interpretation of what was actually happening in the participant's mind when the learning behaviour was recorded, no matter how many coders are used and whether they agree with each other.

To counter such subjectivity, *member-checking* of data is essential (Gu, 2014). Member-checking involves presenting interpretations to the participant to ensure that they agree with the manner in with the data have been interpreted by the researcher.

Improving reliability and validity

Time constraints

The timing of retrospective think-aloud protocols and stimulated recall protocols is directly connected to the quality of the data collected. As with any retrospection, the more time that passes between the event and the reporting of that event, the more problematic the data. For retrospective think-aloud protocols, data collection should occur immediately after the completion of the task. If this is not possible, then a researcher should select stimulated recall as the preferred methodology or at the very least bring some artefacts from the event to aid recollection (see Azaz, 2017).

Stimulated recall typically involves an amount of time between the event being researched and data collection; thus, reliability of data is affected by this length of time (Vandergrift, 2010). Where possible, researchers should ensure data collection occurs as soon as possible after the task or event has taken place, which will enhance reliability of the data. Dörnyei (2007) suggests a maximum of 24 hours, but Gass and Mackey (2000) state that 48 hours' can still result in good data. Longer times can be rationalized so long as the researcher can provide a convincing argument that strong stimuli have been used. As a rule, the stronger the stimulus, the better the participant can recall past events over a sustained period. While researchers may need time to prepare the stimulus between the recording of the event and the stimulated recall interview, this should not be at the expense of time. While good stimuli will result in good data, it would be better to use hastily prepared segments of stimuli to interview participants on the same day than to prepare ideal segments of stimuli and conduct interviews days later. Good piloting will inform a researcher of the best balance between time and good data.

Researcher interference

In introspective and retrospective data collection, the researcher may fall into the trap of 'leading the witness'. Accordingly, the format of think-aloud protocols and stimulated recall protocols should involve as little input from the researcher as possible to minimize researcher bias. The role of the researcher during introspection should be limited to the questions like those in the stimulated recall procedure in Table 3.1. For a discussion on researcher interference during data analysis, see the 'Data analysis' subsection in this chapter.

Reactivity of the protocol

An oft-discussed issue in introspective data collection techniques surrounds the interference of researcher-led protocols on the validity of data. Namely, researchers can become concerned that the act of verbalizing thoughts can have an impact on the object being researched. As noted:

> The validity of thinking aloud as a data-elicitation method has been clouded by controversy over its potential reactivity, that is, whether the act of simultaneous reporting might serve as an additional task altering the very thinking processes it is supposed to represent and keep intact. (Yang, Hu & Zhang, 2014: 52)

In response to this concern, Yang, Hu and Zhang (2014) investigated the effects of thinking aloud on the completion of a writing task, using three groups of students – two of which engaged in different types of think-aloud protocols and one with no think-aloud protocol. The researchers found no evidence that thinking allowed seriously affected the writing processes of the students, except for a prolonged time required to complete the task, and a slight decline in fluency. The researchers concluded that so long as allowances are made in the research design to counter the prolonged effects of thinking aloud and on fluency, there is little evidence to support reactivity of the protocol on second language writing processes in general.

Similarly, Egi (2008) explored the reactivity of stimulated recall on other forms of data collection in a research design. The researcher sought to investigate whether the use of stimulated recall before a post-test would have an influence on participant performance on the post-test. The study has important implications for when stimulated recall protocols are used in experimental designs (because stimulated recall works best as soon as possible after an intervention, which is generally before post-tests are conducted). Egi (2008) found no evidence of reactivity concerns that could be attributed to the stimulus used in stimulated recall. She also found no evidence of reactivity surrounding the verbalization of thoughts by participants during data collection, concluding 'that more accurate stimulated recall comments may be gathered before the completion of post-tests without reactivity concerns' (Egi, 2008: 228).

Bowles (2010) conducted a meta-analysis of studies to explore the effects of reactivity in think alouds. Her results show that research on reactivity in L2 research mainly focused on reading tasks, and there needs to be more research into reactivity in conjunction with verbal tasks. Moreover, the issue of whether students use the L1 or L2 in the task needs to be problematized in terms of reactivity, as at the moment little is known about reactive effects of L2 proficiency in think-aloud data collection.

Thus, although researchers still need to exert caution in the design of think-aloud and stimulated recall protocols to minimize impact on the language processes being investigated, there is a lack of strong evidence for reactivity. Indeed, we would argue that carefully planned protocols can have minimal effects on the research context, so long as an argument can be made that verbalization does not impede performance of the given task. While think-aloud protocols may be useful for second language writing processes, retrospective think-aloud or stimulated recall protocols might prove more appropriate for speech production tasks. If think-aloud protocols are used during language processing tasks, then adjustments to time may be necessary to ensure participants have enough time to complete the task and pause the task for the purposes of thinking aloud.

Addition of direct measures: Eye-tracking and keystroke logging

An important innovation for introspective and retrospective research is the use of eye-tracking technology. Conklin and Pellicer-Sánchez (2016) argue that eye-tracking is becoming increasingly popular in applied linguistics research to explore topics that were traditionally done via think-aloud protocols. As they further explain:

> Many researchers interested in language processing make use of eye-tracking technology to monitor the eye when reading and when looking at a static scene or video while listening to auditory input. Eye-tracking is primarily used to detect and measure an eye's movements (saccades) and stops (fixations), as well as movements back in a text when reading (regressions). (Conklin & Pellicer-Sánchez, 2016: 454)

While eye-tracking has been used in numerous studies to provide a direct measure of learner attention during a task (e.g. Pellicer-Sánchez, 2016), the technology can be used to gather additional data to corroborate think-aloud data. For example, data collected in a think-aloud protocol could be triangulated with data collected via an eye-tracker during the think aloud to add further empirical evidence. Further to this, eye-tracking data can be used as the stimulus for stimulated recall. A study by Stickler and Shi (2017) is presented in the following section to illustrate the use of eye-tracking as stimulus.

Keystroke logging technology is a further technological innovation which allows the online tracking of writing on a computer. As Hyland (2016: 118–119) notes, 'this logs and time stamps keystrokes, pauses, cutting, pasting, and deleting and mouse activity, allowing the researcher to reconstruct text production processes'. In most applied linguistics research, keystroke logging is used as a direct measure of the writing process as a source of data collection in itself. However, there are opportunities to use keystroke logging alongside introspective data collection methods to triangulate data collection. Leijten and Van Waes (2013: 366) argue that 'the combination of observation methods opens up perspectives to deal with research questions that relate to components in the writing model that are difficult to address via keystroke logging solely'. For example, keystroke logging might be used to complement retrospective think-aloud data to confirm or refute participants' interpretations of their thoughts and actions during a task. Like the Stickler and Shi (2017) study, keystroke logs could also be used as the stimuli in stimulated recall protocols where the participant can explain to a researcher what they were doing and thinking during language production, being prompted via the keystroke log record. For a more detailed look into innovative uses of keylogging in writing research, see Leijten and Van Waes (2013).

Example studies in applied linguistics

There have been numerous studies in second language research which have used forms of introspection and retrospection. A range of studies within applied linguistics are shown in Table 3.2, including studies that primarily use think-aloud, retrospective think-aloud and stimulated recall protocols for data collection. Two of these studies, which are methodologically innovative in their combination of direct and indirect measures, are then discussed further in more detail (Schrijver, Van Vaerenbergh & Van Waes, 2012; Stickler & Shi, 2017).

In Stickler and Shi (2017), the researchers report on the use of eye-tracking alongside stimulated recall interviews in two related studies. The first study involved the use of eye-tracking to investigate reading via synchronous computer-mediated communication. The study explored the use of *pinyin* in the reading process of ten students of Chinese during an online tutorial. Videos taken from the eye-tracker were shown to the learners during a stimulated recall protocol in order to better understand the reasons why the students used the *pinyin*. The approach was complementary, in that eye-tracking data showed what the learners focused on during the tutorial, while the stimulated recall protocol allowed the researchers to understand why and how students used the *pinyin*. The second study in Stickler and Shi (2017) explored the teachers' perspective. In this study, three modern foreign language teachers taught an online language class while having their gaze tracked on the screen in a recording. Immediately after the session, each teacher 'watched the gaze plot video with a researcher, recalling what had happened, explaining, commenting and reflecting on their teaching' (Stickler & Shi, 2017: 168). The researchers conclude that the use of eye-tracking during stimulated recall is a powerful way to engage participants

Table 3.2 Examples of introspective and retrospective protocols in applied linguistics research

Researchers	Topic	Participants	Research design	Data collection method
Azaz (2017)	Meta-linguistic knowledge of grammatical feature of Arabic	English-speaking learners of Arabic ($n = 38$)	Grammatical task	Retrospective think aloud
Polio, Gass and Chappin (2006)	Native speaker perceptions in native-nonnative speaker interaction	Preservice ($n = 11$) and experienced ($n = 8$) teachers	Experiment	Stimulated recall
Schrijver, Van Vaerenbergh and Van Waes (2012)	Transediting (translation and editing)	Dutch masters-level translation students ($n = 4$)	Translation task	Think aloud with key capture
Stickler and Shi (2017)	Teachers' attention during online language tutorials	MFL teachers ($n = 3$); MFL learners ($n = 10$)	Case study; ethnography	Stimulated recall with eye-tracking
Vandergrift (2003)	Second language listening strategies	School-aged students of French ($n = 37$)	Listening tasks	Think aloud

with interpretations made regarding their thought processes, 'thereby making reflections potentially more powerful and more meaningful' (Stickler & Shi, 2017: 172).

Schrijver, Van Vaerenbergh and Van Waes (2012) used keystroke logging alongside a think-aloud protocol to examine 'transediting' (translation and editing) processes used by participants during a translation task. In this study, the participants engaged in a think-aloud protocol while writing up their translations on a computer, which was also logged via keystroke software. The researchers argue that keylogging data on their own are insufficient to understand the full picture of the writing process but used together with a think-aloud protocol provide a robust understanding of processes used when transediting. The researchers conclude that the think-aloud protocols revealed strategies in planning and revision that would have been difficult to infer from logging data alone, such as providing explanation for pauses or reasoning behind edits made. Thus, the combination of both direct and indirect measures provided a more comprehensive understanding of thought processes. For a study which uses keylogging with a retrospective think-aloud protocol, see Leijten, Van Waes and Janssen (2010).

These two studies are innovative in their combination of direct and indirect measures; however, robust data can be collected with data triangulation from other sources. For exemplary studies that use think-aloud protocols and retrospective think-aloud protocols as the main source of data collection alongside other data collection methods, see Vandergrift (2003) and Azaz (2017), respectively. For an example study which uses stimulated recall using traditional methods of video recordings, see Polio, Gass and Chappin (2006).

Implications for researchers

As much second language learning research is concerned with better understanding of language learning and language use processes, introspective data collection techniques will continue to play an important role in applied linguistics research. In terms of understanding how or why learners engage in certain cognitive behaviours, the only way to gather this data is to collect verbalized data from the learners themselves. We as a field have benefited from a number of studies that have explored the efficacy of think-aloud and stimulated recall processes as a method for conducting research (e.g. Egi, 2008; Yang, Hu & Zhang, 2014), and the results confirm the methods to be robust if applied correctly with an awareness of the protocols' strengths and limitations.

When choosing an introspective data collection method, researchers must be cognizant of the effects of the protocol on the task being researched. If verbalization is deemed to negatively affect the task, a retrospective protocol will be necessary. If time is seen to cause memory deterioration between the task and the act of retrospection, strong stimuli might be required to ensure adequate recollection of the task.

As introspective data go through two steps of interpretation (the participant's and the researcher's), steps should be taken to remove researcher bias both during data collection and during data analysis. To minimize the effect of research bias, researcher input during data collection should be minimized, and researcher interpretation during analysis should be member checked where possible. Data analysis should also consider the fact that coding of introspective data is an etic activity imposed on emic data.

Interpretations of introspective data can further be confirmed via the addition of direct measures in a study's research design to achieve data triangulation at the level of data collection. Innovations such as eye-tracking have provided new means to explore thinking processes, but they do not tell the full story of a learner's thoughts or behaviours. The best designs make use of the strengths of a combination of perspectives. Some of the more innovative research designs in applied linguistics now combine the strengths of introspective data collection with the strengths of direct measures afforded by technological advances. The innovative researcher is encouraged to continue research in this vein.

Post-reading activities

Reflect

This chapter has suggested that innovations such as eye-tracking can help to add direct measures to language processes. Gu (2014) contends that eye-tracking has shown that think-aloud protocols are a valid measure in their own right. Do you think that introspective research needs to be accompanied by direct measures such as eye-tracking?

Expand

Individually or in small groups, choose one study from Vandergrift (2003), Azaz (2017) or Polio, Gass and Chappin (2006) to read and critique. After reading, consider and discuss: (1) How appropriate was the type of introspection for the task being researched? (2) Were time, memory, researcher bias and task reactivity effects accounted for in the design? (3) Were there any aspects of the methodology which could have been improved? (4) In what ways might a direct measure have been used to triangulate the findings from the introspective data?

Apply

Design a study which explores the vocabulary listening strategies of second language English speakers taking a university-level science course in English. You are interested in discovering what students do and think about when they encounter unknown vocabulary during university lectures. Plan a procedure that would be able to collect this type of data and pay particular attention to the following decisions: What format/type of introspection/retrospection would you use? How would you ensure reliability and validity of the data?

Resources for further reading

Gass, S. M., & Mackey, A. (2017). *Stimulated recall methodology in applied linguistics and L2 research.* New York: Routledge.

This is the definitive book on the use of stimulated recall methodology for applied linguistics researchers. It builds on previous editions and similar books from these two authorities on the methodology. It provides researchers with a comprehensive guide on using stimulated recall protocols in applied linguistics and second language research, including up-to-date studies. The first two chapters explore the greater scope of introspective data collection techniques, before diving deep into stimulated recall methodology and considerations for using this method in L2 research. It includes an excellent chapter on data analysis – an area that some researchers (Gu, 2014) have observed as lacking in think-aloud literature. It also includes an up-to-date final chapter which explores the use of stimulated recall with additional forms of data collection such as eye-tracking data.

Zhang, L. & Zhang, D. (2020). Think-aloud protocols. In J. McKinley & H. Rose (Eds.), *The Routledge handbook of research methods in applied linguistics.* Abingdon: Routledge.

This chapter explores issues surrounding the use of think aloud as a research method for investigating the cognitive processes of learning. It foregrounds the debates surrounding the accuracy and reactivity of the protocol in the fields of psychology, second language education and applied linguistics. These two concerns continue to be sticking points regarding the practicality of using think-aloud protocols as a data collection research method. In this chapter, they make a convincing argument that research findings point to the utility of think aloud as a robust data collection technique if applied appropriately. In this chapter the benefits and pitfalls of think-aloud protocols are carefully scrutinized, providing clear avenues for researchers to apply the protocol successfully for the purposes of examining second or foreign language learning processes.

Bowles, M. A. (2010). *The think-aloud controversy in second language research.* New York. Routledge.

Bowles has an entire book which explores the controversies in think-aloud protocols in L2 research. The book particularly focuses on issues surrounding reactivity, which is essential reading for researchers who plan to use think-aloud protocols to explore elements involving language processing. The book also explores more general considerations of think-aloud data collection methodology, such as ethics, recording, transcriptions and coding.

4

Validated Tests and Measures

Pre-reading activities

Think
Before reading this chapter, think about your answers to the following questions: What does *validation* refer to in terms of data collection tests and measures? How do you know if a test or measure has been validated, and validated well? Where there are multiple validated tests or measures of a construct, how should you decide which one to use?

Discuss
In small groups, or as a class, discuss the following: (1) What are the advantages of using validated tests and measures to collect data about language learners? (2) In what kinds of situations might you choose *not* to use a validated test or measure? (3) Under what circumstances might you make changes to a validated test or measure?

Imagine
Imagine you are conducting a cross-sectional study examining the relationships between working memory capacity (WMC), receptive vocabulary knowledge and second language listening comprehension. You are interested in determining whether and how WMC interacts with vocabulary knowledge in predicting listening comprehension. Briefly review articles that have measured WMC and/or tested receptive vocabulary knowledge and think about the following questions: Are you able to rank the tests and measures by extent of validation? What information do the articles include that allow you to do this? Is there information that you need about the measures that is not reported in the articles?

Introduction

Validated tests and measures abound in applied linguistics research. The terms *test* and *measure* are often used synonymously; however, strictly speaking, *measure* is an umbrella term referring to any procedure designed to obtain data that enable rating or ranking of participants (e.g. a questionnaire designed to measure extent of foreign language anxiety). *Test*, on the other hand, refers to a specific type of measure, one which purports to provide an indication of a test-taker's real-world ability or competence in a particular domain (e.g. the International English Language Testing System or IELTS).

When we talk about a *validated* data collection tool, in basic terms we are referring to the existence of a convincing body of evidence that the test or measure actually does what it claims to do and that the scores or ratings it yields can be used in a meaningful way. We might assume that a test or measure used in published research has undergone a thorough process of validation, but this is not always the case. Even where validation information is in the public domain, there are differing types and degrees of validation that might indicate that one previously developed test or measure is more appropriate to use in a particular research context than another.

There are many benefits of using a validated test or measure in your research. First, doing so means that you save the time on the complicated process of creating your own. Second, using existing measures can facilitate a strong link between the research sphere in which a construct is measured (i.e. your study) and the real-world sphere in which that construct has significance, thereby enhancing the meaningfulness of the research. For example, using a validated test of second language proficiency that was developed so that scores can be mapped onto the Common European Framework of Reference (CEFR) should provide an indication of what a score means in terms of what the sample can actually do in the second language (i.e. beyond the study). Third, using a validated test or measure is a key conduit to drawing links between the findings of one study and those of other studies that have used the same or similar tests or measures: this is particularly helpful to the process of writing the discussion section of a dissertation, thesis or paper because the scores act as a lynchpin for comparison. Another benefit is that validated tests and measures have strong appeal to the general public (including potential research participants). Generally speaking, the public view validated tests as highly authoritative and important and place trust in their scores. Thus, the administration of a validated test or measure can act as an incentive for recruitment to a study because participants may be curious to find out where their scores place them according to the norm and/or scoring criteria, and can lend weight to a study's findings in the eyes of researchers, practitioners and policymakers alike.

Despite the many benefits of using a validated test or measure, they may not always be straightforward to apply in your own research. One common difficulty is that standardized measures are often proprietary (i.e. owned by a publisher) and as such to use them, you (or your institution) will need to pay for them. One such example is the Peabody Picture Vocabulary Test (PPVT), which is copyrighted by Pearson. Whether or not an existing measure is proprietary, it is crucial to read in detail articles/chapters which describe its use in empirical studies so that a judgement on the extent of the instrument's validity and reliability and its applicability to your study can be made. Sometimes, scholars do not describe in detail their process of instrument development and validation – most likely to due to limited word count in published materials – and thus it may be necessary to read a large amount of material (and in some cases to contact the original author directly) in order to obtain the requisite information. Furthermore, it is fair to say that the majority of validated tests and measures of linguistic knowledge pertain to knowledge of English: for example, while standardized tests of L2-English vocabulary size abound, comparatively few exist to measure L2-Mandarin lexical knowledge. Similarly, the lion's share of psychometric measures (e.g. questionnaires measuring attitudes/motivation/anxiety) has been developed and published in English. As such, if the language of focus in a particular study is not English, or if your sample is not proficient in English, it may be necessary to translate existing measures, which is not a straightforward endeavour.

This chapter lays the theoretical groundwork for using validated tests and measures, outlining key concepts and issues before showcasing examples of sound use of validated tests and measures in applied linguistics research.

Key concepts

In this section, we explore the fundamental concepts underpinning the use of validated tests and measures in applied linguistics research.

Types of tests and measures

There are a number of different ways in which validated tests and measures are classified. *Psychometric measures* – such as aptitude tests and IQ tests – are for the most part designed to measure the extent to which an individual has a particular characteristic in order to distinguish individual differences among a sample. *Edumetric measures*, on the other hand, are designed to measure changes in knowledge, skills or ability, usually as a result of intervention (such as second language instruction or naturalistic exposure to a target language).

In *direct tests*, respondents are required to engage directly in the behaviour that is being tested. For example, a test of oral communicative competence in which the respondent must carry out a speaking task with someone else is a direct test. If oral communicative competence is tested via a discourse completion task (i.e. responding in writing to 'what would you say in this situation?'-type questions), then it is an *indirect test*, because the test-taker is not actually engaging in oral communication. Direct tests have more *ecological validity* than indirect tests because their scores/results can be better generalized to real-world skills and situations.

Tests and measures can also be classified by *test format* (e.g. multiple choice, cloze, free-write), which is intricately linked to how items in a measure are marked/scored. Some measures utilize *subjective scoring* (i.e. scoring determined by the subjective judgement of humans) with examiners receiving training on how to match test-taker performance to a rating scale or a set of marking criteria. For example, in the IELTS speaking test the examiner listens to the test-taker's spoken production and gives them a score between levels 1 and 9 in four key areas using descriptors that describe what the test-taker should be able to do at each level. A more restricted type of subjective scoring is the *partial credit model*, whereby the examiner makes a judgement about the value of a response (e.g. 'perfect' = two points; 'acceptable' = one point; 'unacceptable' = zero points). For example, C-tests of language proficiency (a specific type of cloze test in which parts of a text are erased consistent with a fixed rule) often apply a partial credit scoring method. In objective scoring, only one possible response is deemed correct. For example, if an examiner (or machine) is marking a multiple-choice test, they follow a key of correct answers in doing so. Keep in mind, though, that even objectively scored tests carry a modicum of subjectivity in that the test developer has themselves decided what constitutes the correct answer.

Going beyond the scoring of individual test items, it is also pertinent to consider how the overall score on a test is expressed. Some tests' overall scores are *criterion-referenced*, meaning that scores are reported as an indication that the test-taker has achieved a given level in the ability being tested against a set of criteria (as in the IELTS). Other tests' scores are *norm-referenced*, whereby a score places the test-taker in a rank order of all other takers of that particular test. For example, the Test of English for International Communication (TOEIC) expresses test-takers' norm-referenced scores as percentiles, so if a learner scores in the ninetieth percentile, they have outperformed 90 per cent of the people who took TOEIC within a given time period.

Another way of categorizing measures is via the ways in which their scores are used. The outcomes of *high-stakes tests* are used to make important decisions about test-takers, such as whether they gain entry to a particular institution, organization or position. The ramifications of high-stakes testing can therefore be very serious, resulting in penalties, restrictions and/or loss of status (e.g. job loss, educational grade repetition). The results of *low-stakes tests*, on the other hand, do not carry critical consequences and are usually only of importance to the individual student, the teacher (e.g. as a means of formative assessment) or the researcher (e.g. as a contribution to their dataset).

Validity

Validity is arguably the most important feature of any test or measure. Deriving from the Latin *validus*, meaning 'strong', *validity* pertains to the ability and appropriacy of a measure actually to test the construct it is intended to, in the context in and for the purpose it is used. Validity is important because without it, we are unable to trust in the results of the test or measure and nor, therefore, in any inferences made about a respondent based on his or her scores. Validation of a test or measure involves a process of evidence accumulation over time: there are many different types of validity, each of which can be determined in different ways (see 'Procedures and practicalities' section) to establish the extent of the evidence of validity (rather than to yield one specific value).

Reliability

Reliability refers to the consistency and stability of a measure. Reliability is crucial, but not sufficient, to attaining validity (Robson, 2002) in that reliability is a type of validity evidence. Bryman (2016) divides reliability into three facets: (1) *stability*, whereby if the same measure is administered to participants at different times (to investigate a stable construct, e.g. language aptitude), the results should not vary; (2) *internal reliability/ consistency*, pertaining to the notion that the items in a measure should be related to each other and indicative of what the researcher is measuring; and (3) *inter-observer consistency* (*inter-rater reliability*), whereby when an element of subjectivity exists in the test scoring procedure, using more than one observer/rater and then calculating the consistency between the observers' ratings can go some way to cancelling it out. Threats to reliability as noted by Robson (2002) include *participant error* (e.g. the performance of a participant on a measure may vary due to, for example, fatigue or illness) and *participant bias* (when participants modify their responses in some way because they know they are being studied and want to give a certain impression). Additionally, *rater error* and *rater bias* may occur for similar reasons.

Procedures and practicalities

In this section, we focus on the processes and procedures inherent in using validated tests and measures in applied linguistics research. We look at how to find and select measures, when and how to adapt them, how to administer them and how to analyse data yielded via them.

Finding validated tests and measures

The first step in deciding whether to use a validated test or measure is to gather information about existing measures that have been developed to address the construct of interest and to inspect the measures themselves. Finding a copy of a validated test or measure is not always as straightforward as one might expect: while standardized measures can usually be obtained from the publisher (typically at a price) or via your institution library (if an institutional licence is held), it is often the case that full versions of the tests or measures used in empirical studies and reported in journal articles are not published as part of the article (e.g. in the appendices). If this is the case, it is worthwhile consulting online repositories of research instruments, such as IRIS (https://www.iris-database.org/) and MIDISS (http://www.midss.org/). If it is not possible to find a particular measure in the library or online, then the developer of the measure can be contacted directly to ask if they are willing to share a copy. Researchers are generally open to this kind of request because it means that their measure is having an impact beyond their own research.

Choosing validated tests and measures

Where there are multiple validated measures of a construct from which to choose, selecting a measure can be challenging. As Alderson and Banerjee (2002: 82) state, 'Most published studies of language test development are somewhat censored accounts, which stress the positive features of the tests rather than addressing problems in development or construct definition or acknowledging the limitations of the published results.' However, when faced with incomplete or euphemistic information about a particular measure there are some key criteria that can be applied to help decide if it is the right choice for a particular study. According to Bachman and Palmer (1996), there are six important questions to consider:

1 Is the measure *reliable*? Reliability here pertains to measurement (in)consistency. That is, if test item A and test item B are designed to measure the same skill or knowledge domain, and these two items differ in only incidental ways, then the score a test-taker obtains should be the same for both items.

2 Does the measure have *construct validity*? This question speaks to how well the scores from a test indicate test-takers' skills or ability as regards the construct that the test purports to measure. Is the test really measuring what it claims to? Is the current theoretical understanding of the construct accurately and comprehensively addressed in the measure? A test of language proficiency, for example, has low construct validity if it fails to measure things we know contribute to proficiency (e.g. speaking competence, listening comprehension).

3 Is the measure authentic? In other words, to what extent do the tasks in the test correspond to things L2 users actually have to do in the target language? *Authenticity* is an important quality for a measure to have because it allows researchers to generalize score interpretations beyond the test itself and say what they mean a respondent can do with language in real life.

4 Is the measure *interactive*? 'Interaction' in this context refers to interaction between the individual and the task: to what extent do the test tasks draw on test-takers' knowledge/ability? Their topical knowledge (i.e. of real-word situations)? Their affective schemata (e.g. is this type of task motivating for the individuals it is designed to test)?

5 Will the measure have *impact*? Tests have impact at the macro level (e.g. society, educational systems) and at the micro level (i.e. on individuals). As such, care must be taken to consider exactly what impact the use of a test in a given context might have. At the micro level, these kinds of questions might include: (how) will feedback be given to test-takers, and how might this feedback affect them? What decisions will be made about test-takers based on their scores? How might these decisions influence them?

6 Is the measure *practical*? This criterion is critical for researchers: it asks whether more resources (e.g. time, money, people, materials) are required to design, develop and/or use the test than are available. If so, the test is not practical and the researcher should look elsewhere.

Bachman and Palmer (1996) recommend that evaluation of the usefulness of a particular test in a particular context should be based on the combined effect of these criteria, as opposed to considering their effects independently of one another. They do not indicate whether any one criterion should carry more weight than another in a given situation as this balance is likely to shift depending on the testing aims and context.

Once a researcher has chosen a test or measure to use in their research, they will need to check that they have consent to use it: if the measure is in the public domain (e.g. in an online repository, in a library), then it is usually openly available for use so long as the developer(s) is cited appropriately. If the measure is not in the public domain, researchers should contact the developer to obtain their written permission to use it in their research. This can be daunting especially if the developer is a 'big name' or someone they have never met, but researchers are generally very keen for their instruments to be used and developed and will readily give their consent (and sometimes also some very useful tips).

To adopt or to adapt? That is the question

Validated tests and measures may either be administered in their original form or adapted in some way to better suit the context and population of a study. *Test adaptation* may be necessary for a variety of reasons. For example, if a researcher intends on administering a battery of measures to their sample in one testing session, they may decide to truncate some measures as a means of combating participant fatigue. Likewise, some test items may be inappropriate for a different population; for example, a test of L2-English vocabulary that includes American English words (e.g. diaper, sidewalk) will not be appropriate for learners of English varieties that do not share those words (e.g. British English). It is important to note that if a researcher alters a validated test or measure in any way for use in their own research, investigating and thoroughly reporting the reliability and validity of the adapted measure is imperative (see 'Data analysis' section).

The most common way in which tests and measures are adapted in applied linguistics research is via *translation*. It is fair to say that the vast majority of validated tests and measures are developed in English, and this means that if a scholar is researching a population which does not have strong proficiency in English, the respondents' (possibly inaccurate) comprehension of the items is a threat to reliability in the study. Translation is an available option to combat this threat. However, constructs can vary in meaning across cultures. Therefore, a key first step is to consult experts who know both languages and both cultures well to ascertain from them whether the definition of the key construct and its associated terms in the original instrument have exactly the same meaning in the target language and culture. If so, then there is a strong argument for translating the measure. If not, a researcher may need to look for instruments developed in the target language to measure the culture-specific meaning of the construct of interest or to develop their own measure in that language.

Once a preliminary *forward translation* has been done (by someone who knows both the target language and culture well), it can be checked by another translator and any disagreement between them on the accuracy of the translations can be discussed and resolved. Then *backtranslation* (that is, translating the measure back from the target language to the original language) can be carried out (ideally by a third translator) to ensure that the meaning and difficulty of the items have been maintained across versions. The advantage of backtranslation is that if the researcher is not proficient in the target language, they are still able to judge the comparability of the two original-language versions. Hambleton and Zenisky (2011) proffer a useful checklist of questions to consider at this stage, which were compiled from common problems that arise in practice. Finally, we recommend thorough *piloting* of the translated version prior to its use in any study: the pilot sample needs to be as closely matched to the main study sample as possible, and the pilot data should be analysed for reliability and validity (see 'Data analysis' section).

Data analysis

Depending on whether and to what extent a researcher has adapted a validated test or measure, they may need to carry out *a priori analysis* (i.e. analyses carried out on pilot data before administration of the measure in the main study). One commonly used type of a priori analysis is *item analysis*, whereby individual test items are scrutinized to ascertain how they are performing in terms of their difficulty (item facility*)* and their ability to discriminate between test-takers who perform well and less well on the test overall (item discrimination). *Item facility* is an index of the proportion of test-takers who gave the correct response to a test item. To calculate item facility, the sum of correct responses to that item is divided by the total number of test-takers, and the statistic yielded is known as the p value. A p value of 0 denotes that nobody answered the item correctly and a p value of 1 denotes that all test-takers responded correctly. Item facility at these extremes tells us that the item is not measuring individual differences (e.g. L2 proficiency) so may not be appropriate to include in the test. Generally speaking, p values in the middle third (i.e. 0.33–0.67) are acceptable, unless the item is measuring a highly specific feature of knowledge or where the test developer deliberately wishes to include items that are less or more challenging. It should be noted that item facility values are only relevant where the pilot sample is truly representative of the main study population (Fulcher & Davidson, 2007).

The proportion of correct responses to an item is a function not only of the item difficulty but also of the skill, knowledge and/or ability of the test-taker. *Item discrimination* is therefore useful in a priori analysis because it reveals how individuals who performed well or less well on the test overall responded to a particular item. There are a variety of formulae for calculating item discrimination. One method is to take a percentage of the high and low scoring participants on the test overall – usually around 28 per cent from both ends of the spectrum (Henning, 1987), although this proportion may be lowered for a large population. Item discrimination is then calculated by taking the number of correct responses to an item by the high group only and dividing this number by the sum of the number of correct responses to the item by the high and low groups combined. In this method, any item scoring <0.67 should be rewritten (and re-piloted) or excluded from the test. Fulcher and Davidson (2007: 103) outline a different method whereby point-biserial correlation is used to calculate item discrimination: this method yields the correlation between test-takers' responses to a given item and the total scores on all other test items with correlations of $r > 0.25$ considered acceptable.

If a test or measure employs *multiple-choice format* items, another form of a priori item analysis available is *option analysis* (also termed *distractor evaluation*). Option analysis reveals the percentage of test-takers who select each option in the multiple choice format, and can be calculated via a simple frequency table. If very few test-takers select a particular distractor, this means that the option is implausible and should be rewritten or replaced (and re-piloted) or removed.

A posteriori analyses are conducted after a researcher has administered the final version of the measure in the main study and serve to monitor the validity and reliability of the test and its items in the operational phase. There are a range of a posteriori analyses that can be performed to yield evidence of the validity of a test or measure. To establish *content validity*, which refers to the extent to which the items in a measure adequately represent the theoretical representation(s) of the construct being measured, researchers can employ *expert review*, whereby subject matter experts are tasked with reviewing the measure and flagging up items that might need to be added, omitted or modified. Expert review is therefore particularly useful when researchers have modified a validated test or measure.

Construct validity of a test or measure, which is the extent to which the measure represents an unobservable variable (i.e. the construct of focus), cannot be fully established in one study because it entails an accumulation of evidence over time and across research settings. There are, however, a number of analyses that can be carried out that will assess validity and contribute to this accumulation of evidence. *Group differences analyses* involve sampling two or more groups of people who can reasonably be expected to differ on the construct, and then comparing their scores (e.g. using *t*-tests or ANOVAs). For example, on a test of L2 receptive vocabulary size, one would expect a group of learners who have had 10 years of L2 instruction to significantly outperform a group of learners who started L2 instruction less than a year ago. *Correlation matrices* and *factor analysis* (explanatory or confirmatory) are also useful means of exploring construct validity: if a researcher is using a validated test or measure, they may wish to use *confirmatory factor analysis* (a type of *structural equation model*) to determine whether the factor structure in their data corresponds to theory and matches the structure found in other studies that have used the same measure. Such analyses require a large sample size, so researchers intending to apply this type of analysis to their data must be sure to conduct the relevant power calculations in advance of their data collection to ensure they have adequate power.

Convergence and *divergence* are other means of establishing construct validity and are particularly useful where more than one means of measuring a given construct are employed. *Convergent validity* deals with the extent to which scores from one measure converge on scores from different types of measures of the same construct or other constructs which are, or should be, theoretically linked. For example, if a researcher measured L2 vocabulary via a size test and via analysis of the lexical diversity/density/sophistication of spoken production data, they would expect scores from these two measures to be highly correlated. *Divergent validity* (sometimes termed *discriminant validity*) techniques take the opposite approach, whereby correlations with scores from measures of theoretically unrelated constructs are computed, and insignificant correlations taken as evidence of validity.

Criterion-based procedures also contribute to construct validity. In *criterion validity*, a well-established test or measure is used as a comparison point (the criterion) against which scores from another test or measure can be assessed. Therefore, criterion validity is particularly helpful to establish where a researcher has adapted a validated test or measure. The two types of criterion validity are concurrent and predictive validity: *concurrent validity* is assessed through the simultaneous administration of the two measures of the same construct. If the scores on the measures correlate well, evidence for concurrent validity is established. For *predictive validity*, the adapted measure is not administered simultaneously to but rather sometime after the criterion measure with correlation used to determine whether the results of the first measure are able to predict with some strength the results of the second.

There are also various means by which the reliability of a measure can be explored in the data analysis phase. The statistical test usually used to measure *stability (test-retest reliability)* is *Pearson's correlation coefficient*: to establish stability, a measure can be administered to the same group of people on two different occasions and the scores from time one and time two correlated. If there is a significant correlation ($p < 0.05$), then there is evidence pointing to stability of the measure. Internal reliability (or internal consistency) is usually established using *Cronbach's alpha coefficient* (α), a statistical value which establishes the degree of correlation between participants' responses. The alpha statistic is applied to groups of items that measure the same construct so if a researcher is using a questionnaire that yields scores on two different things (e.g. anxiety and self-efficacy), they should calculate the alpha for each scale separately. There is a lack of agreement over what is deemed an acceptable level of internal reliability, although as a rule of thumb, the higher the value, the better. Some scholars have posited that $\alpha > 0.7$ is acceptable (e.g. Nunnally & Bernstein, 1994), with $\alpha > 0.8$ considered a good level. If $\alpha = 0.7$, this means that 30 per cent of the variability in the scores is a result of random error and 70 per cent is due to true individual differences between respondents. The more variability explained by individual differences, the better. Yet, recent work in L2 research (e.g. Brown, 2014; Plonsky & Derrick, 2016) suggests that consistency estimates vary according to a number of factors, such as the reliability index used, the L2 proficiency of the sample, the skill or domain being tested, or features of the instrument employed. As such, we recommend that internal reliability values are interpreted with reference to the broader field of research that has measured similar constructs in a similar way and among comparable populations.

Correlation can also be used to explore the internal consistency of a measure. *Average inter-item correlation* involves isolating all items that measure the same construct (e.g. anxiety) and correlating scores for every pair of these items (e.g. item 1 → item 2; item 2 → item 3, item 3 → item 1) and then taking the average of these paired correlations to find the average inter-item correlation. A further correlational option is *split-half reliability*: this calculation determines whether there is a statistically significant relationship between scores on two halves of items that measure the same construct. Let's say an instrument has six items to measure anxiety: to determine split-half reliability the researcher would administer the complete measure to a group of people and then calculate the overall score for items 1–3 (the first set) and the overall score for items 4–6 (the second set). The correlation between set one and set two is then calculated, thus yielding the split-half reliability statistic.

Inter-rater reliability, which is the degree to which different raters' or observers' scores converge, can be assessed via a number of different indices and can be calculated on most statistical packages (e.g. SPSS). If a study employs only two raters, the most straightforward means of expressing inter-rater reliability is to report the percentage of agreement between them. However, this method, termed *joint-probability of agreement*, is subject to the number of categories the raters use to judge the participants' responses: if there are only two or three categories, then the percentage of agreement will be higher due to chance. To overcome this, another option is *Cohen's kappa* (for two fixed raters) or *Fleiss' kappa* (for 3+ raters who are randomly sampled from a population of raters), in which agreement due to chance is factored out. If the rating data are ordinal (e.g. derived from a Likert-type scale), then it is appropriate to use a *weighted kappa* statistic or a *Spearman rank-order correlation*. If a researcher has continuous data (i.e. interval or ratio variables), Pearson correlation coefficients can be calculated (See Chapter 8 for a detailed discussion of types of variables). If the data are grouped (e.g. if the raters did not all rate the same participants' responses), then *intra-class correlation* can be used. It should be noted that while correlation is a useful and common means of calculating inter-rater reliability, a correlation coefficient does not indicate the extent to which raters' scores match but rather the extent of their parallel variation.

Writing up

Even when researchers have used a validated test or measure that is extremely well known in the field, they must include the relevant information about the measure in the write-up of the study. In the Methodology section of the dissertation, thesis or paper it is customary to state who developed the instrument and when, to describe how it has been validated and shown to be reliable (reporting past studies' Cronbach's alpha statistic is not uncommon), and to outline the populations and samples with whom the measure has been used to date. If a researcher has adapted the instrument in any way, description of and justification for every alteration must be provided, accompanied by a detailed reporting of the investigations into the validity and reliability of the adapted measure.

Improving reliability and validity

Now that we have explored some of the practicalities of using validated tests and measures, our attention turns to specific means by which researchers can improve the validity and reliability of measures they employ in their research.

It is vital that the administration of a validated test or measure is done in such a way that the validity and reliability of the measure are maximized. At the most basic level, this denotes that measures should be administered to all respondents in the same way, ideally at the same time of day and under *test conditions* (i.e. in a quiet place free from distractions and external sources of information and, where necessary/possible, under the watchful eye of an invigilator). It may be possible to test multiple participants simultaneously, which is ideal in terms of time efficiency, but doing so may pose a threat to validity and reliability if large groups are likely to distract one another from the task at hand. It is a good idea to consult previous research which has used the measure to determine whether it is appropriate to administer in groups. If it is, careful consideration should be given to seating arrangements in the room, such that it is not possible for one participant's responses to influence another's.

Instructions to test-takers should be explicit and clear (ideally presented in the L1 or both the L1 and L2): *piloting* is instrumental in determining whether participants are easily able to understand the task or are spending valuable test time trying to work out what they have to do. Individual test items should also be unambiguous, which is another possible threat to reliability that piloting will help to assuage. If the format of the measure is unfamiliar to the sample population, the researcher might consider including an example item at the start of the test (or at the start of specific sections of the test) so that participants are acclimatized to the task in advance of providing data that will be included in the analyses.

Where the scoring procedure for a measure involves an element of subjectivity or inference (e.g. a direct test of speaking proficiency), researchers may consider providing raters with training, standardization procedures and/ or detailed score descriptors. In any measure where scoring is subjective, multiple blind ratings of data should be utilized (and inter-rater reliability calculated), and it is recommended that test-takers' data are labelled by number rather than name, such that any *implicit bias* on the part of raters is mitigated. Raters should be randomly assigned to data and participants, and the outcome of the random allocation checked to ensure no patterns have emerged by chance (e.g. female raters rating only female participants' data).

Case studies of validated tests and measures in applied linguistics research

Such is the prevalence of validated tests and measures in applied linguistics research that there is a wealth of high-quality studies from which to choose

Table 4.1 Examples of validated tests and measures in applied linguistics research

Researchers	Topic	Participants	Research design	Data collection method
Briggs (2015)	Vocabulary gain during study abroad	Adult ESL learners in the UK ($n = 241$)	Longitudinal; repeated measures; multiple regression	Vocabulary Levels Tests
Jin and Dewaele (2018)	The relationships between a positive outlook, perceived English teach/peer support and foreign language anxiety	Chinese ESL university students ($n = 144$)	Cross-sectional; regression	Foreign Language Classroom Anxiety Scale (FLCAS)
Khabbazbashi (2017)	The effects of background knowledge and topic in high-stakes speaking tests	Adult L1-Farsi EFL learners in Iran ($n = 81$)	Cross-sectional; parallel forms test administration	IELTS speaking tasks; C-test of L2-English proficiency
McCray and Brunfaut (2018)	Processing and performance in gap-fill tasks	L1 and L2 users of English at a UK university ($n = 28$)	Cross-sectional; eye-tracking; correlation	Pearson Test of English (PTE) Academic
Saito, Suzukida and Sun (2019)	The influence of aptitude on the development of L2 pronunciation	L1-Japanese EFL university students ($n = 40$)	Longitudinal; repeated measures	The LLAMA aptitude tests
Smith, Briggs Pothier and Garcia (2019)	The environmental and individual factors that contribute to executive function diversity	Spanish-English bilingual young adults in the US ($n = 50$)	Cross-sectional; regression	Delis–Kaplan Executive Function System (D-KEFS) trail-making and colour-word inhibition subtests
Vandergrift and Baker (2018)	The variables that determine L2 listening success	L1-English child learners of L2-French in an immersion programme in Canada ($n = 84$)	Cross-sectional; regression	The Peabody Picture Vocabulary Test (PPVT); Échelle de vocabulaire en images Peabody (ÉVIP)

as case studies. To narrow the scope, we have selected a collection of studies that showcase the measurement of a range of key variables in applied linguistics, which are detailed in Table 4.1. From this selection, we choose two to focus on in more detail.

The Khabbazbashi (2017) and McCray and Brunfaut (2018) studies illustrate the use of high-stakes language tests in applied linguistics research. Khabbazbashi (2017) sought to determine the extent to which scores on the IELTS speaking module are affected by task topic and test-takers' background knowledge. To do this, she administered a C-test (to measure general English language proficiency) and a questionnaire (measuring background knowledge) to a sample of eighty-one L1-Farsi L2-English learners in Iran. Two parallel versions of an IELTS speaking test (each comprising five topics) were administered under test conditions and rated by four trained raters using the IELTS speaking band descriptors. Data were analysed using Rasch and regression modelling. McCray and Brunfaut (2018) used eye-tracking methodology to investigate whether learners' processing of gap-filled text is related to levels of performance. They employed the Pearson Test of English (PTE) Academic, which is a standardized, computer-based measure of academic English covering the CEFR A1–C2 range (i.e. from beginner to advanced proficiency), and tracked the sample's eye movements as they completed the gap-fill tasks. The task items were dichotomously scored and correlated with seven variables derived from the eye-tracking data. Results indicated that low scorers on the test tended to rely more on lower level cognitive processes when completing the task.

Briggs (2015) and Vandergrift and Baker (2018) are included as examples of studies that have utilized validated measures of L2 vocabulary knowledge. Briggs (2015) used versions of the Vocabulary Levels Tests (Laufer & Nation, 1999; Nation, 1990) to measure the receptive and productive lexical gains of 241 adult study abroad learners in the UK. Vandergrift and Baker (2018) employed the PPVT and its French equivalent, the Échelle de vocabulaire en images Peabody (ÉVIP) to investigate the role of L1 and L2 vocabulary knowledge (among a wealth of other variables) in L2 listening success among children enrolled in a French immersion programme in Canada. The PPVT and ÉVIP present target words orally (thus corresponding to the skill of listening) and respondents indicate their knowledge of meaning by selecting the corresponding picture from a choice of four. As such, these tests were administered individually to each of the eighty-four children in the sample.

The final three studies, Saito, Suzukida and Sun (2019), Smith, Briggs, Pothier and Garcia (2019), and Jin and Dewaele (2018), are showcased as examples of applied linguistics research that makes use of standardized measures of individual and group differences: language aptitude, executive function and anxiety, respectively. Saito, Suzukida and Sun (2019) explored the influence of aptitude and L2 learning experience on the development of L2 pronunciation among Japanese EFL students. An oral picture description task was administered three times over an academic year with data analysed for pronunciation proficiency. Participants took three subtests from the LLAMA aptitude test battery (Meara, 2005) after the third oral production task and completed an L2 learning experience questionnaire. Analyses revealed that aptitude uniquely predicted pronunciation gains between the three time points. The Smith, Briggs, Pothier and Garcia (2019) study sought to determine the variables that explain differences in executive function (i.e. cognitive control) among a homogeneous sample of Spanish-English bilinguals in the United States. To measure executive function, the researchers utilized the Delis–Kaplan Executive Function System trail-making and colour-word inhibition subtests, which measure a range of cognitive abilities (e.g., inhibition, flexibility, switching). Scores on these tests were explored via regression modelling in light of a range of possible control and predictor variables – many of which were also measured via administration of standardized tests – including working memory capacity, reading comprehension, non-verbal IQ and language contact. The test battery in this study was administered via Pearson Q-Active tablet, which enabled fast and accurate administration of the many measures employed, as well as real-time scoring.

Jin and Dewaele's (2018) study explored the relationships between a positive disposition, perceived support from teachers and student peers, and foreign language classroom anxiety among English language majors at a university in China. They administered a Chinese translation of the Foreign Language Classroom Anxiety Scale and questionnaire-based measures of positivity and perceived support.

We choose now to showcase two studies to focus on in detail, both of which are longitudinal in design: one employed two validated measures of L2 vocabulary size (Briggs, 2015) and one used three validated measures of language aptitude (Saito, Suzukida & Sun, 2019).

Briggs (2015): A longitudinal study of vocabulary acquisition during study abroad

Briggs (2015) used the Vocabulary Levels Tests (Laufer & Nation, 1999; Nation, 1990) to measure the receptive and productive lexical gains of 241 adult study abroad learners in the UK and analysed these data against responses to a questionnaire that probed her sample's contact with and use of English outside of the classroom during their sojourn in the UK. She hypothesized that (1) the sample would make lexical gains during their stay in the UK and (2) that the type and amount of contact with English experienced by the sample would be predictive of their gains. While the sample did improve their vocabulary size (particularly those who stayed in the UK for a longer period of time), Briggs's second hypothesis was not borne out, possibly as a function of her participants engaging most frequently in L2 contact situations that were not facilitative of varied lexical input or opportunities for production of newly encountered lexis. It is possible that testing only one facet of vocabulary knowledge (size) may have obscured any relationship between language contact and gain in this study: one could argue that depth and/or automaticity of knowledge is influenced by experience in the target language community – something only a more comprehensive battery of vocabulary tests could reveal.

To enhance reliability, Briggs (2015) administered the Levels Tests under test conditions and randomized the test items for the time two administration to mitigate any practice effect. She concedes that an L2–L1 translation test is a more reliable means of measuring knowledge of the form-meaning link than the L2-only tests that she employed but highlights that with a sample of various L1s, L2-only testing was the only feasible option. The receptive Levels Test data were marked solely by the researcher because there is only one possible correct answer for each lexical item in this multiple-choice test. The productive Levels Test data were double-blind marked by the researcher and an inter-rater and Cohen's kappa statistic reported as evidence of inter-rater reliability.

Saito, Suzukida and Sun (2019): Language aptitude and L2 pronunciation development

Saito, Suzukida and Sun (2019) selected three of the LLAMA aptitude tests for use in their study because these tests use natural language (a Central-American language and a British-Columbian indigenous language) rather than symbols and digits and are therefore a more ecologically valid test of aptitude for learning a second or additional language. In order to enhance reliability in the data collection phase, the authors administered the aptitude tests in a specific order designed to prevent participants from guessing the purpose of the tests and thereby to preclude any effects of explicit or intentional learning. Scores on the tests were converted into z scores: the z score is a means of standardizing scores whereby the mean score is subtracted from the individual score, and this figure is then divided by the standard deviation. This allows individual scores from different normal distributions to be compared. Saito, Suzukida and Sun (2019) used the z scores to calculate correlations between scores on the three tests and found no statistically significant relationships between them: the authors use this finding as evidence of validity, given that Meara (2005) posits that each subtest in LLAMA measures a different cognitive construct (phonemic coding, associative memory, sound sequence recognition).

One possible issue with the validity of the use of the LLAMA subtests in this study relates to LLAMA-B, which is a test of associative memory. In LLAMA-B, respondents are visually presented with a large number of lexical strings and their corresponding visual representations and are tasked with memorizing these paired associates. Then, twenty strings are selected at random and the test-taker must match the strings with their paired visual. There is a mismatch, therefore, between the target word presentation in LLAMA-B (visual) and the predominant focus of the study (pronunciation development). However, Saito, Suzukida and Sun (2019) found that associative memory as measured by LLAMA-B weakly predicted prosody and fluency development between the first two time points of data collection (i.e. over one academic semester) and the authors use this finding as justification for their employment of the test in two ways: they state that (1) the relationship found between associative memory and fluency adheres to theory, specifically Skehan's (2016) aptitude-acquisition model, and that (2) even non-linguistic tests of cognitive ability have been found to predict L2 phonological competence. Thus, justifications for the construct validity of LLAMA-B in Saito, Suzukida and Sun (2019) were established both pre and post the data collection phase.

Implications for researchers

One key implication from the discussion in this chapter is that when a validated test or measure is used – even without being adapted in any way – the researcher is in a position to contribute to the accumulation of evidence as regards its validity and reliability. It may be that the test or measure adopted has never been used in the new research context before or that it is being used with a new research population. If so, the researcher is obliged not only to draw on previous studies' use of the measure to justify its validity and reliability a priori the data collection (i.e. in the Methodology section) but also to present results from the study that speak to the validity and reliability of the measure in the new research context (i.e. in the Findings section). If researchers make fundamental adaptations to a measure for use in their study, then the process of accumulating validation evidence for that adaptation begins with the study itself: if they are able to provide clear evidence in the study that the adaptation is valid and reliable, then it is more likely that other researchers will use the adapted measure and thus further contribute to the evidence of its validity, and so on and so forth.

It is also important to note that there is no 'perfect' measure of any construct, regardless of its strength of reliability and validity: no test or questionnaire is above critique (and even if a perfect test existed methodologically, the very act of 'objectively' measuring constructs such as 'L2 proficiency' can be questioned from an ontological and epistemological perspective). As outlined in Chapter 1, measures of a dependent variable are almost always proxy measures of the true constructs of interest to the researcher. So, just as important as generating evidence for the validity of a given measure is the careful consideration of the limitations of that measure. Limitations may be addressed in the study design phase (e.g. planning to collect data about a construct via more than one means) and/or at the writing-up stage (e.g. including balanced critique of the measure(s) in the 'Methodological Limitations' section), but they must be considered in recognition of the fact that as social science researchers we often deal with nebulous constructs and rely upon human interpretation, and therefore our measurement of the world around us may be subject to imprecision and construal.

Post-reading activities

Reflect

This chapter has suggested that a lack of clarity in test instructions and/or items is a threat to the validity and reliability of a test or measure. Under what circumstances might you use a test or measure that is written in your participants' L2? What conditions would need to be met for you to be confident that doing so would not threaten the validity and reliability of your data collection?

Expand

Individually or in small groups, choose one of the studies in Table 4.1 to read and critique. After reading, consider and discuss: (1) Which of the measures employed in the study are validated measures? How do you know they are validated measures? (2) What (if any) information do the authors provide to assert the validity and reliability of the measure(s) they used? (3) Were there any aspects of the methodology which could have been a threat to validity and/ or reliability?

Apply

Design a longitudinal study to investigate the effects of a 3-month study abroad period in the UK on adult L1-Thai L2-English learners' receptive vocabulary size. You intend on measuring vocabulary size at the beginning and end of the study abroad period. Review the literature on testing vocabulary and make a list of possible validated tests of L2-English receptive vocabulary size. Consider the following questions: which test is best suited to your study and population, and why? What (if any) adaptations might you make to your chosen test for administration in this study, and why? How and where would you administer this measure? How might your data contribute to the accumulation of evidence supporting this test as a valid and reliable measure of L2-English vocabulary size?

Resources for further reading

Fulcher, G., & Davidson, F. (2007). *Language testing and assessment: An advanced resource book*. Abingdon: Routledge.

This book is an excellent resource for any student or researcher wishing to develop theoretical and practical knowledge of language testing and assessment. Divided into three sections (introduction, extension, exploration), the volume examines a broad range of topics in depth from test development and classroom-based assessment to validity and testing ethics. Interspersed throughout each section are a number of activities and reflective tasks designed to develop practical skills and aid understanding of the key concepts.

O'Sullivan, B. (Ed.) (2011). *Language testing: Theories and practices.* Basingstoke, UK: Palgrave Macmillan.

This edited volume is written for research students and independent researchers who are interested in language testing theory and practice. The chapters offer a broad range of perspectives on language testing across four key themes: language testing theory, the application language testing theory, language test development and language test use. The final two chapters (which focus on language test use) are of particular relevance to the present chapter and include a useful discussion of the employment of validated tests and measures alongside more qualitative means of data collection.

5

Observations

Pre-reading activities

Think
Before reading this chapter, think about your answers to the following questions: (1) What are the advantages of using observations to investigate various aspects of language education? (2) Are there any aspects of language learning that this data collection technique could prove quite useful? (3) How about for other areas of enquiry in applied linguistics?

Discuss
As we read earlier in Chapter 1, there are different ways a researcher can position themselves in field research from a complete participant to a detached observer. In small groups, or as a class, discuss the following:

- How should the researchers position themselves in relation to those being observed? Why?
- Are there any types of research where one approach would be better than another?
- What should a researcher do before evaluating what they observe?

Imagine
Imagine you are investigating the language used during legal consultations between solicitors and clients in a free community legal centre. You want to investigate differences in talk time, turn-taking and the use of legal jargon between lawyers when conversing with native- and nonnative-speaking clients. Due to ethical reasons you cannot record the sessions so need to observe the consultations in real time. How will you ensure accuracy of data collection during the observation and minimize your bias in recording the data? How could you minimize your impact on the observed setting?

Introduction

Observations in social research are the actions of watching, recording and, in qualitative approaches, interpreting and reflecting on human activity and behaviour. In applied linguistics research, they are naturally occurring ethnographic activities often situated in the theorizing and sensitizing stages (e.g. 'I noticed the students are struggling with this'; 'The language on these warning signs must be unclear'). As a data collection method, they can sometimes be oversimplified and undervalued. For example, in mixed methods studies, the observation might be reduced to a method used only to provide a description of the research setting or as the basis for generating the research question. But such reductionism is passing up the rich opportunities observations afford us. In this chapter, we argue that observations and their associated analytical frameworks are in need of significant shaping and nuancing in applied linguistics research.

In the research methods literature, observations are often placed alongside ethnographic field research and thus are contrasted with experiments in terms of their qualitative and quantitative approaches to research. Observations are often thought of as interpretivist, designed to capture descriptions and reflections, although observation data can and are often quantified using observation schemes, discussed later in the chapter. Like interviews (discussed in Chapter 6), they are another data collection method positioned within the naturalistic inquiry or field research approach. One key difference with observations is that there are varying levels of engagement with the participants, ranging from the insider, with direct involvement, to the outsider, who maintains separation from participants. This means there is a great deal to consider about the type of observation that best suits the sociocultural context of the research inquiry as well as the research questions.

The other big difference between observations and other ethnographic data collection instruments such as interviews is the action involved. Interviews are created situations, where data are collected as reported by participants, whereas observations are done (usually) of naturally occurring activities, where a researcher has an opportunity to collect data directly from the research context, albeit often interpretatively. The presence of an observer risks creating an inauthentic situation known as the Hawthorne Effect, discussed later in the chapter, in which those being observed modify their behaviour, consciously or otherwise.

Objectivity and subjectivity in observations vary depending on the observer's role and position. Objectivity might be best achieved by taking an outsider position, if that is a possibility. Thanks to wide usage of the internet, we also have options of taking a fully outsider position by conducting what Androutsopoulos (2014) calls *online observation*, ideal for exploring computer-mediated communication. Alternatively, subjectivity may be desired and best achieved by taking an insider position. At its extreme, it is even possible to do *self-observation*, which completely collapses the divide between the researcher and that being observed, and is perhaps the most critical form of observation.

Arguably the most used collection of interpretive observation data is in the form of *field notes*. Field notes can take many forms and are not exclusive to observations. The idea is that they provide a record of any information that could be useful to responding to the research questions. For observations, this includes details about the research site and participants, the researcher's descriptions, as well as thoughts and reflections. Field notes may be taken during and after the observation (this may be dependent on the researcher role or type of observation). The use of recording devices can be advantageous for enhancing the detail of the field notes, whether audio only or video. However, the introduction of recording devices might add to the already unsettling feeling of being observed, potentially contributing to what is known as the Hawthorne Effect.

While in this introduction we have problematized observations, we move now to the key concepts of this data collection method to highlight the diverse ways observations can add to the strength of a research design.

Key concepts

We have highlighted five key concepts regarding observations: reasoning, research roles, self-observation, field notes, and observation types and schemes. Each of these concepts is put forward to encourage applied linguistics researchers to be innovative with this data collection method, as we challenge existing approaches to suggest there are ways of shaping and nuancing observations in the field.

Reasoning

First, inductive reasoning is the use of a premise as the basis for an investigation for which there is no hypothesized conclusion but rather leads to a non-predetermined probable conclusion. It is a form of bottom-up logic. Inductive reasoning is the most common in qualitative applied linguistics research, and it allows us to use observations as a starting point from which we can then build our research inquiry. Induction is the most basic and the most common form of scientific activity. We constantly observe our surroundings to learn how to function in them. We watch, discover patterns, draw conclusions and make predictions. For example, a researcher who wants to examine code-switching in the workplace might observe interactions in a factory of multilingual employees and record instances of code-switching, the languages used, and the reasons it has occurred. They could then later try to make sense of the data by coding it and categorizing it into elements such as the length, language and function to be able to say something substantive about code-switching and how it is used. While this seems a valid process, it is not perfect. The conclusions we draw are limited by the observations we make. A small number of observations could result in a unique, rather than representative conclusion.

Deductive reasoning starts with an existing premise or theory, and observations are made to test that theory. The theory to be tested is stated as a hypothesis – one that could be shown to be true, or false, depending on what is observed. In empirical quantitative applied linguistics research, this approach is commonly used, as there are many asserted 'problems' in the field that can be challenged or tested by conducting observations. Hypothesis testing in the field is often discussed in terms of quantitative research, such as frequency observations (see e.g. Norris et al., 2015). For example, the same code-switching researchers might apply taxonomies of code-switch functions derived from previous research to provide a framework to analyse what is observed and would then seek to categorize what they observe to refute or support the type of code-switching they hypothesize should occur. This approach also may encounter limitations as some observations might not fit neatly into predefined theory, or the constraints of theory might cause us to miss something important.

Alternatively, applied linguistics research has done very little in exploring the possibilities of *abductive* reasoning, used when pursuing theories to help explain observations, that is sometimes discussed in relation to grounded theory (see e.g. Timmermans & Tavory, 2012). Like inductive reasoning, it involves bottom-up logic, but this alternative approach allows for theory construction in ways that provide foundations for understanding and anticipating observations. In some ways, they may be more honest framings of the work we do in qualitative applied linguistics research, rather than inductive, which is in truth often informed by some theory. Abductive reasoning, for example, allows us to perceive a phenomenon in relation to other observations with different senses such as a hidden cause and effect, a familiarity of the phenomenon based on previous experience, or in simply making new descriptions of the phenomenon (Timmermans & Tavory, 2012). The reasoning we choose to apply is dependent on our social and intellectual positionality – a crucial aspect of our roles in the research.

The importance for a researcher to understand what type of approach to reasoning they are applying to the observation cannot be overstated, as this impacts our choice of type of observation and our roles within it. This in turn impacts the nature of the inquiry, as the research questions should be written to point clearly towards a particular reasoning. An inductive study will inquire about a premise pointing towards a probable outcome, while a deductive study will test the premise. Alternatively, an abductive study will be based on an imagined premise that can be used to explain the observations.

Researcher roles

In applied linguistics observations, there are several possible researcher roles, ranging from detached observer to complete participant observer. Researcher positionality, as an insider (known as an *emic* approach when regarding the researcher as within the same culture of what is being observed), outsider (*etic* approach) or somewhere in between, needs to be firmly established before conducting observations. Figure 5.1 outlines various roles available to the researcher when conducting an observation. As an outsider, a detached role may be most desirable. The non-participant, detached or complete observer is positioned to be *unobtrusive* – unnoticed by those being observed. In crowded places, this might be more easily achieved than in classrooms, where the participants being observed may be more aware of the presence of the researcher. If a researcher wants to maintain detachment from a researched classroom context, it may be more advantageous to review video recordings than to be physically in the classroom. However it is done, this role is by far the least complex, as there is no interaction between the observer and observed. Also at this end of the spectrum, we identify the standard *observer*. This position is one in which those being observed are aware of the presence of the observer, but there is no or very little interaction between them. In much field research,

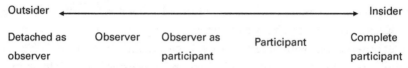

Figure 5.1 Observer role spectrum

this might involve a researcher sitting in the back of the room, where they can minimize their impact on the activities being observed. In the middle of the spectrum sits the *observer as participant*, who may be positioned somewhere out of the way but will occasionally interact with those being observed, possibly asking or answering questions. In classroom research this might involve a researcher sitting at the same table with learners. In other naturalistic research contexts, the researcher might physically sit with those being researched but only participate in activities in a minimal way, and only when required. This is a position moving towards a more natural observation space.

An insider would occupy the other end of the spectrum, taking on the role of either the *participant* (engaging in activities but still taking notes) or *complete participant* (fully engaged with all notes taken after the observed phenomena), which raises several complex issues as this position is *obtrusive*. The insider researcher is reliant on an element of trust within the observed community; the role can be difficult to balance as feelings of the observed being evaluated or judged can create undesirable conditions that could invalidate the study. In most cases, full disclosure and open communication and both ethical and advantageous, as the researcher can observe without concern of keeping any secrets from the participants or the participants raising any suspicions. Power relations can be a major concern where participants feel their behaviour is being evaluated, particularly in classroom research where the observer may sometimes also be a teacher. Again, full disclosure is the best approach, and information sheets and consent forms should clarify the full intentions of the involvement of the researcher(s) and participants.

In the centre of the spectrum we find a role somewhere between observer and participant, what we refer to as *observer as participant*, that raises various issues. In applied linguistics research, as gaining access to a research site might require the establishment of some relationship prior to the study, relationship dynamics can vary widely. There are advantages to establishing an in-between role, as the complete detached observer might be either completely unnatural to the setting, which will cause the observed to alter their behaviour, or might be so outside the community that many otherwise observable phenomena are missed. In the same way, the complete participant observer might be too involved or too close to the action to catch important observable phenomena. So finding a position in between offers the opportunity for the observed to recognize that they are being observed, without any concern about the observer's possible occasional involvement, and the observer can 'dip in and out' of the action as is natural to the occasion, allowing sufficient distance from the phenomena to effectively take note of them in real-time field note recording. Of course, this will all depend on what is being researched, as some research questions will require more, some less, involvement in the observed activities.

Self-observation

The observation of our own uses of language is as old as naturalistic inquiry itself. In applied linguistics research, the term 'self-observation' first appeared in publications in the 1960s, with William Norris (1970) questioning its value as a practice, but it was the work of Andrew Cohen in the late 1970s and early 1980s (building on uses of the Self-observation Scales developed by the National Testing Service in the United States) that helped the concept to take shape. Cohen (1984) divided self-observation of language behaviour into two categories: introspective, when we can observe our language use in short-term memory; and retrospective, when the observations occur anywhere from an hour (more complete) to weeks (less complete) after an event. In applied linguistics research, self-observational studies might include having the researcher (as participant) keep a reflective journal or diary on language learning (see Casanave, 2015, discussed further in Chapter 7) or engage in think-aloud protocols (see Chapter 3). There is sufficient evidence available to support our abilities to rely on our memories for both introspective and retrospective self-observation (Cohen, 1984).

In classroom-based research, teacher-researchers have the ideal opportunity to take critical approaches to classroom observation by observing their own practices. In his discussion of the knowledge base of L2 teacher education, Richards (2009) raises the importance of reflective teaching and action research, seeing them as central concepts in postgraduate studies in applied linguistics. As an example of how to support the concept of the researcher-practitioner who practices reflective teaching, classroom research and action research, Richards points to a proposition by

Kumaravadivelu (1999) known as 'critical classroom observation', in which teachers theorize and reflect on their own classroom practice by conducting a self-observation of a lesson that is compared with students' observation and that of an additional observer of the same lesson. Such observation is the most critical form in the field from an epistemological perspective, as it is insider investigation in its truest sense.

Field notes

In the introduction to this chapter, we explained that field notes are a record of information that can be used to respond to research questions. This indicates that in many cases, more information is collected than used in the study. Field notes are, by definition, notes taken in the field. But they might also be notes taken from audio or video recordings. They are, for the most part, qualitative in nature and are a data source themselves. Field notes are often found in ethnographic studies that involve observations. They are records of the setting, participants and their conversations, as well as the researcher's impressions and reflections of the phenomena observed. These field notes serve as primary data and are coded for analysis. To ease the process for coding, field notes should be planned, systematically and carefully taken (i.e. they should be structured; for highly structured observation notes see *observation schemes* below). While it is acceptable for the observation field notes to be less structured in the beginning, they should become more focused and more selective as the researcher progresses in their understanding of the research context.

For observations without audio or video recording, field notes are the only data the researcher can rely on. In this case, the field notes should be as detailed as possible, providing full descriptions and reflections. These notes should not be used for direct quotes, unless there is absolute certainty words were written down exactly as they were stated. It should also be noted that such field notes are considered interpretive, used solely in qualitative research. Quantitative observation data are best collected using observation schemes and should not be referred to as 'field notes'.

Observation types and schemes

There is great potential for applied linguistics researchers to add originality to their work through adapting or creating new observations frameworks specific to the field. Observations in educational research have been discussed as having a range of structure levels, from structured to semi-structured, to unstructured (Cohen, Manion & Morrison, 2018). Structured observations are systematic, where the researcher looks for and records predetermined actions. Semi-structured observations may also be systematic but allow for flexibility as to what the researcher is looking for.

In applied linguistics research, or more specifically second language research methods, structured observations are more likely to be discussed according to L2 classroom observation frameworks or schemes (e.g. Mackey & Gass, 2015), most that include observer checklists. The most popular of these structured observation schemes date back more than 30 years, including Ullman and Geva's (1984) Target Language Observation Scheme (TALOS), Fröhlich, Spada and Allen's (1985) Communicative Orientation of Language Teaching (COLT) and Nunan's (1989) low-interference 'classroom observation tally sheet'. Mackey and Gass (2015) provide a useful synopsis of each of these frameworks and then raise a discussion around the advantages of using or modifying them. The TALOS is a two-part process; the first is a checklist of classroom interactions, and the second is a rating scale done after the observation. Similarly, the COLT focuses on differences in communicative language teaching; it has two parts, the first for real-time coding of classroom interactions, the second for analysis after the observation. Nunan's tally sheet, like the checklist in the first part of the TALOS, provides thirteen low-interference categories of classroom events involving teacher and/or student action and one category for periods of silence. Such checklists are still often used for peer observation.

In a special issue of *TESOL* quarterly, Spada (1994) referred to the many observation schemes developed for L2 classrooms with differences between types of recording procedures, category type and complexity, and what behaviours were targeted. Some schemes focused on teaching, others on linguistic behaviours, and some both. She explained that we have gained significant insights from the various observation schemes about the variety of approaches, activities and modalities used in L2 classrooms. We now know more about the amount of time teachers and students spend talking, about teachers' approaches to error correction, about interactions between students and about questions raised. All of this has helped to improve teacher training programmes as well as raise awareness of experienced teachers about ways of improving their teaching.

Despite these obvious strengths, observation schemes, with their predetermined categories, have been described by ethnographers as limited and restrictive of observers' perceptions. There are concerns that the schemes, if we consider their categories to be limited or to have questionable valid predictors, lead observers to ignore potentially significant behaviours or features that fall outside the predetermined categories (Spada, 1994). There is also the limitation of the use of observation schemes that are unable to capture extended discourse, treating language as isolated and discrete. Such limitations invite adaptation of schemes to better deal with research inquiries in different contexts.

Indeed, there have been many attempts to develop new schemes over the years, such as Guilloteaux and Dörnyei's (2008) Motivation Orientation of Language Teaching (MOLT) and Weitz et al.'s (2010) Input Quality Observation Scheme (IQOS), but none that have the traction of COLT or TALOS (although arguably, MOLT has gained in popularity in motivation studies). While these schemes are still considered effective for L2 classrooms, there are few commonly used observation schemes for applied linguistics research outside the classroom. Video recordings of language use in natural settings offer plenty of opportunities to conduct careful observational analysis of language use outside the classroom, but it may be the inherent ambiguity and randomness of language use that makes the development of observation schemes so difficult. Classrooms have a wide variety of categorical activities and interactions that can be recorded. Other settings may have categorical activities and interactions, such as those that occur in business, legal or financial settings, but perhaps the variety of those activities is not so diverse that a categorical observation scheme would be needed. We certainly encourage applied linguistics researchers to challenge this, however, as there may be great insights to draw on from various observation schemes that have yet to be developed for contexts outside L2 language learning contexts.

Procedures and practicalities

Observing, as part of the naturalistic/field research approach, involves a series of stages starting with locating the field of study, which requires a justification of choice of setting. Next, the role of the researcher as an insider or outsider (or somewhere in between) needs to be confirmed as this raises issues of how to manage entry into the research context, if required. Next, ethical issues need to be addressed so that participants in the research setting know how their data are being used by the researcher and indeed what the researcher is going to observe. Some projects will require more from some participants than others, so researchers will also need to decide on the sample and subsamples to be observed (see Chapter 9 for more on non-probability sampling). Once participants are confirmed, they are often debriefed on the project using participation information sheets and consent forms to initiate transparency of the researcher-participant and maintain trust throughout the data collection period. From this point, data collection can begin, either with or without a predetermined observation scheme, depending on the chosen approach to the observation.

How to observe

The procedure for observing will depend entirely on the role of the researcher. In traditional observations, the researcher attempts to observe phenomena without intruding in any way, lest the situation be altered by their involvement (i.e. the Hawthorne Effect). Unobtrusive observation may best be conducted with the use of video recording (either set up for the study or taken from security or surveillance cameras where appropriate), without the researcher present. Physical detachment from the observed site may result in contextual details about the setting being diminished, as maintaining a distance in an effort to go unnoticed can also result in fewer details recorded. If physically present, the unobtrusive observer must find a place where they can see as much activity as possible and make as little disruption as possible; this usually involves a seat at the back of the room, making it difficult to see facial expressions or to hear accurately. These are important limitations to anticipate and address, to reduce potential negative impact on the study. To combat this issue, some researchers might deploy multiple recording devices in the observed site to capture unheard discourse or behaviours that are less visible or audible from the researchers' physical location.

For participant observations, involvement with participants raises several complex issues and does little to reduce concerns about loss of detail. While they do allow for a more natural environment (wherein participants are not asked to ignore the person at the back of the room), participant observations likewise cannot be of fully representative events, as the observer's presence ultimately influences them, challenging the validity of the data – what Mackey and Gass (2015) refer to as the 'observer's paradox'. To conduct participant observations, the researcher needs to prepare by informing participants inasmuch is required for their consensual participation, deciding if field notes will be taken during or after the observation and making efforts to reduce any interference that may disrupt the event or reduce the quality of the observation. During the observation, the obtrusive observer participates in events at the level understood by the role, understanding that higher levels of involvement mean field notes must be taken retrospectively – and it is something that should be done as immediately after the observation as possible. Recall of events observed is more effectively done when video or audio recordings have been made.

What to observe

Observing in applied linguistics research may be fairly structured, such as when testing hypotheses about whether particular uses of language occur in certain contexts, or can be unstructured, where the researcher is exploring how language is used in certain contexts with no (or few) preconceived ideas. Observation data might include details about the physical environment of the inquiry, about the people involved in the inquiry, about their interactions with each other or about the overall organization in which the inquiry is set. We might observe how children speak to each other when playing, taking note of what they say, and how, when and possibly why they say it. We can observe how strangers speak to each other in public spaces in which they might typically interact, such as in service situations (e.g. customers in a café or patients in a hospital).

For classroom observations, the observation schemes mentioned in the previous section provide a useful starting point from which to consider what to observe in language use. They provide predetermined categories for researchers to record types of activities and interactions, as well as the amount of time spent on them. Observations can be made of teachers and their teaching behaviours, and/or students and their behaviours. Whatever behaviours are observed, observations alone cannot be used to evaluate the effectiveness of classroom practices, for example, as post-observation interviews with teachers and/or students would be needed to understand the observed behaviours more fully.

What to keep in mind

Ultimately, observations are a powerful data collection instrument that can provide first-hand data to respond to research questions asking what happens when people use language in various contexts. Indeed, observations are the mainstay of many studies in applied linguistics, providing the basis for structuring analyses and providing solid evidence for theory testing. But they are also riddled with significant limitations regarding their reliability, as human behaviour is very difficult to authenticate and is highly likely to be affected or influenced by the realization of being observed. It is, after all, human nature to alter the way we speak, for example, in instances where we wish to be perceived in a particular way, to show that we are part of a group or that we are aware of or well informed of a particular matter. So observations should always be made with this understanding, and these inherent limitations should be addressed in any study in which observations are a primary source of data.

Reliability and validity

Observations in applied linguistics research have a number of conditions that could too easily render them ineffective, so it is imperative to address the limitations and make every effort to overcome them. When observations are used as a qualitative data collection method, reliability and validity may be better considered in terms of credibility. Credibility of observations can be achieved via transparent examples of how observation schemes were applied, such as those described earlier in the chapter for classroom observations. When schemes are not used, the coding process used to analyse the data needs to be accompanied with a thick description so that an external researcher would be able to replicate the methods of data collection and data analysis and (hopefully) arrive at the same results. Beyond this, however, we find most discussions about observations make use of the terms *reliability* and *validity*, which are easily threatened in observations.

Turning for a moment to the related field of psychology, a major foundational field of applied linguistics, we find a common approach which is to have more than one observer, not so dissimilar from Kumaravadivelu's (1999) protocol for self-observation. Having an additional observer offers inter-observer reliability and helps to address issues of researcher subjectivity and bias. The practice involves two independent observers comparing field notes, considering them reliable if they are in agreement. If they fail to agree, the field notes or observation scheme used are considered unreliable. While this seems reasonable, the practice relies on an assumption about observations: that the categories used or values observed are true and fixed, and the observations can therefore be sufficiently similar between two independent observers. But certainly, since observations rely on researcher perception, there may be differences simply due to the fact that the observations were conducted by two different people. While an observation scheme for observing applied linguistics phenomena can be adapted to control somewhat for differences, the practice ignores the ambiguity of human behaviour.

The Hawthorne Effect

Raised several times earlier in the chapter, the Hawthorne Effect, sometimes called the observer effect, is when observed participants modify their behaviour due to an awareness of being observed. The term takes its name from Hawthorne Works, where researchers were analysing whether workers were more productive in various levels of light. They found that productivity improved when lighting changes were made but that once the study was over and the observers gone, the workers were no longer motivated by researchers taking an interest in them, and productivity went down again. It is easy to imagine this scenario regarding language usage, where observed participants may want to impress observers with their language abilities, thus behaving in ways that would otherwise be unnatural to them in an effort, for example, to appear more proficient or engaged.

While this effect seems to suggest it is impossible to conduct truly authentic observations if those being observed are aware of the observation, there is sufficient evidence to show that the effect may be minimal at best and, in many cases, not found at all (Adair, 1984). One of the most popularly used ways to combat the Hawthorne Effect is for researchers to try as much as possible to avoid 'one-shot' observations. If multiple observations are conducted, and analysis reveals a stark difference in observed behaviour in the first few observations compared to later observations, this could be an indicator of the Hawthorne Effect. In such cases, a researcher might decide to discard the first few observations on the basis that behaviour had been modified due to researcher presence and then returned to a more naturalistic state as they became accustomed to being observed.

Improving

With the understanding that human behaviour is ambiguous and therefore difficult to categorize, our efforts to improve the reliability of observations should not be to create an observation instrument that can best do this. Instead, what we can do is acknowledge and address the limitations of our observational abilities and find ways to give ourselves better opportunities to understand the phenomena observed. We suggest two ways: one to improve detached observations and the other to improve participant observations.

First, in the introduction, we briefly mentioned Androutsopoulos's (2014) *online observation* as an approach to conducting detached observations. This approach involves systematic observation of online activities, such as those on social media websites. The degree of detachment here is so far removed that one could argue this is not an observation at all (i.e. we are not seeing the people engaging in the behaviour we are observing). But there is certainly valuable human behaviour to observe online, behaviour that is increasingly common and of great interest to social researchers.

Second, on improving participant observations, we consider the value of *mindfulness*. Mindful observations are usefully described with the acronym ODIS: Observe, Describe, Interpret and Suspend evaluation (Ting-Toomey & Dorjee, 2019). This method argues that before any evaluation, it is best to first be attentive of communication exchanges, both verbal and non-verbal, and describe the interaction regarding specific behaviours, such as eye contact or body position. Based on these notes, multiple interpretations of the interactions are made to try to understand them – maybe there are cultural influences or environmental; maybe there is a power dynamic, or maybe one interlocutor is tired or emotional. It is not necessary to choose one interpretation; instead, we might suspend evaluation by engaging with the different interpretations reflexively to better understand our own ethnocentricity in relation to the observed phenomena.

Ultimately, the improvement of observations as a data collection method relies on our ability to recognize and address the limitations, both of ourselves as reliable observers and of the phenomena being observed – often ambiguous and difficult to categorize.

Case studies in applied linguistics research

Observations are used extensively in applied linguistics research, most often to observe language use in natural settings, from various positions as

Table 5.1 Examples of observations in applied linguistics research

Researchers	Topic	Participants	Research design	Data collection method
Androutsopoulos (2015)	Language practices in social media	Greek background secondary school students in Germany (*n* = 7)	Online ethnography (case study)	Online observations (detached) of online activities, screen data + elicited data
Curdt-Christiansen (2016)	Children's biliteracy environments	Children aged 5–7 in multilingual homes in Singapore (*n* = 3)	Multiple ethnographic case studies	Language audit, interviews with parents + participant observations in homes
Farrell and Ives (2015)	Teacher beliefs and classroom practices	A novice male ESL teacher in a university language school in Canada (*n* = 1)	Case study	Interviews, structured classroom observations (unobtrusive) + teaching journal
Hinds, Neeley and Cramton (2014)	Group dynamics in multinational business teams	Six high-tech multinational company project teams in India, the US and Germany (*n* = 96)	Ethnography	Interviews + concurrent observations (all *observer as participant*
Hofer and Jessner (2019)	Multilingual education effect on young learners' proficiency	Elementary school students recruited from two institutions in South Tyrol, Italy (*n* = 84)	Experimental/ Mixed methods	Classroom observations, questionnaires interviews, various tests and tasks
McKinley (2019)	Contextual literacy in EAP	University students in Japan (*n* = 12)	Action research	'Observer as participant', semi-structured (during) and structured observations (using video) + students' written reflection
Van Praag and Sanchez (2015)	Mobile technology use in L2 classrooms	Teachers in a private English language centre in the UK (*n* = 3)	Multiple case studies	Interviews, non-participant observation (using video) + stimulated recall

outsiders, insiders or somewhere in between. In the following selection of studies that utilized observations, we offer a variety of observation types and approaches. In some studies, observations are the main data source, and in others they are supplementary (see Table 5.1).

In applied linguistics studies that use observations, we show in this selection that ethnographies (Androutsopoulos, 2015; Curdt-Christiansen, 2016; Hinds et al., 2014) and case studies (Androutsopoulos, 2015; Curdt-Christiansen, 2016; Farrell & Ives, 2015; Van Praag & Sanchez, 2015) are common research designs. This is because the research questions in these studies seek to provide descriptions of phenomena or to try to understand phenomena as they occur in *the real world*, so detailed, rich descriptions possible with these designs are needed. In Androutsopoulos (2015), the online observations of seven students' activity on Facebook were used as a fully detached approach to seeing how these students interacted with each other through the popular social media platform. In this ethnographic study, these observations were paired with data elicited through direct contact with the participants. Curdt-Christiansen (2016) observed linguistic behaviour in three different homes of children living in multilingual environments, each one representing a major language group in Singapore. Along with a 'language audit' (a questionnaire for each family to provide basic information about the languages used in the home) and interviews with the children's parents, the home participant observations were made of regular day-to-day activities. Hinds, Neeley and Cramton's (2014) study investigated the effect of differing language fluency in multinational teams of employees of the same multinational company. Observations and interviews were conducted by a team of five researchers to find that in some, but not all cases, observable subgrouping resulted. Van Praag and Sanchez's (2015) study investigated the mobile technology use of three experienced second language teachers in the classroom, conducting preliminary interviews, non-participant classroom observations and stimulated recall interviews.

The other two studies also use popular research designs but not necessarily commonly paired with observations, including experimental (Hofer & Jessner, 2019) and action research (McKinley, 2019). Hofer and Jessner's (2019) study involved observations combined with several other data collection methods to test the effects of multilingual education by testing two experimental groups of students who studied in Italian, German and English, compared with two control groups who studied only in

Italian. Findings showed that the experimental group had greater cognitive advantages. McKinley's (2019) action research study of university students in Japan participating in a 4-week socio-historic role-playing activity involved two stages of observation.

We now take two of these studies as cases, taking Curdt-Christiansen (2016) as a non-classroom-based study in which observations made up one-third of the data collected and McKinley (2019) as a classroom-based study where observations were the main data collection method.

First, Curdt-Christiansen (2016) provides an ideal example of the use of observations in ethnographic studies outside the classroom. The study focuses on three participants who came from a larger study designed to investigate young children's (ages 5 to 8) 'biliteracy environments' as they are impacted by family language policy. As the inquiry was about a real-world environment, observations were an obvious data collection method. Curdt-Christiansen had to conduct *participant* observations, as she needed to engage naturally with the family of each participant in their home while observing their interactions. She used audio-only recording devices to reduce awkwardness and spent time with the families over a period of 6 months, getting to know them, as required for ethnographic research, but also powerful to reduce the impact of the Hawthorne Effect. In the paper, Curdt-Christiansen provides detailed descriptions of each participant's families and their linguistic activity. The level of detail is apparent as necessary to convincingly support her interpretations of the phenomena.

As a classroom-based inquiry, McKinley's (2019) action research study is a good example of how observations can serve as the primary data collection method. The observations in this study were held in two different stages in two different forms, taking the position of 'observer as participant' naturally as the teacher in the class conducting the observations of students' classroom performance. The first stage was semi-structured observation involving real-time field notes. The second stage involved structured observations (using specific criteria for analysis) conducted after class by reviewing video recordings. The depth of familiarity with the phenomena being investigated was aided by the study's design. As an action research study, McKinley had insider information about the students beyond the immediate observations, which helped with the interpretation in the field notes. For triangulation (discussed in Chapter 12), he added students' written reflections which were used to map the field notes.

Implications for researchers

Observations are not an exact science. They are reliant on the observers themselves, their perceptions, biases, subjectivity or simply their presence. This makes observations a risky endeavour, but one that may be appropriate depending on the research questions. The importance of acknowledging and addressing the limitations of this research method cannot be overstated. Social research is messy, and observations are a perfect example of that. But observations in applied linguistics research are not just ideal for some research questions; they are imperative for responding to those questions that require description or first-hand impressions or interpretations of language use.

As a qualitative data collection method, observations require researchers to reflect on what they observe. These reflections are recorded in field notes, as well as a researcher journal, if one is kept. Reflections of observations in this case serve as actual data, as opposed to other types of reflections. Field notes, containing both descriptions and reflections, are coded for analysis like any other written data such as interview transcripts or documents. Structured field notes such as those following observation schemes are essentially pre-coded, making analysis a faster process. However, observation schemes are limited by their own efficiency, relying on the assumption that predetermined categories capture the true value of the communication being observed. We also understand that observation schemes see language as isolated in categorical items, as they do not capture extended discourse. Observation schemes can be adapted for the context and type of inquiry, and we can be flexible to allow ourselves to take additional notes, perhaps after the event with the help of audio or video recordings.

Certainly, technology has greatly added to the potential value of observations in applied linguistics research. Being able to observe video recordings of linguistic behaviour multiple times, or sharing a recording so multiple researchers can 'observe' it, helps us to increase the reliability of the data collection method. We also have the option of conducting observations of existing videos and drawing comparisons between our own research subjects and those in other videos. Taking advancements in digital technology further, we also must consider the potential of online observations as yet another source of observation data – one that targets social media communication, an exponentially growing area of research.

Post-reading activities

Reflect
This chapter states that observations are a common yet problematic method of data collection in applied linguistics research compared to other methods due to the ambiguity of language and the inconsistencies in human perspectives. Do you agree with these statements? Why or why not?

Expand
Individually or in small groups, choose one of the studies in Table 5.1 to read and critique. After reading, consider and discuss: (1) Did the researcher(s) sufficiently justify the use of observations for the study, including the type of observation? (2) Do you think the additional data collection methods were appropriate? (3) Did the researcher discuss their positionality in the research? (3) Thinking of the type of analysis used, were there any aspects of the methodology which could have been improved in design or implementation?

Apply
Imagine you are going to investigate the premise that less shy, more boisterous language students may be more proficient. How would you go about answering this question using observations? Can the amount of engagement and participation in classroom activities be equated with the level of language proficiency?

Resources for further reading

Curdt-Christiansen, X. L. (2020). Observations and field notes: Recording lived experiences. In J. McKinley & H. Rose (Eds.), *The Routledge handbook of research methods in applied linguistics*. Abingdon: Routledge.

In this handbook chapter, Curdt-Christiansen discusses qualitative approaches to observations and field notes in applied linguistics research as tools to collect data about people, language learning processes, linguistic interactions, non-verbal communication and various activities in settings such as the classroom, home domain, workplace and other social contexts. She covers key features of the research methods by reviewing recent development in the field of applied linguistics. By examining empirical data from some existing studies, she also deals with the purpose of using these tools and the stance of the observer, as well as when, what and how to observe. In addition, the chapter illustrates how observations and field notes are used together with other data collection tools.

Mackey, A., & Gass, S. M. (2015). *Second language research: Methodology and design, 2nd edn.* Chapters 7 and 8. London: Routledge.

In this edition of their very popular research methods book, Mackey and Gass do not have a dedicated chapter to discuss observations, but readers are advised to check Chapters 7 and 8 for subsections related to observations. These sections provide valuable overviews of classroom observation schemes, as well as practical guidance for conducting observations of second language learning.

6

Interviews

Introduction

In qualitative applied linguistics research, the most commonly used data collection method is the interview. Interviews allow the researcher to probe participant responses by offering alternative question forms, asking for clarifications, and, depending on the interview, co-constructing knowledge produced in the interaction. In applied linguistics research, interviews are used to investigate such constructs as experiences, identities, attitudes and beliefs. Talmy (2010a) argued that while interviewing has grown in popularity as a qualitative data collection method in the field, inconsistencies in the theorization of interviews have put the reliability of the method at risk. He calls for more *reflexivity* in interviews, which is defined as the act of referring to the self and social influences in investigatory research – an act designed to affect the researcher and inform the research. While this call may have been heeded by many experienced researchers in informing their practice, scholars venturing into interviewing for the first time may continue to rely on popular methodological literature, which remains somewhat conservative and non-innovative in approach (see Chapter 12 for a discussion of innovations). A lack of reflexivity and engagement with the methodological issues of interviewing remains problematic in the reporting of applied linguistics research that too often brushes over the method and analysis, failing to problematize the roles of interviewer/interviewee (see Block, 2000, 2017) as well as the data. Reflexivity allows us, as researchers, to recognize that interviews are more than just data collection instruments – they are a *social practice* (Talmy, 2010b). This understanding sees interviews as collaborative; there is a co-construction of knowledge and development of identity in both the interviewer and interviewee. This co-construction can contribute to the research process when conducting interviews in applied linguistics research.

This chapter will follow similar lines of the discussion surrounding the ideologies of interviews as those found in Block (2000, 2017) and Talmy (2010a, b), as well as Talmy and Richards (2011). This chapter will extend the discussion and challenge and problematize our understanding of the value of conducting interviews. This chapter will also provide an outline of the procedures and practicalities of interviewing, covering issues such as leading questions, the interview environment, interview bias, prompts and follow-up questions, establishing rapport and so on. It will cover essential 'how to' considerations when conducting interviews, including how to structure the question set, how to gain access to interviewees, how to establish an appropriate interviewer–interviewee relationship and how to construct knowledge during and after the interview. As these procedures have been comprehensively covered by renowned scholars in applied linguistics (Richards, 2003, 2009; Richards, Ross & Seedhouse, 2012), education (Cohen, Manion & Morrison, 2018) and the broader social sciences (Brinkmann, 2014; Brinkman & Kvale, 2014; Kvale, 2007), this chapter will also consider newer practices in interviewing in applied linguistics research, such as developments in online interviews.

The decision to use interviews as a method of data collection should be based on a balance of both ideological and practical points. While interviews are generally referred to as a qualitative data collection method, interviewing is commonly paired with other data collection methods, both qualitative and quantitative. When part of a qualitative research design, interviews are powerful tools to provide rich data, such as in case study, ethnography or narrative research. Equally, quantitative designs such as experimental or quasi-experimental research might also utilize interviews as a data collection tool, as too do many survey designs, where interviews are popularly used to follow up quantitative data by providing a more situated and in-depth investigation. Whatever the design or framework, the research question will be written in such a way that an in-depth qualitative approach such as interviewing will provide the necessary data to answer it.

Key concepts

The typology of interviews includes those which differ in structure (structured, semi-structured, unstructured), timing (preliminary, follow-up) or design (focused, stimulated recall, retrospective, problem-centred, theme-centred, in-depth, focus group). Threats to reliability and bias during data collection can vary depending on the type of interviews employed.

Types of interviews: Structural differences

Oft-cited interview types are structured, semi-structured and unstructured, although these types are more appropriately viewed on a spectrum with completely structured at one end, and completely unstructured at the other, and semi-structured interviews occupying the middle territory. There are advantages and disadvantages with each type of interview. The obvious advantage of structured or semi-structured interviews is the opportunity to have all (structured) or at least the most crucial (semi-structured) questions carefully written beforehand. Depending on how complex the questions are, they could be sent in advance to interviewees so they can prepare their responses. The obvious disadvantage, however, is the restriction of getting through the questions in a reasonable and consistent amount of time for each interviewee at the possible expense of forgoing further probing into interesting interviewee responses. For unstructured interviews, the lack of prepared questions might seem daunting for novice researchers, putting a lot of pressure on what is common in narrative interviews – a single prompt. But the obvious advantage here is the allowance for interviewees to develop their own narrative in response to that prompt, coupled with the freedom to explore new ideas and concepts as they emerge.

Structured interviews are also known as standardized open-ended interviews. They are used often in quantitative research, as by asking the same questions in the same order with all participants, the responses can be easily aggregated. Questions can be closed- (like survey questions) or open-ended. Structured interviews are also used in qualitative research when interview schedules are strictly followed with set questions. The consistency of structured interview schedules improves validity and reliability because questions are carefully prepared beforehand, and all participants are asked the same questions in the same order. Follow-up questions help to ensure that the respondent has understood the question correctly and that answers are complete. It is important to keep track of time, as too many follow-up questions could mean insufficient time to ask all the questions. A potential problem to consider for the use of structured interviews in applied linguistics research is the inherent lack of researcher reflexivity. However, this format can be useful if systematicity is vital to the reliability of data, such as if a large team of research assistants are conducting the interviews and must maintain consistency in their approach to data collection.

Semi-structured interviews offer much of the ease of conduct of structured interviews but require a degree of flexibility and careful listening skills to ask further questions about certain responses the researcher finds interesting. This allows for new ideas to form within a predetermined framework of themes. Semi-structured interviews are strictly qualitative and provide more opportunities for reflection. Semi-structured interviews will have an interview schedule like a structured interview, and while these are more flexible, the interviewer still needs to have a clear idea of the topics to be explored. In this way, while new ideas may develop during each interview, they will need to develop within the expected framework. An advantage of the semi-structured interview is some degree of reflexivity to explore topics in varying depths and in varying order for each interviewee.

Unstructured interviews are sometimes referred to as informal conversational interviews or non-directive interviews, as there is no predetermined plan for what direction the interview will take. Sometimes a researcher might just work within a flexible list of topics to guide the interview when needed. Unstructured interviews, while at least targeting a specific topic or topics, are purposely sparsely planned to allow for unexpected outcomes. Depending on the interviewee, it may be that only one question is required, allowing the respondent to tell a story that addresses the main topic but is not otherwise guided outside of an occasional question for clarity or affirmations of encouragement to continue. If the interview is the format of an informal conversation, this means the researcher's thoughts are sometimes also shared in the interview. This helps to contribute to identity development and the co-construction of knowledge, but it is essential to avoid imposing ideas on participants. Sharing opinions is fine, as this can initiate further discussion, but the participants' ideas should almost always be expressed first to avoid leading the interviewee to a desired response.

Types of interviews: Temporal differences

The information provided on interview types is relevant for both short 'snapshot' studies in which single interviews are conducted, as well as longer studies that require multiple interviews with the same participants over a specified period. In these longer studies, depending on the stage in the research process, an interview will be conducted to achieve different outcomes. For example, at the start of the research process, a preliminary interview may be used to gather demographic data and other background information. This data will then be used to inform later interviews, which might be referred to as follow-up interviews, if they are indeed building on previous interviews. For some research projects, the timing of the interview might depend on other data collection techniques, such as pre-observation and post-observation interviews conducted before and after a participant is observed.

Types of interviews: Design differences

Narrowing our presentation of interview types further, we consider several subtypes that may be helpful in justifying the data collection method and making the research more manageable depending on the scope of the project. Additional types include, and are not limited or delineated to, *focused*, where interviews seek interviewee responses to a previously analysed situation (Merton, Fiske & Kendall, 1990); *stimulated recall*, where respondents are given a sample of previously collected data such as an audio or video recording to prompt them to reflect on their thought processes at the time (Mackey & Gass, 2013); *retrospective*, where the interviewee is asked to explain the reasons for their interview responses; *problem-centred*, where interviewees start with a set of well-informed ideas but open themselves to myriad outcomes (Witzel & Reiter, 2012); *theme-centred*, where apparent realities and subvert communications are decoded (Schorn, 2000); and *in-depth interviews*, conducted with fewer participants to allow for more individualistic investigation (Cohen, Manion & Morrison, 2018), among others.

A final consideration of interview type is when interviewing multiple people together in a *group interview*, not to be confused with a *focus group*. These are not the same, as a group interview usually involves the same interview schedule (usually structured or semi-structured) as an individual interview but asked of more than one person at the same time. A focus group requires the interviewer to provide a prompt and then facilitate conversation between group members (usually in an unstructured manner) and is discussed further in Chapter 9.

Bias

Researcher bias may play more of a role in less structured interview schedules but is also prevalent in poorly constructed or poorly conducted structured interviews. Acknowledging bias can be very productive if treated respectfully. Bias can be more than just injecting an interviewer's own perspective into the interview and can manifest as a result of something as innocuous as silence, which can be a difficult aspect of interviewing. Interviewers will be tempted to fill silence, but allowing the interviewee to reflect and think may be key to achieving greater depth and reaching into more complex issues.

Interview bias is very difficult and, depending on the topic and researcher background, impossible to avoid. In post-positivist qualitative research, it is understood that the best approach for a researcher in this situation is to acknowledge the fact that all researchers have bias (McKinley, 2017b). As researchers, we come with our own experiences that will influence our approaches. Given the social nature of applied linguistics research, and the understanding that interviews are most effective when they allow for the co-construction of knowledge and identity development, we understand that our biases make us who we are. But we must not let them restrict the interview. We must ensure that we do not steer respondents towards desired outcomes and maintain respect and openness to interviewee responses. Establishing rapport with the interviewee can help to reduce the impact of interview bias. A pre-interview friendly interaction can be very helpful, especially where it leads to finding common ground with the interviewee. This is especially important in cross-cultural interviews (see Spencer-Oatey, 2004), as well as interviews with children (see Kuchah & Pinter, 2012) and other groups where sensitivity is important (see e.g. Appleby, 2017).

Procedures and practicalities

Conducting interviews requires both careful planning and flexibility regarding procedures and practicalities. In this section, we will address the set-up and conduct of interviews, keeping in mind practicalities of what can be a challenging data collection method but one that, if carried out successfully, can yield rich data in response to important real-world questions in applied linguistics.

Cohen, Manion and Morrison (2018) suggest ten stages of conducting interviews in educational research, which are also relevant for much applied linguistics research. Their procedure is comprehensive, from thematizing, designing and constructing the interview schedule and its carefully formatted questions and decisions regarding response modes, to the conducting of the interview followed by the transcribing, analysing, verifying and reporting. Richards, Ross and Seedhouse (2012) raise important considerations to keep in mind with interviews, which include the time-consuming nature of interviews, the lack of opportunity for generalizability from interviews, the lack of anonymity in the interaction, and the opportunity to use both qualitative and quantitative methods in treating interview results. Further considerations are question construction and delivery, prompts and follow-up questions, recording, note-taking and non-verbal communication, and the interview environment.

Theorizing the interview and formulating the questions

The first step is to establish the purpose of the research (what Cohen, Manion and Morrison refer to as 'thematizing'), identifying the theory supporting the research, aims, potential contribution and reasons for choosing this data collection method. From here, goals should be drafted to clarify specific research objectives in response to a clearly stated research problem that the rest of the study will depend on. Given the criticisms of interviewing that it lacks reflexivity, ensuring consistent theorization of the roles and identities of the interviewer and interviewee is paramount.

Once objectives are clear, interview questions can be formulated. Researchers will need to design questions that yield facts, opinions, attitudes or all of these. The level of specific detail, or depth desired in responses, will be built into question format and order. Questions should reflect the researcher's considerations of both the interviewer's and interviewee's level of understanding, the kind of information respondents will have and the need for structure in respondents' thoughts. Further considerations should be made of respondents' motivation and the relationships that will develop with the respondents. The question formats themselves might be varied so that they are not all necessarily open questions. Some closed questions can help the pacing of the interview as can a mix of direct (yes/no) and indirect (seeking opinions) questions, and specific and non-specific questions. Background questions are usually asked first, as they are quick and can help to put the interviewee at ease. Remaining questions might be descriptive, experiential, behavioural, knowledge-based or designed to target respondents' feelings. Some questions are asked to develop the process or line of questioning; these might include introduction of topics ('Could you say something about … ') or follow-up ('Could you say something more about … ', 'could you provide an example?').

The interview schedules themselves must be meticulously planned, and it is always good practice to review the wording and order of questions with research collaborators, peers or pilot participants. Regarding prompts, word choice should be simple, clear and unbiased. Leading questions, where answers are often what the interviewer wants, are usually best avoided, but there may be justification for using them, if the idea is that they will either maintain a focus on the topic or lead to depths that would otherwise be more difficult to achieve with vaguely worded question formats. There are some questions always to be avoided. Questions that include assumptions about respondents' situations or understanding can be unethical. Also, 'double-barrelled' questions, when interviewers ask two questions at once, can be confusing and can lead to incomplete responses. Questions should be written in such a way to allow respondents to reasonably recall events.

Probing questions should also be prepared in the interview schedule. Scholars have identified multiple types of probes, some less, some more intrusive than others. They might be designed to get more details from the participant or to get the participant to elaborate or clarify their responses. They might be anticipated, spontaneous, conditional, emergent, cognitive, confirmatory or expansive (see Cohen, Manion & Morrison, 2018: 514 for various probe types). Whatever is decided, it is important to maintain reflexivity, and not to overdo probing, as this can reveal unwanted biases in both interviewer and interviewee, as well as interviewee resentment.

Ethics

As with all research conducted with people, ethical approval is necessary to ensure that researchers have taken necessary precautions: to avoid coercing participants, to protect their privacy and identity, to prepare participants by letting them know what is expected of them, and to be respectful always.

Participation terms of agreement should be clear in the consent form. This includes what is the general focus of the interview, what will happen in the interview, how long it is expected to last, that it will be recorded, that the interviewee can stop the interview at any time without question, and that the interviewee will be given the chance to read over the transcription and ask for changes where they feel they were misheard or misrepresented.

Researchers must be honest in writing up results. Given the subjective nature of interview analysis, it is very important to report what really was said, rather than what the researcher hopes or wishes was said, even if the results counter the original argument or are completely unexpected. In fact, it is the unexpected results that can be the most advantageous, adding depth to a study's findings. In reflexive interviewing, conflicting opinions can also facilitate identity development and the co-construction of knowledge and should therefore not only be acknowledged but embraced.

The position of the interviewer in relation to the interviewee raises important issues of power dynamics and ethics. Kubota (2017) describes the process of researching privileged populations (*studying up*), populations that include the researcher (*studying across*) or underprivileged populations (*studying down*) to generate discussion around the importance of acknowledging our position in relation to our participants, as it raises challenges and potential threats to the research that need to be addressed. As establishing an appropriate interviewer–interviewee relationship is essential, working out differences of power and position needs to be done before and throughout the interview process.

It may seem that studying down is the most attractive as it gives researchers the chance to support social justices or impart wisdom as a reward to the interviewees. But studying up is extremely important in applied linguistics research, as questioning key stakeholders in positions of power (heads of institutions, policy- and decision makers) is required when the research inquires why decisions are made. Gaining access should be done with caution, recognizing that those in positions of power may be less willing to participate, possibly seeing academic inquiry as no different from sensationalist journalism. Kubota (2017: 25) concludes her advice about these ethical considerations with the suggestion that we should *study in* 'by critically recognizing our own privilege, which occupies the top of the socioeconomic power hierarchy, and the potential complicity of our work in perpetuating the hierarchy. Exploring ways to overcome this dilemma is imperative in our field'.

Interviewing from a distance

In applied linguistics research, it is a common occurrence that researchers need to access participants who are not local. While in many cases face-to-face interviews offer a more intimate environment for the interview, due to various circumstances, interviewing from a distance may be the only way to conduct the interview. These include telephone interviews, online interviews and the emerging 'multimodal' interview.

Telephone interviews are common in all areas of social research, and many scholars have explored the differences between face-to-face and telephone interviews (e.g. Holt, 2010; Shuy, 2003; Sturges & Hanrahan, 2004). While the telephone may be used for practical reasons, it might also be justified as an appropriate method, where allowing interviewees to sit comfortably in their own environment, without researcher presence, might yield the best results. Indeed, in our increasingly online world, it is not unusual to find a person who feels most natural and willing to participate by being in their own environment for the interview. Of course, measures to minimize distraction should be taken, but telephone interviews can be, in some cases, more productive than face-to-face interviews. Of course, non-verbal cues are missed when the interviewer and interviewee are not in the same room, so the enquiry itself needs to be considered when choosing not to interview face to face. For example, ethnographic studies, requiring a depth best achieved through up-close and personal communication, might be lacking if interviews are conducted from a distance.

On the rise is the *online interview*. This type seems to be open to interpretation, as it has been used to refer to interviews conducted via 'Google chat' (e.g. Kang, Rubin & Lindemann, 2015) and Skype (e.g. Banegas & Busleimán, 2014), involving real-time videoconferencing; the term has also been used by scholars who use it to refer to an open-ended questionnaire accessed online (e.g. Kang, 2015; Staples, Kang & Wittner, 2014). According to Cohen, Manion and Morrison (2018), an 'online interview' could refer to all of the above, from audio and video, audio only, a combination of texts and visuals, or text-based only. Interviews via video chat apps, many that are free, such as Skype, Viber, WeChat, WhatsApp, Google Hangouts, Facebook Messenger, and many more, involve differences in the interaction. Therefore, questions and transcription formats should be devised to show a clear understanding of how the interaction is different. The time of day might be different for the interviewee and interviewer, as is, of course, the environment. All these differences need to be taken into consideration.

There are also very different interactions in interviews that we call 'multimodal interviews'. These interviews involve various modes of either questioning or responding with either the interviewer or interviewee using writing to communicate. These interviews might take place in real time, via online chat or similar, or in delayed time via email or similar. While many will question whether a 'written interview' is indeed an interview at all, this approach is in many cases simply more realistic and, in some cases, more conducive to achieving more in-depth, honest responses to questions. Communication impairment or disabilities may be reason for one or both people in the interview to use writing. Sensitive topics may be easier for respondents to open up about if they can reply to questions in writing via online chat. The need for interpreting services might be alleviated by using online translation, although this raises concerns about reliability. Nevertheless, sometimes, alternative modes for interviews might be necessary, preferred or simply just more convenient.

Recording, note-taking and non-verbal cues

Recording interviews is common practice, but participants must be fully informed of their options regarding the recording, and the recording process should be as unobtrusive as possible. Recording alters interactions, as both interviewer and interviewee are very aware of the recording taking place, knowing their words will be scrutinized later. Consent forms need to clearly state that recording, audio or video, will take place.

Note-taking for non-verbal cues can provide important artefacts in interviewing for later analysis and is often overlooked by researchers. While audio recording and transcribing interviews allow a researcher to go over the full interview repeatedly, catching every word, without video, the researcher may miss some important non-verbal cues. Therefore, note-taking during interviews can be especially crucial to dissect the meaning of interviewee responses. Did the interviewee seem distracted? Did she nod? Rub his eyes? Cross her arms? Shift around uncomfortably in his seat? Smile? Frown in disagreement? These are potential non-verbal cues that may inform the meaning of the response and even dramatically change the literal interpretation of the words said.

Transcribing and transcription models are a significant part of the data collection process that are too often paid insufficient attention. Yes, transcribing is inevitable, and indeed, time is a factor. For every 1 hour of interview recording, as many as 3 hours should be factored in for transcribing. Transcription services should be avoided if researchers expect to understand interviewee responses with real depth. And before interviews are even conducted, a transcription model should be decided, as the notes, especially those referring to non-verbal cues, will need their place in the transcription. If pauses, speed or intonation is important, this should be reflected in the transcription style. Studies on the research topic that have used interviews will often include excerpts from the transcriptions – these can be very helpful for clarifying the transcription model or style and providing justification for choosing it.

Interviewing in multilingual settings

A practical issue common in applied linguistics research is deciding which language(s) will be used in the interview, especially important when conducting interviews in multilingual settings. A researcher must also decide whether to transcribe and analyse data in the language(s) used in the interview or in the language of the write-up. Participants who are given the opportunity to use the language they are most comfortable with may even choose to mix languages if the languages are shared with the interviewer. Transcriptions in another language or in multiple languages differing from the language of the write-up may be best analysed in the languages used so as not to lose meaning. Yet analysing in the same language as the write-up similarly helps to avoid losing meaning in translation and allows greater access to the data by the reader.

The decision of which language to choose for transcription and analysis is ultimately up to the researcher. As it is already not always easy to understand what qualitative researchers actually did during analysis and how they arrived at their findings from the data, the processes of translation and overall treatment of the data should always be stated and justified in the write-up.

Reliability and validity

There has been some debate over the relevance of using the terms *reliability* and *validity* in relation to interviews. Like observations, interviews are common in naturalistic or interpretive studies but supplementary in positivist studies. Quantitative researchers tend to distance themselves from the research, whereas qualitative researchers acknowledge their position and embrace their roles in the research process. But both quantitative and qualitative researchers must test the credibility of the study: it has been suggested that the credibility in quantitative research is dependent on instrument construction, whereas in qualitative research, the researcher is, in fact, the instrument (see Golafshani, 2003). While the term *credibility* could be used in place of reliability and validity of interviews, for consistency between chapters in this book, we address the common terms *reliability and validity*.

Threats to interview reliability and validity

As interviewing is dependent on the people involved, and because every researcher will interpret the interview differently, the reliability and validity of the method, in theory, are always risk. However, we generally accept interviewing as a legitimate research method because 'the person of the researcher as the research instrument is actually a virtue of interviewing and ... due to its dialogicality – may be the most valid research instrument to study qualitative, discursive, and conversational aspects of the social world' (Brinkmann, 2014: 1008).

Regarding interview analysis and coding, 'inter-rater reliability' used in statistical studies is somewhat ineffective; two researchers will not produce the same results, which is an obvious threat to reliability. However, this kind of traditional positivism has no place in such qualitative social research, where social constructivism and social constructionism are at the heart of the research approach (McKinley, 2015). Working with peers to support interpretations of interview data is generally good practice, and differences in interpretations can be discussed to reach a more confident analysis, discussed in detail in the next subsection.

In the introduction to this chapter, we mentioned that inconsistencies in the theorization of interviews have put the reliability of the method at risk. It is very important that researchers are reflexive with interviews and always consider what knowledge is being co-constructed and what developments to the identities of those involved are occurring. While interview schedules can improve validity and reliability, there are always risks to the reliability of interviews due to the environment, mood and other contributing factors. In the act of analysing 'as you go', biases can threaten reliability as leading interviewees towards desired responses becomes harder to resist.

Researchers' opinions, prejudices and other biases always need to be acknowledged and carefully handled when using interviews. Social researchers are not a 'clean slate'. Singleton and Pfenninger (2017: 122) emphasize, 'We cannot necessarily wipe the slate clean, but it is our responsibility to be true to our research in resisting the application of [our biases] in education.' Subjectivity is important; being reflective and conscious of 'who you are' will shape and enrich the study.

Improving interview reliability

At the start of this chapter, we raised one of the biggest threats to interviews as a data collection method – a lack of reflexivity. We contend, as does Talmy (2010a), that interview reliability can be improved by being reflexive and problematizing the design and theory underpinning the data collection instrument. Applied linguistics researchers might be tempted to choose interviews for their convenience in situations where there is easy access to teachers and students. Resulting research from such situations, however, may be severely lacking sufficient conceptualization, as well as lacking justification for choosing to conduct interviews. Just because we have easy access to language learners does not mean interviews are the most appropriate and most advantageous data collection instrument. Reflexivity is achieved by acknowledging both the researcher and social influences in the research, which in turn informs the researcher and the research. This should be the first step in improving interview reliability.

Another way to improve interview reliability, as stated earlier, is with interview schedules. Maintaining uniformity with question forms and order helps to provide more evenness in data collected from different interviewees. Levels of consistency using interview schedules have even been quantified to measure the reliability (see Goodwin, Sands & Kozleski, 1991). But this is not an expected procedure to support interview reliability. If reliability is of particular concern, certainly, structured interviews will be considered more reliable.

A third way to strengthen and improve interview reliability is to work collaboratively. Our subjectivity as researchers is not only important to acknowledge in interview data collection, it is also essential. But as our subjectivity serves as one of the major threats to reliability of interview data, we can greatly improve the situation by taking social constructivism and/ or social constructionism as a conceptual theory in which to situate the research. With these theories, the researcher maintains the understanding that knowledge generated from the research is co-constructed in working with collaborators or peers through the processes of developing the interview schedule and analysing the data. Social constructionism focuses on *what* knowledge is co-constructed, while social constructivism focuses on *how* that knowledge was constructed. These theories support the activity of multiple researchers analysing interview data, comparing interpretations and discussing differences to adjust interpretations that might be overly subjective or biased.

Case studies in applied linguistics research

With the wide variety of approaches to interviewing, the following selection of studies (see Table 6.1) provides examples of some of the more commonly conducted and cited approaches. Notably, several of these studies problematized the interview as a data collection method, which led to a clearer sense of identity development and co-construction of knowledge.

Ethnographic, narrative approaches inherently include interviews as a primary data collection method. Barkhuizen's (2006) study provides an excellent example of a narrative inquiry research design in which in-depth interviews are essential. He sought to gain an understanding of immigrant parents' perceptions of their children's use of language, especially their emotional response to their awareness of their children's linguistic changes, by prompting them to tell their stories. The content analysis employed allowed themes to emerge that were then coded, patterns identified and interpretations made. Similarly, Prior (2011) employed a narrative approach – specifically a narrative constructionist ethnography with a single immigrant participant in exploring self-representation in a complaint narrative. The theory supporting the interview as a data collection method was problematized by prior to extract what we might describe as 'beyond the words'. This longitudinal study involved interviews conducted over a period of 4 years, which was effective in grasping the various aspects of communication beyond simple transcriptions, displaying a strong sense of identity development and co-construction of knowledge.

Effective problematizing of interview theory can be done by conducting interviews in tandem with other data collection methods in a case study research design. For example, Spence and Liu (2013) used interviews as a follow-up to questionnaire data and as support for observation data in their study investigating the needs of engineers in Taiwan using English at work. McKinley (2018) used interviews to support the analysis of Japanese

Table 6.1 Examples of interviews in applied linguistics research

Researchers	Topic	Participants	Research design	Data collection method
Barkhuizen (2006)	Immigrant language use	Immigrant parents (*n* = 14)	Narrative inquiry	Single in-depth narrative interviews
Fang and Ren (2018)	Student awareness of Global Englishes	EFL undergrads in China (*n* = 12)	Mixed method	Single end of year interview in Chinese (plus reflective journal)
Farrell and Ives (2015)	Teacher beliefs	EAP teacher (*n* = 1)	Case study	Multiple interviews over 4-week period
Kuchah and Pinter (2012)	Children's perspectives of L2 education	L2 students in Cameroon (*n* = 5)	Exploratory	Single group interview
McKinley (2018)	Writer identity development	EFL writing students (*n* = 16) and teachers (*n* = 4)	Multiple case study	Monthly interviews over one academic year (plus text analysis)
Prior (2011)	Self-representation in immigrant narrative	Vietnamese immigrant in Canada (*n* = 1)	Ethnography (narrative constructionist)	20 hours of narrative interviews over 4 years
Spence and Liu (2013)	Engineering L2 English needs	Engineers in Taiwan (*n* = 11)	Case study/needs analysis	Single interview (plus questionnaire and observation)
Yan and Horowitz (2008)	Student perceptions of language anxiety	ESL students in China (*n* = 21)	Grounded theory	Single interview of 30–40 minutes, semi-structured in Mandarin

university students' English writing in the introduction of a new framework for analysing their writing. We chose this study to showcase an example of how interviews can be used to supplement other data collection methods, as the main data collection method in this study was the students' written texts (see Chapter 10 for document data collection).

Implications for researchers

Important to maintain throughout the entire research process is the recognition that the answers received in interviews are often superficial: 'what people *say* they do or *should* do in certain circumstances rather than what they actually do' (O'Reilly, 2009: 21). Researchers conducting interviews must therefore be aware that individual realities do not necessarily align with how interviewees present themselves in an interview. This does not necessarily mean that the data are misleading. When analysed critically, this self-reported reality helps a researcher to understand the phenomenon being studied from the level of the individual – their thoughts, feelings and ideas, which make up a community.

A successful interview is contingent on the interviewer's ability to listen to the interviewee and respond accordingly in the form of carefully recorded notes and follow-up questions. No matter how carefully planned the interview, the success of it depends much more on the interviewee's ability to facilitate respondents to speak on topic reflectively and critically. Learning to be an active listener takes practice, as interviewers need to analyse as they go, avoiding all judgement and potential steering of the interview and asking questions in such a way that interviewees *want* to tell them valuable information that they could not otherwise get in a questionnaire. In many ways, it is an art form, and even the most charming individual and engaging conversant needs to consider the greater research project and what the interviews can do to make or break the project.

Researchers using interviews must recognize the power dynamic involved, as an 'interview' is most often associated with a form of evaluation or assessment by the interviewee, although this will depend greatly on whether the interview is a study up, down or across (see Kubota, 2017). If interviewing experts or people in positions of power, consent forms should be very thorough, and negotiable, to establish a trusting interviewer-interviewee relationship. If conducting interviews as part of an ethnographic study, it might be more beneficial to avoid the word 'interview' altogether and use instead 'discussion', 'conversation' or similar. Note that in ethnographic research, the researcher will have established a relationship with the participant. This has implications for ethicality and sensitivity, discussed earlier in the chapter. In any qualitative interview, the researcher must be willing to give up power (perhaps best achieved through reflexivity), to allow interviewees to take the discussion in the directions they want to, and only help guide the discussion where it veers too far off topic.

Post-reading activities

Reflect
This chapter suggests that most interviews require reflexivity. Why do you think the authors have emphasized this so much? How do you strike the right balance between getting consistent data across interviews but also being reflexive to each interviewee's needs?

Expand
Individual or in small groups, each choose one of the studies in Table 6.1 to read and critique. After reading, consider and discuss: (1) Did the type of interview used in the study allow for a level of reflexivity appropriate to the topic? (2) Were there any aspects of the interview type (structure, timing or design) which could have been improved the data yielded? (3) What other data collection instruments could have been used to triangulate the data yielded from the interview, and if none were used, what could have been added?

Apply
Design a snapshot study which explores the language-related challenges of China-based students taking a content course in English for the first time. You are particularly interested in understanding the challenges they face and how challenges vary depending on different aspects of the course. Plan an interview that would be able to collect this type of data and pay particular attention to the following decisions: What format/type of interview would you use? What would you have participants reflect on? What would you reflect on? How would you ensure reliability and validity of the data?

Resources for further reading

Rolland, L., Dewaele J-M., & Costa, B. (2020). Planning and conducting ethical interviews: Power, language and emotions. In McKinley, J., & H. Rose (Eds.), *The Routledge handbook of research methods in applied linguistics*. Abingdon: Routledge.

This handbook chapter provides a clear introduction to preparing for and conducting interviews in applied linguistics research. The authors question power in the relationship between research participant and interviewer and take an ethical approach to the discussion. They raise the significance of working with multilingual participants, highlighting the importance of language choices offered in the interview, and adaptations that will need to correspond to the methodology. Issues of credibility are addressed by identifying our own interviewer vulnerabilities, recognizing the potential for vicarious traumatization and safely navigating working with vulnerable groups. They offer interview strategies such as emotional preparation, embodied reflexivity and self-care for both interviewer and interviewee.

Richards, K. (2009). Interviews. In Heigham, J., & R. Croker (Eds.), *Qualitative research in applied linguistics: A practical introduction* (pp. 182–198). New York: Palgrave Macmillan.

Much of the work of Richards on interviews has been mentioned already in this chapter, but this 2009 overview targets novice researchers, offering clear justifications for the use of this popular qualitative data collection method in applied linguistics research. In addition to the usual instructions about how to conduct interviews effectively, Richards raises some insightful considerations regarding ways of improving the quality of interviews. The pre- and post-reading questions should also prove valuable for novice researchers.

7

Diaries, Journals and Logs

Pre-reading activities

Think
Before reading this chapter, think about your answers to the following questions: What is the difference between a diary and a log? How about a journal versus a diary or log?

Discuss
In small groups, or as a class, discuss the following: (1) What are the advantages of using journals, diaries or logs to collect information from language students about various aspects of their language learning? (2) Are there any aspects of learning for which this data collection technique could prove quite useful? (3) How about for other areas of enquiry in applied linguistics?

Imagine
Imagine you are conducting a 3-week-long study which examines out-of-class contact that language users have with their second language. You are particularly interested in having participants report on out-of-class language use in a journal, diary or log. Plan an instrument that would be able to collect this type of data and pay particular attention to the following decisions: What type of information would your journal include? When would you have the participants record this information in their journal? Can you think of any methodological issues that might arise? How could you ensure that the participants record accurate information?

Introduction

One underutilized data collection technique in applied linguistics is the use of journals. A journal is defined as a data collection instrument, kept by participants, in which they record activities, accounts or thoughts surrounding a specific construct being investigated. In the context of instructed second language acquisition, a journal is defined as 'a regular record of language learning or learning-related activity which is kept by the learner, together with some form of review of that activity in order to inform future action' (Murphy, 2008: 199).

> Data from diary studies can be used to make cross-sectional comparisons across people, track an individual over time, or study processes within individuals or families. The main advantages of diary methods are that they allow events to be recorded in their natural setting and, in theory, minimize the delay between the event and the time it is recorded. (Krishnamurty, 2008: 197)

As journals are kept by participants themselves, they can be extremely effective to collect data related to language learning or use, which may otherwise be hidden from an outsider researcher. Journals can be a powerful research method to gain insight into learner practices and thoughts that may be impossible to elicit using other data collection methods (Dörnyei, 2007).

Journals can provide a valuable and systematic vehicle for reflection and learner introspection in autonomous learning (Porto, 2007). Bolger, Davis and Rafaeli (2003: 580) state that diaries and journals, as 'self-report instruments used repeatedly to examine ongoing experiences, offer the opportunity to investigate social, psychological, and physiological processes, within everyday situations'. A further strength is that journal methods facilitate the examination of event, behaviours and experiences in their normal, spontaneous settings, offering insight not achievable by many other methods (Reis & Gable, 2000).

A further strength of journals as a data collection instrument is that the participants themselves are given agency to present their own thoughts, behaviours and actions as data for analysis. Dörnyei (2007: 157) argues that a strength of journal studies is that 'the participants become co-researchers as they keep records of their own feelings, thoughts or activities'; thus, it is by its very nature 'an insider account'. If journal studies are designed well, they can provide highly contextualized and personal insights into the phenomenon being studied, and they minimize interference from external researchers.

Good journal studies can be used to collect meticulous information on the construct being studied, should not be overburdensome for participants and should produce data primed for analysis. Bad journal studies can collect invalid, messy or even missing data, which a researcher will have trouble to analyse when they apply their analytical frameworks to answer their research questions. This chapter lays the theoretical groundwork for journal studies, outlining key concepts, before showcasing examples of sound journal research in applied linguistics.

Key concepts

In this section, we explore key differences between journals, diaries and logs as well as key types of journals which can be used for research purposes. In this chapter, we do not discuss in-depth journals in their oft-used functions as pedagogic tools for learning, as outlined in early work such as Bailey (1983) and Howell-Richardson and Parkinson (1988). We also do not discuss heavily journals as tools for reflective practice in teacher education (e.g. Jervis, 1992) vis-à-vis examples of practitioner reflection for action (Schon, 1983). This pervasive use of journals in language education has pedagogical – not research – functions at its core. Borrowing terms from Bartlett and Milligan (2015), there is a difference between solicited journals, which serve a clear research purpose and unsolicited journals which are produced for other reasons. While data from unsolicited journals can also be used for research purposes (such as outlined in Parkinson and Howell-Hutchinson, 1990), they are best viewed according to their primary function rather than as data collection instruments. In this chapter, we explore the use of journals for the specific purpose of data collection in applied linguistics research.

Differences in format: Journals, diaries and logs

The terms *journal, diary* and *log* are often used interchangeably both within research methods and in daily life. However, this chapter makes a small, but important, distinction between the three.

In this book, we use the word 'journal' as the generic term to refer to any document which records specific activities and events, usually at a pre-established time in order to maintain a record for later use. Typical journals usually require participants to write very specific and targeted information related to the constructs being investigated. Journal entries can use a combination of written and categorical answers to set items or questions to capture the information required for analysis by a researcher.

We use the term 'diary' as a self-opinionated record, which can contain one's thoughts, reflections, moods and emotions and is written in the author's own time and usually by their own volition. According to Ma and Oxford (2014: 104), a diary 'is a form of learner narrative'. Oxford et al. (1996: 20) further define it as 'a type of self-report which allows learners to record on a regular basis numerous aspects of their learning process'. Our use of the term diary to describe this type of personalized writing is also in keeping with the style of 'diary methods' used in second language education, which now spans decades (e.g. Bailey, 1983; Casanave, 2012; Hall, 2008; Jervis, 1992; Oxford et al., 1996). Diaries usually include subjective, personal accounts of the construct being studied and thus involve a degree of creative freedom by the writer.

In contrast to the narrative style of diaries, a log is a more constrained version of journal, which often collects only specific information, usually in the form of numbers or words in predefined categories. Logs might require participants to enter specific information related to time, context, language use or interlocutors. They can embody a questionnaire-like structure, within which participants log their feelings and experiences on scales or other measures.

These differences can be further delineated via an illustrative example of a research project in applied linguistics, which aims to investigate out-of-class informal language contact of second language learners. A typical journal could be used for learners to record specific moments of language contact along with their reactions to these events. A diary might be used to explore learners' more personalized thoughts and reflections on these experiences. A log could be used for students to only record moments of language contact after each occurrence in predefined categories such as length of contact (in minutes), difficulties in communication (on a Likert scale), nationality of the interlocutor (within set categories) and purpose of communication (in short word format). Thus, while all of these documents could be referred to as journals, the term *diary* can be used to specify documents which require more self-opinionated introspection by the participants. Likewise, the term *log* could be used to signal that a journal seeks to maintain a record of pre-specified information.

Thus, all journals including diaries and logs are used to keep a record of events and are usually maintained by a person who can offer a first-hand account of the event being documented. However, in this chapter we use the term *journal* to describe the typical form of this document, but we use diaries and logs to respectively describe the more personalized and impersonalized formats of journals.

Types of journals

Journal methods can be categorized into the three types of design: interval contingent designs, signal contingent designs and event-contingent designs (e.g. Wheeler & Reis, 1991). Bolger et al. (2003) group interval and signal contingent designs into a single 'time-based' type as both are organized according to temporal factors. They argue: 'As we see it, diary studies serve one of two major purposes: the investigation of phenomena as they unfold over time, or the focused examination of specific, and often rare, phenomena' (Bolger et al., 2003: 588). Using this time-based category, they also outline an additional form of a time-based journal referred to as a variable-scheduled journal. By contrast, event-contingent journals are organized to occur with a particular experience and thus temporal elements do not dictate their use by participants.

Interval contingent journals require participants to write in their journals at set intervals, for example, at 10 a.m. and 3 p.m. each day, the end of each class, or on Fridays every week. This design can be useful to systematically investigate a topic. For example, in-service language teachers might be required to reflect on their lessons at the end of each day in order to collect data on how constructs taught in teacher education programmes affect teacher cognition. Similarly, newly arrived EAL immigrants might be required to record their language anxiety in a log using items on a Likert scale. Likewise, EFL learners might be required to report at the end of each week any informal out-of-class language contact they have had with speakers of the target language. While interval contingent journals might be useful for our trainee teacher example as a means to have them reflect on their lessons, they could prove more problematic for the language contact study, especially if the time between the event and the record-keeping is long. This may impact on the accuracy of the event being reported (discussed later in the section on validity and reliability). Likewise, an interval-based design would be especially problematic for our language anxiety study. As language anxiety can fluctuate depending on the activity in which the L2 user is engaged, a record of anxiety at the same point of each day may not be reflective of users' overall patterns of anxiety at different time periods. Perhaps at the end of the day the participants in the study will be most relaxed, because they are at home in a supportive environment, and the anxiety experienced during the day (when they were entrenched in the L2) has faded away.

A *signal contingent journal* requires participants to write in the journal at variable and randomized times. Signal contingent designs require participants to use the journal only when signalled to do so. They can be useful if temporal factors are seen to have an impact on the topic being researched. The timing of these signals is randomized by the researcher to capture maximum variation of construct being studied. In the past, researchers have signalled participants via a pager, a text or a phone call. These days, with the growth of mobile technologies, researchers are able to send mobile alerts, where participants can even log their experiences on their phones after receiving the signal to do so. As stated, this design is useful when randomization of time is important, especially if the construct you are measuring may change throughout the day. Thus, for our language anxiety study, this approach could potentially be a more valid design. A disadvantage of this design is that participants may be busy when they receive the signal and therefore may be unable to record extensive information in the journal. Due to this issue, signal-contingent designs often work best with log-type journals, which can be filled out quickly by the participants. Bolger et al. (2003) refer to an off-shoot of this journal design as a *variable-scheduled journal*, where a researcher instructs participants in advance to adhere to a certain response schedule, thus discarding the need for a signal to achieve variability in time. Both designs require participants to write entries at potentially inconvenient times, so researchers may have to provide a degree of flexibility for participants to use them (e.g. within 2 hours of the signalled or scheduled time).

Event-contingent journals require participants to write in their journals after they experience or complete the event being studied. They are useful to measure participant reaction to, or completion of, a task. As event-based designs centre around a specific behaviour or action, it is probably of most relevance to our illustrative language contact study. In this example, participants could be asked to answer questions in their journals directly after they have engaged in an incident of informal language contact. As Rose (2015: 428) observes, 'This format helps to minimize the time between the event and the report, thus avoiding the problems of other retrospective data collection methods, but adds structure to a research project more so than a narrative account.' Thus, an advantage of this format is that it helps to minimize the time between the event being studied and the participants' reporting of it. This is unlike interval-based designs, which may require a good degree of retrospection, especially if time has passed between the event and the journal-writing activity.

Design innovation

It is important to note that interval, signal/variable-scheduled and event-based designs are not mutually exclusive. In fact, 'Mixed or combination schedules can markedly strengthen a study design' (Bolger, 2003: 591). We would extend this observation to also cover broader journal formats. For example, a good journal data collection method might consider mixing the personal writing of diaries with the impersonal record-keeping of logs and thereby collect data primed for both qualitative and quantitative analysis. Returning to our hypothetical language contact example, a powerful journal design might mix diary types to have learners record essential information in an event-contingent log (such as brief descriptions of the context, topic, purpose and interlocutor) after each experience of language contact but also have students write more personal reflections on this language contact in an interval-based diary every two of days. The mixing of journal type and format can allow for a richer understanding of the phenomenon being researched. Mixing of journal formats can also save participants time. A single journal entry could potentially contain items where a participant can simply plot information on predetermined scales or categories in addition to providing lengthier written answers to set questions.

Procedures and practicalities

Time commitments

When a researcher decides to adopt journals as a data collection instrument, she must think carefully about the demands on the participant. Journals require a huge time investment of participants, so it is essential that participants are well informed of the time commitments of taking part in the study. In contexts where the researcher is exploring a classroom-learning activity, there may be pedagogical value to the exercise of journal keeping by learners (Bailey, 1983; Oxford, 1996). If so, there may be opportunities where the journals could be integrated within the curriculum, which is especially useful for the teacher-researcher. This gives the researcher more control over how the journals are implemented and adopted by the learners. Learners are also more likely to take their journal seriously as it becomes part of their language learning practice, which indicates value to their own language development. However, if the teacher-researcher wants to use these journals for research purposes, consent must still be sought from learners to use them in this way.

Another practical concern is that participants usually need comprehensive training to ensure that they fully understand the correct protocols of the journal's use (Reis & Gable, 2000). Nothing can be more frustrating to a researcher at the end of a journal study than to discover many of the journal entries contain the wrong type of information, due to being completed in unexpected ways. This can render data unreliable and a study incomplete. A good training session will also reduce the time and literacy demands of the journals on the participants (discussed later), as they will better understand how to use the journals and what information to record. A good journal should also have a clearly worded protocol attached to it so that participants can refer to it later. In a paper-based journal form, this could appear on the first page. In an electronic journal, this should be available at the click of a button.

Technology

Bartlett and Milligan (2015) argue that digital, web and social networking technologies have afforded the diary method with continued, and even enhanced, flexibility in collecting rich data from a wide range of participants. Even simple forms of technology can be useful in having students record their journals electronically. Electronic journals can also ensure that the information is kept confidential under password protection and that the journals will not get misplaced by participants. Good electronic journals should also ensure that participants can access them by any mobile or computing device, especially in the case of variable-scheduled, event-based or signal-based designs when participants are required to complete the journals 'on-the-move'.

A further advantage of an electronic journal is that entries are primed for data analysis as the researcher avoids a need to convert hand-written entries into type-written documents for analysis. This can be especially time-saving in diary studies, where each participant may produce thousands of words of lengthy written reflections. Nevertheless, there may be certain contexts where a paper-based journal is preferable either due to a lack of access to technology or a lack of functionality. These more traditional designs, however, will place more burden on the researcher during analysis.

Data analysis

Journals, like any data collection instrument, can be analysed in numerous ways, depending on the study's analytical framework and research questions. As shown in Chapter 1, research design, data collection research methods and data analysis are independent constructs. Nevertheless, some types of journals lend themselves to certain types of analysis. Narrative-style journals are usually analysed for their themes and content, either quantitatively via corpus linguistic methods or qualitatively via qualitative text analysis (Kuckartz, 2014), sometimes called qualitative content analysis (Mayring, 2000).

Logs on the other hand can produce data primed for statistical analysis, applying similar techniques as in the analysis of questionnaire content. In the field of psychology, journals are often used to obtain aggregate measures of a phenomenon over time, and journal data can be analysed via advanced statistical data analysis, such as multilevel modelling and structural equation modelling (Bolger et al., 2003). Thus, considering the strong connections between journal methods and quantitative analysis in psychological studies, journals in the other social sciences should definitely not automatically be relegated to qualitative methods. In most applied linguistics research thus far, journals have been used to mainly yield narratives for qualitative data analysis, and thus our field lacks good models of quantitative research using this method. Motivated quantitative researchers may, therefore, need to delve into the psychological research literature for further guidance.

Well-planned and -executed data analysis is important to navigate data collected via journal studies, as data can be quite voluminous. Plans for data analysis can also help to inform the design of the journals themselves. If a researcher has a clear understanding of how they plan to code and handle the data, they may be able to adjust items within the journals. For example, they may be able to replace certain questions with targeted short-answer responses, which are better formatted for analysis. If a researcher knows that they plan to analyse textual responses in journals in predefined categories, short-answer responses may be reduced into drop-down menus or multiple-choice items. This has an added advantage to reduce the time and literacy demands on the learner – a topic discussed in the next section.

Improving reliability and validity

Now that we have explored the practicalities of implementing journal studies, our attention turns to factors which may threaten reliability and validity of the information recorded in journals during data collection. Major threats to reliability and validity of journal data centre on the time, memory and literacy demands on participants which can sometimes lead to incomplete, ill-timed or inaccurate entries.

Memory deterioration and retrospection bias

Like any other form of retrospective data collection (see Chapter 4), it is essential that journal studies are sensitive to the time between the event or behaviour being researched and the writing up of it by a participant. As many researchers have noted, retrospective data are susceptible to being negativity affected by the memory capacity of the participants (Carson & Longhini, 2002; Oxford et al., 1996). It is also quite well established in research methods literature that the longer the time period between the event and the documentation of it, the more likely the record will be diminished in accuracy and detail. Unlike stimulated recall (discussed in Chapter 4), due to the autonomous nature of journal writing, the researcher is not in a strong position to help arouse the participants' memories.

Memory deterioration is especially problematic in interval-contingent designs, where substantial time may have passed between the concepts being studied and the recording of them in the journal. Interval contingent designs are sometimes used when it is not possible for participants to use their journal immediately during the language use or learning activities being studied, such as when learners have to report at the end of a busy school day on a learning activity which occurred in the morning. In these cases, researchers need to become more creative to solve issues surrounding memory deterioration. For example, to reduce effects of memory deterioration in a diary study conducted by Ma and Oxford (2014: 103), the participant 'kept a notebook during the classes to write down useful notes, and as soon as possible wrote the diary entries based on the notes'.

Memory deterioration can also be problematic for other designs as well. Signal contingent designs are dependent on having participants log their entries after receiving a signal to do so. This can be difficult for participants who are mobile at the time of receiving the signal or are engaged in other activities. For this reason, signal contingent designs may work best when the writing demands are lessened for the participants, so they can log their entries even when engaged in other activities. A foreign language anxiety study might, for example, merely have participants log their anxiety level of a sliding scale on their phone as soon as they receive a signal.

Likewise, event-contingent designs require the documenting of an event after it has occurred. The simplest solution to prevent memory deterioration is to reduce the time as much as possible between the incident being researched and the journal writing activity. While good in the theory, it can be difficult in reality, where participants are busy people and may often have to delay their entries until they have time. The effect of memory deterioration is also somewhat dependent on the topic:

> Retrospection bias may be a more pronounced problem for some phenomena than for others. Concrete, objective events (e.g., number of caffeinated beverages consumed) may be less susceptible to recall bias than are transient subjective feelings. (Bolger et al., 2003: 589)

Thus, journals which require records such as 'descriptions of interactions using the target language' might be less prone to memory deterioration than more affective constructs such as 'anxiety felt when using the target language'.

Time and literacy demands of the diary

Journal methods require a substantial time investment for participants. 'In order to obtain reliable and valid data, diary studies must achieve a level of participant commitment and dedication rarely required in other types of research studies' (Bolger et al., 2003: 592–593). As we state earlier in this chapter, it is possible to reduce the time demands of some journal content by replacing open-response questions with log-type items so that the time required for each journal entry is reduced. A detailed understanding of what type of data is needed for coding and analysis can feed into these decisions.

In applied linguistics, there is an added threat to reliability and validity compared to other fields in the social sciences, and that is the literacy demands of journal research methods. In applied linguistics research, our participants are often second, foreign or additional language users. Moreover, when participant populations come from a variety of L1s, data collection often occurs through the L2 or target language. Low-proficiency language users may struggle with the literacy demands of journal writing, particularly if the personalized diary format is used. As a result, participants may not write reliably (e.g. their entries may be infrequent and varying in length and quality of description), or they may not represent themselves validly (e.g. they may not be able to fully articulate a nuanced entry which truly reflects their thoughts, actions or behaviours).

To circumvent the literacy demands of journals, researchers have several options. First, they can allow students to write in their L1s (which repositions the literacy demands from the participants in data production to the researcher in data analysis). As Hall (2008: 119) observed in his diary study of twelve English language learners in the UK:

> it is possible that writing in English possibly affected the quality and quantity of the data, as might the daily collection of the diaries, and it would be interesting in a future study to explore these concerns through, for example, alternate L1/L2 entries.

Second, they could apply flexible guidelines to the journal writing task, allowing participants to use flexible language norms, translanguaging or multimodality in their expression (e.g. by allowing audio recordings of journal entries, use of drawings and so forth). Third, as with the reduction of time demands, researchers could reduce the literacy demands for L2 users by integrating scales, short responses and multiple-choice responses into the journals in place of open-ended response items.

Case studies in applied linguistics research

There have been numerous studies which have used journals as their data collection instrument, but compared to other methods it is still a rather underdeveloped approach. Furthermore, compared to other disciplines

Table 7.1 Examples of diaries, journals and logs in applied linguistics research

Researchers	Topic	Participants	Research design	Data collection method
Aubrey (2017a)	Flow in EFL classrooms	Japanese EFL learners ($n = 42$)	Quasi-experimental	Event-contingent journal completed after a set task, requiring five short answer items, completed on ten occasions
Casanave (2012)	Japanese language learning	Participant-researcher ($n = 1$)	Autoethnography	Interval contingent diary, requiring narrative accounts of learning
Galloway and Rose (2014)	Global Englishes exposure	EFL learners in Japan ($n = 108$)	Quasi-experimental (classroom intervention)	Event-contingent journal requiring four short answer items, completed on ten occasions; interviews
Goh (1997)	English language listening strategies	ESL learners in Singapore ($n = 40$)	Classroom intervention	Interval-based journals (weekly), completed on ten occasions.
Hall (2008)	Reflective language learning	Teacher ($n = 1$); EAL learners of German L1 ($n = 12$)	Ethnography	Unclear diary design completed over 4 weeks
Jervis (1992)	Teacher education	In-service teachers ($n = 15$)	Ethnography of teachers in 3–4-month teacher education course	Interval-contingent (weekly) reflective diaries over 3–4 months
Ma and Oxford (2014)	Learning strategies	Participant-researcher ($n = 1$)	Autoethnography/ Ethnography	Interval contingent diary, requiring narrative accounts of learning
Parkinson and Howell-Richardson (1990)	Activity and anxiety of language learners	General English learners ($n = 74$)	Survey design of use of English language use and anxiety	Interval-contingent journals (two-sides of A4), completed daily over 7–10 days

such as psychology, journal studies in applied linguistics are rather underutilized. Nevertheless, there have been notable studies over the years which serve as examples of journal-based studies. A small selection of these is outlined in Table 7.1. From this selection, we choose two to showcase in further detail.

The Jervis (1992) and Hall (2008) studies are showcased here to provide examples of typical 'diary' studies in applied linguistics research – which were heavily informed by earlier literature in teacher education (e.g. Bailey, 1990). These studies, while high in educational value and knowledge creation, are not necessarily the best examples of journals used for robust data collection due to this alternative purpose. Hall's (2008) study appears to adhere to no discernible study design and had learners and teachers reflect on classroom activities over a 4-week period. A daily interval point was established of which only 7–8 students frequently met. With a lack of structure or clear research focus, it is unsurprising that he found the method to be 'extremely problematical' (Hall, 2008: 121). Both the Hall (2008) and Jervis (1992) discuss problems fitting their diary studies into clear research designs, perhaps because they were grounded in pedagogy and reflective practice, rather than research. Nevertheless, we present them here to highlight the flexible ways in which journals are used especially when researching topics related to the language learner and the language teacher as reflective agents.

Goh (1997) and Parkinson and Howell-Richardson (1990) highlight the use of diaries to yield targeted constructs for research in language classrooms. Goh (1997) had a group of Chinese learners of English in Singapore keep listening journals in which they recorded occasions of listening to English, strategies used to comprehend the language heard, and thoughts and opinions on the task. The study by Parkinson and Howell-Richardson (1990) explored the language use in and outside of the classroom of general English learners ($n = 74$) across two cohorts. Journal entries consistent of targeted log-type and diary-type items organized on a single A4 piece of paper. Participants completed a journal entry each day, over 7 days for one cohort and 10 days for the other. This study further highlights a second study of modern languages students.

The Ma and Oxford (2014) and Casanave (2012) studies are examples of using a 'personal diary' to collect data in the form of learner narratives within an autoethnographic study design. As outlined in Chapter 1, autoethnography is a research design which draws together the features of autobiography and ethnography (Paltridge, 2014). Thus, the participant in each of these studies was also an author on the published article. Ma and Oxford (2014) used an interval-based diary to record activities surrounding a learner's conscious use of language learning strategies. The participant-researcher used notes throughout the day to minimize retrospection bias. Casanave (2012) used personal diaries to analyse her autobiographical journal as a second language learner of Japanese, an experience she further elaborated on in a methodology-focused paper (Casanave, 2017).

The Aubrey (2017a) and Rose and Galloway (2014) studies highlight the use of event-based journals, which are connected to specific classroom-based tasks. In Aubrey's (2017a) study, 208 journal entries were collected from 42 Japanese EFL learners. The entries were connected to specific intercultural and intracultural tasks set by the teacher, who was also the researcher. Additional data were also collected via questionnaires and transcripts from the tasks, although these were reported in a separate article (Aubrey, 2017b).

We choose now to showcase two studies to highlight the various formats of journals used for research (journals, diaries and logs), as well as the types of journals (interval, signal and event-contingent) with each study offering insight into a different combination of these dimensions.

Galloway and Rose (2014): An event-contingent journal-type study

In Rose and Galloway's (2014) study, 1,092 journal entries were collected from 108 Japanese EFL learners, which explored learner reflections on a listening activity of exposure to Global Englishes. The listening activity was an assigned homework task for students and formed part of their English language course curriculum. As the researchers describe, the 'journals served as a pedagogical task, and as a research instrument' (Galloway & Rose, 2014: 386). Listening journals most often take form of an event-contingent design – that is, these journals only require participants to make an entry into the journal after the event being studied. Event-contingent journals such as listening journals often require learners to record specific information rather than lengthy narratives and thus avoid some of the pitfalls of other types of journals, which include time and literacy demands on the participants, outlined previously in this chapter.

Drawing on this design, the researchers required students to listen to ten self-selected audio samples of Global Englishes and record in their journals: the speaker's nationality, the reasons for choosing that particular audio sample and an extended reflective comment on the listening activity. The task resulted in 1,092 journal entries collected from 108 learners over 4 classes, which were coded for qualitative analyses, of which some codes were further reduced to counts of frequency.

Important to note in this study was that one of the researchers was also the teacher of the learners, which reveals both advantages and disadvantages of the research design. As the journal activity was fully integrated into the curriculum, the researchers could obtain a sizeable data set, which was largely produced by the students. The integration of the journals into the curriculum also meant there were few to no missing entries from participants. To obtain a data set of 10 different time points from each of 108 participants would normally require a huge time investment from researchers using other methods (e.g. interviews). This study highlights a clear advantage of diary methods in harnessing the 'participant-as-co-researcher' role. A disadvantage of having the journals serves a dual research and learning purpose was that the journals needed to be written in English by the students, which increased the literacy demands placed on them. This decision may have also reduced participants' ability to fully communicate nuances in their reflective comments, as suggested by Hall (2008). This may, in part, explain the simplistic stereotypes in reflections, which were noted by the researchers (see Galloway & Rose, 2014).

Casanave (2012): A variable-scheduled diary-type study

A second illustrative study is by Casanave (2012) which is representative of a more informal diary study used to capture unstructured reflections on one's learning experiences. In this study, the author draws on her own personal learning diaries spanning 8 years of Japanese language learning. While it is clear from Casanave's thick narrative descriptions that her journal was of a diary format, it is unclear whether these diaries fall into a formal categorization of research diary type. Interval-based design usually necessitates a degree of systematicity in terms of the time points of journal entry – a feature not entirely apparent in this study. The use of the diary at varying intervals over the 8 years could mean we could broadly categorize it as a variable-scheduled diary, albeit with a very loose schedule. However, we would argue that variable-scheduled diaries require the researcher to predetermine entry times for the participants. Nevertheless, the approach was used within an autoethnographic research design in which the researcher was also the participant, and thus it is perhaps the best way to categorize its design.

Years later Casanave (2017) discusses her experiences publishing the findings of her diary study, which she states to have necessitated twenty drafts before having it successfully published in *TESOL Quarterly*. While she chalks up much of this difficulty due to the challenges of presenting one's own story as research, she does allude to the fact that the diaries had been written for a different purpose, and only later did she decide to reimagine them as a 'piece of autoethnographic "research", in the tradition of the diary studies' (Casanave, 2017: 239). Thus, an alternative way to look at this study as a research method is that it is not a pure diary study at all but rather the content analysis of a diary as a textual artefact. That is, the existence of the diary was external to, and independent from, the reported study.

The use of Casanave's (2012) diary is also highly removed from the use of dairies in much psychological research, as too is its analysis, which is connected to narrative inquiry – a burgeoning field in applied linguistics (see Barkhuizen, 2014). Nevertheless, Casanave's (2012) narrative study shows how journals, as vessels of data collection, can be used to produce highly nuanced and personal data for in-depth qualitative analysis. Her data analysis is very different from the impersonal frequency counting and thematic analysis of the Galloway and Rose (2014) study, highlighting the broad spectrum of data yielded by journal methods. Casanave's (2012, 2017) study further highlights how journals can be applied in creative and novel ways to a wide variety of social research topics which fall under the applied linguistics umbrella.

Implications for researchers

If journals are such a powerful way to collect data, then why do we not see more good journal studies in applied linguistics? One explanation may be that early, and influential, diary studies in the field (e.g. Bailey, 1983) took a somewhat constrained view of journals and presented them as the stereotypical 'dear diary' instruments in which participants were free to record their feelings and reflections. A general trend in using diaries in this manner can be tracked over time, especially in terms of research related to teacher and learner reflection (e.g. Casanave, 2012; Hall, 2008; Jarvis, 1992). While such diaries might be useful for reflective research, they offer a very narrow illustration of how journals can be used by applied linguistics researchers. Looking at the bulk of journal methods over the decades in applied linguistics, it is no wonder that the method has developed a reputation for not being terribly robust. In fact, Bartlett and Milligan (2015) note that most highly regarded and popular research methods books make little to no mention of the method.

For this reason, we have intentionally elected to adopt the term *journal* in this chapter instead of the typical term of *diary* used in other social science disciplines. By using the term *journals*, we hope to distance this method from images of personal diaries in order to position journals as the highly contextualized and powerful data collection instruments that they are. While diary-type studies remain useful to continue the tradition of collecting reflections and narratives in language education studies, they offer just a glimpse of the possibilities of how this method is applied in other social science research disciplines. Unshackling the data collection method from this constrained function and diving into the psychological research on journal studies will further open the possibilities to use this method for a range of applied linguistics topics, including those in the cognitivist, social and psychological domains.

It is an understatement to write that journal studies have not been fully realized as a methodology in applied linguistics research. This fact is especially egregious considering many of our researchers work alongside large cohorts of language learners, who are in a prime position to record in such journals due to their dual function as a research instrument and pedagogical tool. In fact, in the Galloway and Rose (2014) study, the use of journal data for research purposes was ancillary to its production as a homework task for the participating students, but it nevertheless achieved a substantial sample size due to its integrated function. Thus, there is huge potential for carefully planned journal studies to yield wider ranging and targeted data than this chapter has been able to showcase in its highly limited examples. As a discipline we have merely scratched the surface of the potential that this research method has to offer.

Post-reading activities

Reflect

This chapter suggests that journal methods have not been fully developed in applied linguistics compared to other disciplines such as psychology. Why do you think this is so?

Expand

Individual or in small groups, choose one of the studies in Table 7.1 to read and critique. After reading, consider and discuss: (1) Did the type of journal design chosen in the study match the research aims of the study? (2) Were there any aspects of the methodology which could have been improved in design or implementation? (3) What other data collection instruments could have helped to triangulate the data yielded in the study?

Apply

Design a 3-month-long study which explores the language-related challenges of UK-based French language students going on a short-term exchange in France for the first time. You are particularly interested in understanding the challenges they face and how challenges decrease or increase in intensity throughout this period. Plan an instrument that would be able to collect this type of data and pay particular attention to the following decisions: What format/type of journal would you use? How would you have participants record information in the journal (i.e. what items would be included)? When would you have the participants record this information in their journal? How would you ensure reliability and validity of the data?

Resources for further reading

Bolger, N., Davis, A., & Rafaeli, E. (2003). Diary methods: Capturing life as it is lived. *Annual Review of Psychology, 54*: 579–616.

Although this resource is based in the field of psychology, we think it is one of the best articles which delineates journal research explicitly and unambiguously. It is the source of many key concepts in this chapter including the types of journals and threats to validity and reliability when using them for data collection. With more than 3,000 citations within the broader academic literature, it is the most referenced article on the method within the social sciences (source: Google Scholar). Note that the authors of this paper use the term *diary* in the same way that we use *journal* in this chapter, and it refers to targeted, rather than highly personalized, writing.

Bartlett, R., & Milligan, C. (2015). *What is diary method?*. Bloomsbury Publishing.

This book provides an accessible and concise introduction to the diary method in social and health sciences. It is aimed at novice researchers and postgraduate students and offers useful guidance on diary design, practicalities, use of technology, ethics and control over reliability and validity of the method. At just 136 pages, it is a simple go-to resource for people venturing into diary studies for the first time.

8

Questionnaires

Pre-reading activities

Think

Before reading this chapter, think about your answers to the following questions: Have you ever filled out a questionnaire for market research or an academic study? What was the questionnaire measuring (e.g. facts, behaviours, attitudes)? Did you enjoy completing the questionnaire? What made the questionnaire easy/difficult/engaging/frustrating to complete?

Discuss

In small groups, or as a class, discuss the following: (1) What are the advantages and disadvantages of using questionnaires as a data collection methodology relative to using, say, interviews? (2) What kinds of data can a questionnaire yield? What kinds of data are questionnaires less capable of generating? Are there topics/situations/populations for which using a questionnaire would be inadvisable? (3) What features of a questionnaire might influence the quality of the data it collects?

Imagine

Imagine you are designing a study that aims to explore the attitudes of EFL learners in Spain towards task-based language teaching. Briefly review articles in which questionnaires were used to probe language learners' attitudes towards L2 pedagogy and think about the following questions: How were the key constructs defined and applied in the instrument design? How and when were the questionnaires administered, and why did the researchers choose this approach? How do the researchers address the issues of validity and reliability of their findings?

Introduction

Questionnaires are a hugely popular choice of data collection research methodology among applied linguists. Variously termed *surveys, inventories, scales* and *profiles*, Brown (2001: 6) defines questionnaires as 'any written instruments that present respondents with a series of questions or statements to which they are to react either by writing out their answers or selecting from among existing answers'. Dörnyei (2003) identifies three types of questionnaires based on the type of data elicited:

1 Facts (e.g. date of birth, language learning experience)
2 Behaviour (e.g. language learner strategy use, self-regulation)
3 Attitudes (e.g. evaluations, values, opinions, beliefs, interests)

Arguably, however, most questionnaires will be a combination of at least two of these types because researchers generally collect demographic (factual) information about their respondents in tandem with measuring their behaviour or attitudes.

At face value, questionnaires are a 'quick and dirty' data collection methodology, enabling time-efficient data collection from large numbers of people, even at a distance. Questionnaire data are increasingly easy to collect and process, as an abundance of web-based tools (e.g. Qualtrics, Bristol Online Survey Tool, SurveyMonkey, Mechanical Turk, Google Forms) offer phone and tablet-supported administration and direct data exports to Microsoft Excel, SPSS and other data analysis packages. Questionnaires are also a flexible research method, as they can be applied to both qualitative and quantitative research and to a wide range of topics, populations and situations. The anonymity offered by questionnaires is another of their advantages: unlike, say, interviews, focus groups and other self-report methodologies, questionnaires provide participants the opportunity to respond to a topic 'unseen', which is likely to encourage honest and frank responses.

Despite their many advantages as a data collection tool, questionnaires – if developed and administered without the requisite care – can yield data of very poor quality. This means that sufficient time needs to be devoted to designing and piloting them before the main data collection phase of a study, thereby belying the face value of ease and speed. Questionnaires are subject to the same limitations as other types of self-report methodology, in that individuals vary in their capacity for introspection and retrospection. Also, the data that questionnaires yield can be affected by *bias*: factors or conditions beyond the study's focus that influence respondents' answers. For example, questionnaire items and response scale labels, such as the difference between 'sometimes' and 'frequently', can be interpreted differently by different participants, leading to an element of subjectivity in the data collection procedure that often remains unacknowledged in the discussion of findings. Furthermore, while anonymity may lead to greater honesty, there are no means of establishing how truthful participants' responses actually are.

Questionnaires are enticing to many novice researchers, as they deceptively seem like an easy way to collect a large volume of data. In reality, questionnaires can easily lead to poor quality and unusable data, if correct procedures are not followed or satisfactory precautions are not taken. This chapter lays the theoretical groundwork for using questionnaires in applied linguistics research, outlining key concepts and issues before showcasing examples of sound use of questionnaires in the literature.

Key concepts

In this section, we introduce validated questionnaires and original questionnaires and discuss their benefits, limitations and implications.

Original questionnaires

If there is an existing measure for the construct of interest that is theoretically supported, reliable, well validated and appropriate to use with a certain population (see Chapter 4 for discussion of the processes involved in locating and obtaining copies of validated measures), then we would argue that there is no point in a researcher 'reinventing the wheel' by designing a novel instrument. However, where there are no existing instruments appropriate for use in a study, the task of questionnaire design and development must be undertaken. This does not mean, however, that reference to existing measures should be entirely abandoned. Far from it: where an original tool is being designed, it is common practice for researchers to 'borrow' quality questionnaire items from existing tools. One of the key benefits of original questionnaire design and administration, therefore, is that if it is carried out in a principled and meticulous manner, the resulting tool is not only beneficial in terms of yielding valid and reliable data for a study but is also a contribution to the field at large as a useful tool for others to adopt or adapt in future research.

Validated questionnaires

Some questionnaires have been so influential in applied linguistics research that the questionnaires themselves have formed the basis of journal articles. These include Oxford's (1990) Strategy Inventory for Language Learning (SILL) and the Language Contact Profile (LCP) developed by Freed et al. (2004). Using existing questionnaires can be very beneficial for research, both in terms of the time and resources saved in creating an original tool and for enhancing comparability between the findings of the study and other research that has investigated a similar topic using the same tool. Yet it is often the case that a validated questionnaire will need to be adapted in some way for use in another study; for example, for use with a different population, or for a slightly different 'take' on a given construct: in cases such as these, the principles of original questionnaire design should be kept in mind and rigorously applied.

We would thus argue that whether the researcher designs an original questionnaire, adapts an existing questionnaire or administers a validated questionnaire without adaptation, the procedures and practicalities outlined in this chapter are equally important to consider. In original questionnaire design, the researcher is applying these principles for him- or herself. In using a validated instrument, the researcher is evaluating the application of these principles by the original questionnaire developer. In adapting an existing measure, the researcher is combining personal application with evaluation of others' application of these principles.

Procedures and practicalities

In this section, we focus on the processes and procedures involved in using questionnaires in research. We look at defining and operationalizing a construct, writing and selecting appropriate items and response scales, formatting and sampling, and piloting, administration and analysis.

Constructs

Questionnaires commonly measure *constructs*: that is, phenomena that are not readily observable and that may comprise a number of subcomponents, for example personality, values or anxiety. For a questionnaire to measure a construct, the construct must first be *operationalized*: in other words, measurable indicators of the construct should be developed. Some constructs are very easily operationalized. For example, the construct of 'age' is operationalized by simply asking respondents to state their date of birth. Others are infinitely more complex. For example, one indicator of L2 motivation might be how positively a person feels about the second language, but L2 motivation might also be evidenced by how much time an individual spends studying the language or their future goals for using the language: in the case of L2 motivation, therefore, there are multiple indicators that its operationalization needs to encompass. For complex, multidimensional constructs, it may be necessary to develop subscales in a questionnaire such that there are items measuring each of the construct's components. Consideration should be given to whether the components are equally weighted: that is, theoretically speaking, are some components more important indicators of the construct than others? If so, it may be reasonable to analyse the data from components separately or to assign different weights to items in different subscales.

Item writing

After defining and operationalizing the constructs of interest, one of the first steps in questionnaire development is *item writing*. Questionnaire items can broadly be categorized as either open or closed. Open items require participants to 'free-write' their response. While open items are useful in enabling respondents to express their opinions in their own words, they are very rarely the only type of item in a questionnaire. It is more common to combine closed and open items, with open items included to allow respondents to explain or justify their choices on a closed-type item. This is because open items take longer to complete, thus limiting the number of items that can be included in the questionnaire. They are also complex to transform into any meaningful numeric code and can thus be difficult to analyse.

Closed items force respondents to choose the response that best matches their viewpoint from a set of options. Closed item response scales can be dichotomous (e.g. Yes/No) or include more than two options (e.g. Never/Sometimes/Always). One of the most prevalent graduated closed item response scales is the *Likert scale*, which requires the respondent to read a statement and then choose one of usually five or six options from 'Strongly disagree' to 'Strongly agree'. Another prevalent graduated item type is the *semantic differential scale*, whereby the participant marks their response between two bipolar labels, one at either extreme of the scale. For example, self-reported L2 proficiency might be measured by asking respondents to mark a point between 'Highly proficient' and 'Not at all proficient'. *Numerical rating scales* require the participant to assign a 'score' out of a possible total for each item to indicate the extent to which they agree with the statement.

The advantage of using closed items is that, through the restriction of respondents' answers, the item is arguably more easily and quickly answered by the respondent, and the resulting data are easily and quickly coded by the researcher. Using closed items can also boost the total number of items that can be included in a measure: because they are quick to complete, more closed than open items can be answered in a given time period. However, restricting response options may introduce bias into the data, in that respondents are forced to select a response even where there may not be an option that truly matches their viewpoint. Similarly, the questionnaire developer may have offered response options that would otherwise not have occurred to the respondent. Another issue with closed items is a lack of depth: the respondent is not able to explain or justify their response option selection and is forced to 'place all their eggs in one basket'. For example, in response to a frequency-based scale, it may be the case that the respondent 'Always' behaves in a particular way in a given context yet if the context changes would only behave in that way 'Sometimes' or 'Rarely'.

Two questions that often arise when considering an appropriate response scale for a set of closed questionnaire items are: (1) how many scalar points to include and (2) whether to opt for an even or odd number of points on the scale. Regarding the first question, Menold and Bogner (2016) posit that the greatest validity, reliability and differentiation are attained with five to seven scalar points and further argue that a five-to-seven-point scale is more favourable to respondents and easier for the researcher to verbally label. The latter question is more complex to answer: if an odd number is employed, there is no guarantee that a respondent who selects the scale midpoint harbours a neutral viewpoint. For example, their choice might represent an unwillingness to answer the question, a lack of opinion on the topic or an issue with comprehension of the item. On the other hand, if an even number is employed, the respondent is forced either to agree or disagree. This is problematic because of *acquiescence bias*, which refers to the propensity of people to agree with statements about which they are undecided or unsure. On balance, we recommend using an odd number of scalar points to avoid forcing participants' hands. However, care must be taken in the *item analysis* phase to determine whether certain items have yielded a disproportionate number of mid-point responses. Where this is the case, the items in question might usefully be omitted or reworded and re-piloted to establish whether it is the topic of the question itself or rather the wording of the item that is leading participants to the central point.

When investigating a *latent construct* (i.e. an unobservable phenomenon, such as motivation or aptitude), it is recommended that *multi-item scales* are used. A multi-item scale is the use of more than one item to measure the same construct (or sub-construct). Multi-item scales are useful because they reduce the potential for bias carried by the wording of individual items. While there is no set number of items for a multi-item scale, Dörnyei and Csizér (2012) recommend a bare minimum of four per (sub)construct, such that if one of the items on the scale performs poorly at the *item analysis* stage, there are still multiple viable items remaining for inclusion in the final version of the instrument.

Formatting

Once an initial item pool has been arrived at, then the researcher's task is to arrange the items in a format which is clear and engaging for piloting with the intended population. There are some useful rules of thumb to apply in formatting a questionnaire. First, researchers should try to use the minimum possible number of items to avoid any *fatigue effect*, which could lead to non-completion of the tool and thus a lower response rate, especially if the questionnaire is administered remotely (i.e. online). Fatigue may also lead participants to respond to items, particularly those towards the end of a questionnaire, with a lack of care. Therefore, factual items (e.g. date of birth, gender) should be placed at the end of the instrument: this is so that the items that measure the construct of primary interest are responded to when the participants' attention is 'fresh'.

Items are usefully grouped by topic with each new topic introduced by a linking sentence (e.g. 'This section asks about contact with English outside of the classroom'), and by format, with each new section preceded by clear instructions on how to answer (e.g. 'Please tick one box next to each sentence'). In addition, Dörnyei (with Taguchi) (2010) advises against placing items from a multi-item scale consecutively after one another as a means of avoiding repetition.

Sample size

In questionnaire-based research, *sample size* matters. In simple terms: the bigger, the better. However, determining an exact minimum or optimal number of participants should be driven by consideration of the types of analyses that will be conducted on the data. This means that the analytic approach needs to be decided upon in advance of consideration of sample size. A basic rule of thumb, posited by Hatch and Lazaraton (1991), is that a sample size of thirty participants is the minimum number required to achieve normal distribution of a variable (i.e. when the distribution of values resembles a perfect bell-shaped curve), which is a primary assumption of parametric inferential statistics (the most powerful statistical tests that enable generalization to the population and the testing of hypotheses, such as *t-tests* and *multiple regression*).

Where group comparisons are to be made, the rule of thumb of a minimum sample size of thirty should be applied to each group in the sample. For example, if a researcher intends to compare the foreign language classroom anxiety of beginner, intermediate and advanced proficiency learners, every group (beginners, intermediates, advanced) should include at least thirty cases. However, in order for true group differences or relationships between variables to be confidently detected (i.e. to reach statistical significance), a minimum sample size of 50 per group is recommended (Dörnyei (with Taguchi), 2010). Additionally, certain statistical analyses require a far greater number of participants than thirty or fifty: for example, the sample size for factor analysis is posited to be an absolute minimum of $n = 100$ (Gorsuch, 1983; Kline, 1994).

Sampling strategy

A good sample is one which is truly representative of the population: in other words, that matches the population on all characteristics that may have a bearing on the construct(s) that a questionnaire is designed to probe. Sampling strategy is important because the extent to which a sample is a true representation of the target population dictates the *generalizability* of the questionnaire findings. Sampling strategies can be dichotomized as either probability based or non-probability based. *Probability-based sampling* refers to procedures that include random selection of participants to the sample from the population. Random selection is important because by reducing systematicity in the selection of participants, the potential influence of any peripheral variables on the key construct in the study is diminished. Some prevalent probability-based methods are *simple random sampling* (whereby all members of the population are represented by a number and a random number generator is employed to determine which numbers to include), *systematic random sampling* (whereby all members of the population are randomly given a number and every 'nth' (e.g. seventh) number is selected for inclusion) and *stratified random sampling* (whereby the population are divided into rational groups, usually based on more than one key characteristic, and simple random sampling is used to select participants within groups).

It is often the case, however, that the researcher does not have access to all of the people she or he is interested in researching (i.e. the entire population) and is therefore unable to ensure that every member of the population (or of a group within the population) has known odds of being selected into the sample. As such, *non-probability sampling* methods are very commonly used. Some prevalent non-probability sampling methods are purposive sampling, convenience sampling, snowball sampling and quota sampling. *Purposive sampling*, as the name suggests, involves purposive selection of participants on the part of the researcher. That is, the researcher deliberately selects certain individuals to include based on the purpose of the study. This process involves the predetermination of a set of exclusion and inclusion criteria (e.g. over a certain proficiency threshold, from a specific L1 background). Purposive sampling may target individuals who are likely able to provide the most information on a given phenomenon (*critical case sampling*), who have expertise in the phenomenon (*expert case sampling*), who have idiosyncratic characteristics in relation to the phenomenon (*extreme case sampling*), who are likely to represent a wide array of perspectives on the phenomenon (*maximum variation sampling*) or who are purported to represent the 'standard' perspective on or experience of the phenomenon (*typical case sampling*).

Convenience sampling (also termed *opportunity sampling*) is another non-probability method. It involves sampling based on convenience of access: that is, sampling members of the population who are geographically proximal to the researcher(s) and who are willing to participate. *Snowball sampling* begins with purposive sampling, in that the researcher first selects an individual or group of individuals who meet the inclusion criteria for participation. Then, this initial group of participants is asked to recommend or contact other people like them, who are also likely to meet the inclusion criteria. *Quota sampling* involves the use of a priori fixed quota to non-randomly select participants from the population. *Proportional quota sampling* describes the practice of deriving fixed quotas for the sample related to the proportions of certain key characteristics in the population. For example, if pupils who study French in the UK school system are 60 per cent female, and a sample size of 100 pupils is the target, then a proportional quota sampling approach would mean that only 40 boys are recruited to the study, even if there is potential access to a greater number of boys who meet the inclusion criteria. In *non-proportional quota sampling*, however, the researcher predetermines how many participants will be recruited in each category (e.g. fifty boys and fifty girls), usually on the basis of ensuring that there are sufficient numbers in each key category for group comparisons to be made. One key consideration in quota sampling is the choice of population characteristics on which to focus: just as in purposive sampling, the researcher must ensure that the characteristics selected are those that will yield a strong match between sample and population.

Piloting

It is crucial to pilot a questionnaire prior to its administration in the main phase of a study. This tenet holds for both validated questionnaires and original questionnaires. When using a validated measure in its original form, the process of *piloting* is likely more focused on the experience of the pilot participants, who should be as representative of the population as the main study sample. For example, to determine the length of time it takes them to complete the measure, to pinpoint any items or formatting issues (e.g. font size) that cause difficulty and to gauge the utility of the response scale from the respondents' perspective. In this regard, it is useful to pilot a questionnaire in person, such that a critical discussion of the tool can be held with the pilot participant during or immediately after completion of their responses. In applied linguistics research specifically, the issue of comprehension of questionnaire instructions and items is particularly important where a measure is administered in the respondents' L2. If the L2 proficiency of the sample is not sufficient to adequately comprehend the language used in a questionnaire, it is recommended that problematic items are simplified or that the tool as a whole is translated into the mother tongue (see Chapter 4 for a detailed discussion of translating validated measures) and then re-piloted in its simplified or translated form.

Piloting original questionnaires involves a greater number of steps and considerations than piloting validated measures. The initial piloting will not only encompass the practical experience of the pilot participants as described above but also serve to generate data for a priori statistical exploration in the form of *item analysis*, whereby the ability of individual items to discriminate between respondents is scrutinized. Piloting will also test the *internal consistency* of the questionnaire, whereby the degree of correlation between participants' responses is calculated (see Chapter 4 for a detailed discussion of the procedures for conducting item analysis and establishing internal consistency). For this reason, we recommended a pilot sample size of at least thirty for original questionnaires, mirroring Hatch and Lazaraton's (1991) guideline for sample size for inferential statistics. Once the measure has been adapted on the basis of these initial analyses, it must be piloted again with a new pilot sample and subjected to the same analyses to determine whether the *item discrimination* and internal consistency are now improved and ensure that any issues of formatting and clarity have been resolved.

Administration

Once a sampling size and strategy has been decided, the success of questionnaire-based research hangs on administration: the tool must be administered to the target sample in a manner which maximizes the response rate while minimizing any threats to the validity of reliability of the findings. In applied linguistics research, questionnaires are most commonly administered on a one-to-one basis (i.e. the researcher sitting with the participant while s/he completes the measure), to groups of participants (e.g. in-tact classes of L2 learners) or online, via email or using web-based programmes such as Survey Monkey or Qualtrics. See Dörnyei (with Taguchi) (2010: 67–72) for a detailed discussion of the strengths and limitations of each approach and recommendations for enhancing response rate, reliability and validity.

Data analysis

The first step in analysing questionnaire data is *coding* of the responses into numerical values that will yield variables. Questionnaire data commonly yield one or more of three types of variable: (1) *nominal*, whereby categories that cannot be meaningfully ordered or ranked are arbitrarily assigned numerical values (e.g. 0 = 'Male'; 1 = 'Female'); (2) *ordinal,* whereby a fixed number of ordered/ranked categories are assigned numerical values (e.g. a frequency scale from 0 = 'Never' to 5 = 'Always'); or (3) *continuous,* whereby the respondent provides a value from a potentially infinite range of responses (e.g. number of hours of formal L2 instruction). Note that where negatively worded items have been used with ordinal response scales, the resulting data should be *reverse coded* before analysis such that an assigned high value represents the same sentiment as for positively worded items.

Frequency-based descriptive analyses are commonly applied to nominal variables (e.g. calculating the proportions of men and women in a sample), for which the *mode* (the most commonly occurring value) is the central measure. The most widely reported measure of central tendency for ordinal data is the *median* (middle) score and for continuous data the *mean* (average). Parametric statistical tests (e.g. *t*-tests, ANOVAs) assume that the dependent variable is continuous and normally distributed, so non-parametric alternatives (e.g. Mann–Whitney *U*, Kruskal–Wallis) should be used with nominal and ordinal data or with continuous data that are subject to outliers or extreme values. Although Likert-type data are firmly ordinal, it is not unusual for researchers to calculate the mean instead of the median (or mode) from this type of response scale and to use the resulting measure in parametric analyses. Briggs Baffoe-Djan and Smith (2020) suggest that this practice is only defensible where the mean is derived from a multi-item ordinal scale comprised of a high number of individual items.

Data reduction

As questionnaires usually include large numbers of items, it is common for researchers to apply *data reduction* techniques such that there are a smaller number of more concentrated variables to work with in the data analysis phase. One technique in this regard is to take the mean (or sum) of items on a multi-item scale; however, the *internal consistency* of the scale in measuring the underlying construct must first be established. To do this, a reliability analysis in the form of *Cronbach's alpha* can be run (see Chapter 4 for a discussion of interpreting alpha values). Cronbach's alpha coefficient should first be calculated on pilot data prior to the main study questionnaire administration in order to pinpoint and amend/omit low-performing items in advance (see Chapter 4 for a detailed discussion of *item analysis).* Alpha should then be run again on the main study data, and it is this a posteriori coefficient that is reported in the write up of the research (usually in the Methodology section of the document where the instrument is detailed, rather than in the Results section). An alpha statistic should be reported for each of the multi-item scales in a questionnaire.

Another commonly applied questionnaire data reduction technique is *factor analysis*, which is a statistical procedure that seeks to identify patterns in responses to questionnaire items on a given construct via *intercorrelation*. Where a cluster of large correlation coefficients is detected, the items yielding the cluster are grouped together into a factor. Each factor is deemed to represent an underlying dimension (or *latent variable*) of the original construct – a dimension that may or may not have been accounted for in the item writing phase of the questionnaire development. For example, a series of items designed to measure awareness of L2 vocabulary strategies may have been written with a skill focus in mind (e.g. strategies that involve writing, listening, speaking and reading), yet factor analysis of the data might yield factors that group the strategies by function (e.g. to determine meaning, to memorize) or by context (e.g. interactional, individual). For each factor yielded, a *factor score* (i.e. a calculation of the score that respondents would have received for the factor had it been directly measured) can be estimated and used in other analyses (e.g. as a predictor variable in regression modelling).

There are two main types of factor analysis: *exploratory factor analysis* (EFA) and *confirmatory factor analysis* (CFA). The former serves to detect interrelationships in the data where there are no firm preconceived theoretical assumptions about the latent structure of the observed (i.e. measured) construct. The latter, however, is a much more sophisticated statistical procedure which seeks to test (i.e. confirm) a hypothesized latent set of factors. As such, EFA can be seen as way of characterizing the data and contributing to theory development, whereas CFA uses data to directly test theory (and therefore contributes to establishing construct validity). While EFA can be computed using SPSS alone, CFA is run via the SPSS add-on package AMOS (analysis of moment structure) or via a more sophisticated package such as R. Another analytical procedure in the factor analysis family is *principal components analysis* (PCA), which is often erroneously conflated with factor analysis: PCA yields *components* rather than *factors*, where components are derived from analysis of all of the variances in the data and factors derive from shared variance alone. In simple terms, the key difference is that PCA simply summarizes the dataset whereas EFA and CFA go beyond the data to cultivate and evaluate theory. For a detailed discussion of EFA, CFA and PCA, see Tabachnick and Fidell (2014).

Improving reliability and validity

Now that we have explored the practicalities of using questionnaires, our attention turns to factors which may threaten reliability and validity during data collection. One primary threat to the reliability and validity of questionnaire data is bias: in other words, the existence of extraneous factors which have a systematic influence on the data collected. There are a number of ways that potential bias can be mitigated at the item level in questionnaire research. Dörnyei and Csizér (2012) proffer five helpful strategies in this regard:

1 Length: items should be written in concise a manner as possible
2 Language: the language used should be simple and natural
3 Clarity: an item should be devoid of ambiguity
4 Construction: negative constructions (e.g. 'I don't do X'; 'I never feel like Y') are to be avoided
5 Focus: double-barrelled questions (e.g. 'Do you like eggs and ham?') should also be avoided

Leading questions (i.e. items that make an assumption about the respondent's viewpoint or behaviour) and the use of technical jargon should also be avoided, as should items which may lead the participant to respond in a socially acceptable (but not necessarily truthful) way (e.g. 'How often do you read to your children?'). While negative constructions are not recommended, using negatively worded items (e.g. 'I find taking notes in class unhelpful') is a useful technique to enhance variety by probing the construct of interest from an alternative perspective.

At the questionnaire design stage, *order effects* (i.e. the order in which items are arranged in a questionnaire) can introduce bias because preceding items serve to establish a context which may influence responses to later items. For example, where a respondent is asked to self-rate their proficiency, and then directly afterwards asked to rate the quality of the L2 instruction they have received, the former response is likely to have primed the latter. To avoid order effects, formatting should take account of the possible relationships between the topics probed: items are usefully grouped by topic, but topics that are highly related should be separated by unrelated topics (with randomization of topic order another possible option).

Response rate to a questionnaire (i.e. the proportion of people who completed the measure from all those who could have completed it) is an important issue to plan for, report and consider. This is because the lower the response rate, the higher the risk of bias in a sample: sampling strategies are designed to systematically include individuals in a sample based on key characteristics relevant to the study, but if response rate is low, it is likely that the resultant sample is biased towards those individuals who were willing to participate, which is not (usually) a characteristic around which sampling strategies are devised. Another form of bias deriving from administration of a questionnaire is *recall bias*, that is systematic error in the data derived from a confounding influence of participants' memory. Recall bias is a particular threat to questionnaires that probe behaviour in retrospect (e.g. asking study abroad learners about their L2 exposure and use after they have returned to their home country). To avoid recall bias, an instrument is best administered during (or very shortly after) participants' experience of the phenomenon of interest.

Case studies of questionnaires in applied linguistics research

Table 8.1 comprises summaries of six applied linguistics studies that have utilized questionnaires as a data collection methodology. From this selection, we go on to showcase two studies in more detail.

Two studies which made use of behavioural questionnaires in second language research are Briggs (2015), and Teng and Zhang (2016). Briggs's (2015) questionnaire was an adaptation of the Language Contact Profile (LCP) – originally developed by Freed et al. (2004) – used to measure the informal L2 contact (exposure and use) experienced by adult study abroad learners of English in the UK. Administered to learners from a variety of L1 backgrounds and with a range of L2-English proficiency levels, the informal contact data were used as a primary independent variable in multiple regression analysis to determine whether informal contact predicts vocabulary gain over sojourns of various lengths. Teng and Zhang's (2016) study aimed to validate The Writing Strategies for Self-Regulated Learning Questionnaire (WSSRLQ) – an original instrument they had developed to measure the self-regulation behaviour of learners of English when engaged in L2 writing. The WSSRLQ utilized a seven-point Likert-type scale with the anchors 1 ('Not at all true of

Table 8.1 Examples of questionnaires in applied linguistics research

Researchers	Topic	Participants	Research design	Data collection method
Briggs (2015)	Vocabulary gain during study abroad	Adult ESL learners in the UK (*n* = 241)	Longitudinal; factor analysis; regression modelling	An adaptation of the Language Contact Profile
Briggs, Dearden and Macaro (2018)	English medium instruction (EMI) teacher cognition at secondary and tertiary levels	EMI secondary and tertiary teacher in various non-Anglophone countries (*n* = 167)	Cross-sectional; comparison of means	Online questionnaire on beliefs about English medium instruction
Hessel (2017)	The role of individual differences on L2 proficiency gain during study abroad	German Erasmus students on a study abroad exchange in the UK (*n* = 96)	Longitudinal pre- and post-tests of L2-English proficiency; regression modelling	Online questionnaire measuring psychological factors and background characteristics
Iwaniec (2014)	The L2-English motivational properties of Polish upper secondary pupils	15–16-year-old Polish *gymnasium* pupils in southern Poland (*n* = 236)	Cross-sectional mixed methods; factor analysis; regression modelling	Questionnaire measuring 12 key motivational factors, plus background characteristics
Teng and Zhang (2016)	Validation of models of self-regulated L2 writing strategies	L1-Chinese undergraduate EFL students (*n* = 790)	Cross-sectional; structural equation modelling	Writing Strategies for Self-regulated Learning Questionnaire
van der Slik, van Hout and Schepens (2015)	Gender differences in L2 Dutch acquisition among immigrants to the Netherlands	Adult immigrants to the Netherlands with various L1s (*n* = 29,767)	Cross-classified multilevel regression modelling	Background characteristics questionnaire

me') and 7 ('Very true of me') and was administered to 790 undergraduate students in China, who also completed an IELTS writing task. Regarding the strategies questionnaire, three hypothesized latent structure models were tested using CFA. The results indicated that self-regulation is a higher order construct that explains the relationships between the nine individual writing strategies as lower order constructs. In terms of the L2 writing measure, multiple regression analysis revealed that six of the nine individual strategies were significant predictors of L2 writing proficiency.

Factual questionnaires are often used in applied linguistics research to collect data on key independent variables in a study. One study which utilized an existing factual questionnaire in this regard is van der Slik, van Hout and Schepens (2015). The research aimed to determine the effect of gender (among other individual differences) on L2 acquisition of Dutch among a very large sample of immigrants to the Netherlands. This aim was achieved via *secondary data analysis* of test scores on the State Examination of Dutch as a Second Language – a proficiency test targeted towards immigrants wishing to enter the Dutch higher education system – over a 9-year period. The researchers analysed the test data against data on background characteristics (such as date of birth, gender, country of origin, date of entry to the Netherlands), which was gathered via a factual questionnaire administered automatically upon subscription to the exam. The study found that – controlling for all other factors – women significantly and substantively outperformed men on L2-Dutch speaking and writing, whereas no gender gap was found in reading and listening scores.

The Briggs, Dearden and Macaro (2018) study is included here as an example of the use of attitudinal questionnaires in applied linguistics research. The researchers designed an original, web-based survey that aimed to elicit beliefs about English medium instruction (EMI: the teaching of content subject disciplines – such as science or mathematics – through the medium of L2-English in non-Anglophone contexts) from EMI teachers in the secondary and tertiary educational phases across the globe. The questionnaire adopted a teacher cognition theoretical framework and utilized a five-point 'how true of me' response scale with gradation rating from 1 ('This sounds a lot like me') to 5 ('This sounds not at all like me').

One example of a mixed-type questionnaire comes from Iwaniec (2014), who developed a 103-item survey to investigate the 'general motivational properties' of her sample of 236 Polish EFL learners who were state gymnasium pupils aged 13–16. A five-point Likert scale was used to elicit data on the learners' L2 self; knowledge orientation; international orientation; peer group pressure, motivated and self-regulated behaviour; self-efficacy; and parental engagement inter alia. Hessel (2017) also employed a mixed questionnaire – covering both psychological (including attitudinal) factors (e.g. self-efficacy, foreign language anxiety) and background characteristics (e.g. study abroad placement details, L2 learning history) – which she administered to German study abroad students before and after a 3-month sojourn in the UK. A C-test was administered at the same time points to determine L2-English proficiency gain. Of the factual data collected, only gender showed a significant association with proficiency gain. The final regression model (which held time 1 proficiency constant) explained 45 per cent of the variance in the C-test scores and indicated that any initial influence of gender was superseded by the predictive power of the psychological factors.

We choose now to showcase the two behavioural studies outlined above to highlight the principled use of original and validated questionnaires in applied linguistics research.

Briggs (2015): Informal L2 contact and vocabulary acquisition during study abroad

The first study of focus is Briggs (2015), who explored the relationship between behaviour – in the form of informal L2 contact (i.e. exposure to and use of the L2 outside of the L2 classroom) – and vocabulary gain among study abroad learners of English in the UK. In order to measure informal L2 contact, Briggs adapted the Language Contact Profile (LCP), a behavioural questionnaire which was originally developed by Freed et al. (2004). The original LCP measures the type and amount of informal L2 contact experienced by L1-English learners of L2-Spanish. It contains two parts: (1) a 'pre-study abroad' section – to be administered in the home country before the study abroad has begun – which requires respondents to indicate the frequency with which they experience different types of L2 contact in their home country (from 'Almost never' to 'Daily') and (2) a post-study abroad section – to be administered after the sojourn has finished and the respondent has returned to the home country – which asks for similar information but with a greater level of frequency information (the respondent must indicate how many days per week and hours per day on average each type of L2 contact was experienced).

Briggs (2015) adapted the LCP in two key ways. First, she changed the response scale from a frequency-based scale to a 'how true of me' scale (i.e. 1 = 'This is not at all true of me'; 5 = 'This is very true of me') in order to avoid cumulative treatment of frequency scales of items of a different nature. The second adaptation related to recall bias: rather than administering the second section of items after the respondents had returned to their home country, Briggs altered the instructions such that the part 2 items pertained to *current* experience of informal contact and administered the questionnaire while the participants were still living in the UK. The adapted measure was administered in English to a convenience sample of $n = 241$ study abroad learners with various L1s – a feature that may have affected the reliability of the findings given the proficiency threshold for participation was relatively low at CEFR B1. However, the Cronbach's Alpha coefficient suggested a high level of internal consistency ($α = 0.816$) of the scale, and three clear informal contact factors emerged from the EFA.

Teng and Zhang (2016): Validating a writing strategies questionnaire

Teng and Zhang's (2016) study is showcased here as an example of questionnaire-based research in applied linguistics in which the very focus of the study is validation of an original questionnaire. A large convenience sample of undergraduate L2-English students in China was recruited to complete the Writing Strategies for Self-Regulated Learning Questionnaire (WSSRLQ) to test – via CFA – the veracity of three hypothesized latent structure models derived from self-regulated learning theory. The initial WSSRLQ item pool was generated from (1) focus group data, where pilot participants had been asked to discuss the strategies they use when writing in English, and (2) reference to items in existing questionnaires of L2 writing strategies. To enhance construct validity at the item writing stage, experts in the field were employed to evaluate the initial forty-five-item pool against the operationalization of the key constructs to be measured (self-regulation; language learner strategies), and five items were omitted based on the outcome of this procedure. The seven-point, Likert-type 'How true of me' scale was selected to mirror the response scales used in other validated measures of self-regulation and language learner strategies, and the use of multi-item scales was the justification for cumulative treatment of these ordinal data. Translation of the measure into Chinese was employed to heighten the reliability of the participants' responses and subsequent backtranslation to English used to ensure parallelism between the L1 and L2 versions. The WSSRLQ was administered to the sample after they had completed an L2 writing course as a means of mitigating the effects of recall bias. Prior to the CFA, data were analysed for any evidence of systematic response bias and missing values, resulting in the deletion of a small number of individual cases.

Implications for researchers

As a discipline we have long been critical of questionnaires as a data collection methodology. For example, Reid (1990) aired the 'dirty laundry of ESL survey research', highlighting the many pitfalls of questionnaire design for the novice researcher, and Luppescu and Day (1990) argued strongly against 'blind acceptance' of survey findings without requisite attention to validity and reliability. It has taken some time since these early papers, but in recent years, a proliferation of publications on questionnaire validation in applied linguistics has emerged (e.g. Petrić & Czárl, 2003; Teng & Zhang, 2016). There is now a strong obligation for scholars and consumers of applied linguistics research, therefore, to go beyond a focus on questionnaire findings and weigh these in light of a detailed and critical eye on issues of methodology, validity and reliability. In doing so, the focus on quality in questionnaire research within our field is likely to continue to improve.

Critical appraisal of questionnaire-based research denotes a solid level of statistical literacy among applied linguists, and recent research (e.g. Loewen et al., 2014) suggests that while statistical training in the field is widespread, it may not be wholly adequate in the eyes of those who receive it. It is fair to say that statistical competence is a key area of insecurity for novice researchers, who feel they lack the requisite expertise to critically engage with published research, particularly in the quantitative paradigm. Yet this chapter has highlighted that there are multiple avenues to achieving rigour in questionnaire-based research, and we would suggest that a focus on bias mitigation at the item writing, sampling and administration phases is as important a consideration as the application of appropriate statistical procedures in the data analysis phases. As such, novice researchers have a gateway into critical engagement with questionnaire-based research – one which will be further complemented as quantitative know-how matures.

Post-reading activities

Reflect
This chapter has suggested that the quality of the findings of questionnaire research is as much reliant on the development and administration of the tool as it is on the analysis of the data collected. Do you think questionnaires are unique in this respect? What other data collection methodologies are 'front loading' in this regard?

Expand
Individually or in small groups, choose one of the studies in Table 8.1 to read and critique. After reading, consider and discuss: (1) What type of data were collected using the questionnaire? Was a questionnaire the most appropriate method for collecting this type of data? (2) Were there any aspects of the questionnaire design or implementation which could have been improved? (3) (To what extent) Did the researchers consider the potential for bias in their data? If so, how? If not, how might they have done?

Apply

Design a cross-sectional study into language teachers' beliefs about grammar instruction. You are particularly interested in determining whether and how teachers' beliefs about grammar instruction are related to their experience of (1) L2 grammar learning and (2) teacher training related to grammar. Design a questionnaire to collect these types of data and pay particular attention to the following decisions: How will you operationalize your constructs of interest? How many items will you include for each construct? What type(s) of items and response scales will you use, and why? How will your instrument be formatted? What steps will you take to ascertain whether your instrument is a valid and reliable measure of beliefs about grammar instruction among your population? How will you administer your questionnaire, and what are the strengths and limitations of this approach?

Resources for further reading

Dörnyei, Z. (with Taguchi, T.) (2010). *Questionnaires in second language research: Construction, administration, and processing* (2nd edn.). London: Routledge.

This second edition of Zoltán Dörnyei's seminal volume on the use of questionnaires in applied linguistics research is a key resource for students or independent researchers interested in designing, developing, adapting and/ or administering a second language-oriented questionnaire. This edition is particularly helpful for those involved in the process of questionnaire development because it charts the development of a questionnaire according to the principles laid out in the book. The volume is also updated to include coverage of the issues inherent in translating existing questionnaires and using software to administer questionnaires online.

Dörnyei, Z., & Csizér, K. (2012). How to design and analyze surveys in SLA research? In A. Mackey & S. Gass (Eds.), *Research methods in second language acquisition: A practical guide* (pp. 74–94). Malden, MA: Wiley-Blackwell.

This chapter provides a concise and practical summary of the key considerations and issues in questionnaire design and analysis. Of particular utility is a checklist of points to include in the write-up of questionnaire research and a list of further resources beneficial for anyone planning a questionnaire-based study. As in Dörnyei (with Taguchi) (2010), the principles discussed are helpfully illustrated with reference to actual practice in the form of 'real life' research projects.

9

Focus Groups

Pre-reading activities

Think

Before reading this chapter, think about your answers to the following questions: What is the difference between a focus group and an interview? How about between a focus group and a group interview?

Discuss

In small groups, or as a class, discuss the following: (1) For what type of research would a focus group with four groups of six people each be preferable to conducting twenty-four individual interviews? (2) If a focus group aims to create group discussion around a topic, what would be the minimum and maximum number of people needed in a single group?

Imagine

Imagine you are conducting a study at a university exploring students' attitudes towards a proposed change in the language entry requirements for university admission. The university has roughly equal numbers of domestic and international students (a variable you believe may impact on attitudes), across three faculties of equal size (arts, sciences and social sciences). You have a budget to conduct and analyse 12–15 focus groups with 6–10 people in each group. Decide how groups should be organized (e.g. how many groups, and what their composition will be of male and female students from each of the three faculties). Be ready to provide a rationale for your decision.

Introduction

Focus groups are 'a way of collecting qualitative data, which – essentially – involves engaging a small number of people in an informal group discussion (or discussions), "focused" around a particular topic or set of issues' (Wilkinson, 2004: 177). While focus groups are often conflated with interviews in research methodology books, it is important to emphasize from the outset of this chapter that focus groups are *not the same as group interviews*. While focus groups may share some characteristics with interviews, they entail much more than interviewing a group of people at one time. Focus groups aim to leverage the group dynamics by taking advantage of the fact that participants exist as part of a larger social community. Rather than treating them as silos of individual knowledge or experience, they try to understand how people co-create knowledge and share their experiences with one another. As Galloway (2020) notes, this interaction distinguishes focus groups from the qualitative interview, as in focus groups the emphasis is on the group, rather than the individual. For applied linguistics researchers interested in examining group interaction, the method can be very powerful.

Focus groups generally involve having groups of participants engaged in a moderated discussion that focuses on a particular topic, situation or phenomenon under investigation (Stewart, Shamdasani & Rook, 2007). When used for research purposes, a focus group is typically moderated by a trained moderator whose identity is socially close to the group members; but they can also be self-moderated under certain conditions. When the moderator is the researcher, efforts must be made to close any power gap between them and members of the focus group.

Focus groups have existed since the 1920s as a tool to probe people's beliefs and responses surrounding key issues and have largely been embraced by the field of market and political research. For market researchers, who are interested in understanding widely held beliefs, they are well known as an effective way to listen to the opinions of key segments of the population regarding the topics, products or innovations being explored. Market researchers have long accepted the notion that opinions are formed within pre-existing social units, in that the opinions of others in this unit affect the opinions of the individual. Attitudes are not formed in a bubble but are rather socially constructed.

While focus group interviewing techniques have existed since the 1920s, and were popular to explore the effectiveness of propaganda videos during the Second World War, they only became formalized as a research tool in the 1950s. However, it is only in recent decades that the method has begun to emerge in the mainstream of social science research, and Galloway (2020) observes that the method is yet to make a substantial impact within the field of applied linguistics. Considering a large segment of applied linguistics research concerns itself with attitudes, beliefs and social practices, focus groups should ideally play a larger role in applied linguistics research methodology.

As Krueger and Casey (2014: 2) note, 'a focus group is a special type of group in terms of purpose, size, composition, and procedures'. Along this line, in this chapter we explore considerations of group size and constituents, as well as the role of the moderator, who is often not the researcher. We also focus on key issues surrounding the use of focus groups to collect data within extant or created social groups. We further explore practical issues surrounding focus group data collection and data analysis, because large group interaction creates specific data analysis needs and opportunities. Finally, we provide an overview of the use of focus groups in recent applied linguistics research, highlighting implications for researchers wishing to apply this complex methodology to their research.

Key concepts

Sampling

As focus groups aim to elicit views from a portion of a community to make a generalization of the target population, sampling decisions are paramount to collecting good data. If group opinions are predicted to be divided according to demographic differences in the population, a sampling technique to capture this difference is necessary. In the case of probability sampling, a *stratified random sampling* technique could be appropriate, where the population is divided into key characteristics, or strata, then the population is randomly sampled within each category. However, due to time or financial resource limitations, a non-probability sampling version of this technique is usually applied, which is referred to as a *quota sampling* technique. This follows the same principles without a need for randomness. For example, if a university population, within which researchers want to explore opinions about a policy change, has unequal numbers of domestic and international students, and this is a variable that researchers believe to impact opinion, they should make sure to recruit representative numbers of domestic and international students within their focus groups to capture this difference. Likewise, if the population is further divided unevenly across three faculties of unequal size (arts, sciences and social sciences), researchers will also want to capture this within their sampling strategy. In creating the quota, it would be essential to also explore the numbers of domestic and international students within each of the three faculties, and to ensure each faculty group is representative of the target population. An example of this sampling is shown in Table 9.1.

In other types of research, representativeness may not be the main sampling criteria but rather a researcher might aim to understand the full range of experiences and opinions within a population. In such cases, a *maximum variation sampling* technique might be useful. In this sampling technique the researcher aims to include the full spectrum of the population. For example, if a researcher were exploring the attitudes of language teachers in Hong Kong of recent policy mandating them to pass a level of language proficiency, a researcher may want to ensure the entire spectrum of the population was included, from teachers of low proficiency to very high proficiency. Even if teachers of a very low proficiency are just a small segment of the population, their opinions nonetheless matter and must be included in the sample. In this case, the researcher's aim is not to gauge 'popular opinion' but to ensure all voices are heard.

In a further example of non-representative sampling, the researcher may only need to target specific pockets of the population in an exploration of a particular phenomenon, in which case a purposive sampling technique may be useful. *Purposive sampling* refers to the collection of data from targeted segments for a refined purpose. For example, if a researcher aimed to explore issues surrounding language maintenance of speakers of endangered

Table 9.1 An example of quota sampling in focus groups

Faculty	Arts	Sciences	Social sciences
Target population	5,000	15,000	10,000
–Domestic	–3,000	–3,000	–5,000
–International	–2,000	–12,000	–5,000
Quota sample	10	30	20
–Domestic	–6	–6	–10
–International	–4	–24	–10
Focus groups	2 groups	5–6 groups	4 groups

languages, who were living outside their L1 communities, then only this specific population would be recruited. The participants are sampled not because they are representative or a larger population, but because they offer something of unique interest to the research questions.

Homogeneous versus heterogeneous groups

Another key consideration in the design of focus groups is deciding which members should constitute each grouping of participants, namely whether groups should be homogeneous or heterogeneous according to variables of interest. For example, if age might be considered a key demographic that divides opinion on a research topic, a researcher might decide to divide focus group membership according to age (e.g. 20–30, 30–50 and 50+). In creating homogeneous groups, the participants aged 20–30 would then discuss opinions surrounding the research topic within their own age band. In many ways, homogeneous groupings are a more realistic reflection of society, where people tend to move in clusters of similar or like-minded people and where opinions are formed within socially bounded communities.

In some societies, key demographic divisions such as social class or power dynamics might also affect the ease with which participants are able to voice their opinions. In some cultures where age is an important socially dividing characteristic, if a researcher were to place younger participants in the same group as older participants, it may affect the ability of more junior participants to voice their opinions. Culturally they might feel obligated to agree with their superiors, or let them speak first. Thus, even if age were not a variable of research interest, it might still be an important consideration when deciding group membership. Further to this point, homogeneous groups can create safe spaces for marginalized populations who cannot articulate their thoughts easily with members outside of these groups, as the method provides them with collective power (Liamputtong, 2011). In such cases homogeneous groups are essential in providing this collective power. Researchers, therefore, need to consider social power relationships, cultural norms and extant sociocultural divisions when deciding whom to include in homogeneous groupings.

Homogenous groups are also useful for pragmatic reasons. For example, in a focus group where participants are required to use a second language to communicate, lower proficiency students might feel intimidated by higher proficiency students. By grouping students according to proficiency, the researcher may create a safe space for participants to communicate.

If enough participants who share an L1 are recruited, the researcher might also consider the advantages of holding the focus group in the participants' L1 to minimize within-group differences. Homogeneous groups, therefore, may counteract such issues.

Heterogeneous groups also have their advantages for certain research topics. If the aim of the research is to create debate and try to find a consensus among diverse groups of people with differing perspectives, a researcher may believe the advantages of creating group dynamism outweigh the advantages of homogeneous groupings. For example, if the aim of a focus group is to explore parents' attitudes towards a decrease in time provided for language education at their child's school, the researcher might want to have a maximum variation sample within each focus group so that people hear multiple perspectives before trying to reach an agreement on the issue. Although participants may feel pressure to agree with the dominant group view (see 'Dealing with silent and dominant voices' section), the focus groups nonetheless give participants an opportunity to listen to a range of opinions, share their own thoughts and help them to formulate their final viewpoint (Morgan, 1997). Heterogeneous groups can therefore help participants to understand more fully how their ideas might affect others outside of their social communities.

Generally, heterogeneous groupings are more suited to problem-solving topics and usually have practical value in that each focus group represents the actual diversity in the target population. Homogeneous groupings tend to create cleaner and more workable data and avoid problems that may emerge when people of different demographics within a group have unequal societal power, thereby silencing members of the group and producing biased data. While the decision to create heterogeneous or homogeneous groups depends greatly on the research topic and target population, whatever decision is made must be methodologically justified.

Group sizes

Group sizes for focus groups can vary, and there is no magic number that is needed to facilitate a good group discussion. As a crude rule, a focus group should be sufficiently large to provide a range of diverse opinions but sufficiently small to ensure that all group members are able to voice their thoughts (Onwuegbuzie et al., 2009). Generally, research methods literature suggests group sizes ranging from four to twelve, although six to eight is more common in applied linguistics studies. Rather than adhering to suggested ranges, a researcher should be able to convincingly articulate how they have ensured the group size best facilitates discussion for all members, while allowing diversity of opinions. Cultural and contextual factors should also be considered when deciding on group sizes, as this might affect the comfort level of participants to voice their opinions in front of large groups of people. Galloway (2020) states that over-recruitment of focus groups is advisable, stating that when members fail to turn up to a planned session, the integrity of group size can be affected, resulting in sessions needing to be cancelled due to low participant membership.

Moderator versus interviewer roles

A feature of focus groups that makes the method distinct from the qualitative interview is the differing role of the interviewer and moderator. In interviews, the interviewee (who is often the researcher) plays an active role in the data collection process, asking questions and leading the interviewee through a set agenda or list of interview questions. The interviewee talks directly to the interviewer. In focus groups, the moderator (who is sometimes not the researcher) plays a passive role in data collection by steering discussion on the topic and introducing new topics when conversation becomes exhausted. The focus group members talk among themselves and not to the moderator, who is a facilitator of discussion but not a participant within it (group interaction is a key characteristic of a focus group, so if all discussion occurs via the moderator rather than between participants, the data collection is better viewed as a group interview). Focus groups are sometimes self-moderated, meaning that the group follows set instructions to guide them through a series of discussion prompts. However, it is more common for a trained moderator to steer the session, as discussions otherwise can become derailed and participants can easily become sidetracked from the main research issues that need to be covered during the session.

Procedures and practicalities

Focus groups require specific procedures to be followed (Krueger & Casey, 2014), and this section focuses on those needed to yield useful data.

Video recording for good record-keeping and multimodal analysis

When conducting focus groups, there is a greater need to video-record, rather than just audio-record, each session. Especially in large groups, where there could be up to twelve people per group, it can be difficult in data analysis to be certain of who is speaking, especially if there is a lot of overlapping conversation. At the start of the focus group, it can be good practice to have each member state their name and other key identifying information to the camera, as this can facilitate their accurate identification later on.

Having a good video record is also essential for multimodal analysis. As focus groups look for group interaction, agreement and dissent, it is important to have a record of and who in the group offers cues of agreement or disagreement to the points raised by other members. Often these come in the form of both verbal and non-verbal cues. When members nod in agreement to a point another member is raising, this can provide important evidence of agreement, and is something that audio records simply cannot capture. If video cannot be taken for ethical reasons, good observation notes may suffice, but it might be necessary to have a second researcher in the room to capture non-verbal cues, as the moderator will often be too preoccupied to do so. Notes should be carefully maintained to keep track of who is speaking throughout the audio recording.

Questioning

Generally, focus group questions are organized around discussion topics, rather than a series of 'interview' questions for participants to answer. In many cases, these topics are in the form of prompts and at times accompanied with contextual or background information to orient group members to the key issues of interest. This information could range from textual materials or even the use of media such as short video clips. Krueger (1998) offers a framework to sequence topics, moving from general to more specific issues, operationalized in five categories of questions: opening questions, introductory questions, transition questions, key questions and ending questions. This is similar to Morgan's (1997: 41) 'funnel approach', which moves from free discussion topics to more structured topics.

When discussion on a topic appears to be winding down, and the moderator is satisfied that new ideas are becoming exhausted, they then introduce the next topic for discussion. It is important for the moderator to balance a need for all voices to be heard with the time limitations of the session, as all topics need to be covered by all groups for consistency of analysis. As a general rule, it is better to have fewer topics of exhaustive coverage than a larger number of topics which fail to elicit a full range of opinions.

Data analysis

While there is 'extensive advice on how to conduct focus groups, there is relatively little in the focus group literature on how to analyse the resulting data' (Wilkinson, 2004: 182). To fill this gap, we outline some popular data analysis techniques in the field of applied linguistics that are highly suitable for focus group data analysis. Commonly, qualitative content analysis is used to capture the content of transcribed focus group data in the form of key topics organized around emergent themes. This type of analysis follows the same format as when used for other types of texts or transcribed data for their content (e.g. see Chapter 6). Downe-Wamboldt (1992: 314) describes content analysis as 'a systematic and objective means to make valid inferences from verbal, visual, or written data in order to describe and quantify specific phenomena'. Qualitative content analysis is powerful in the exploration of *what* is being said in the focus group data but is relatively weak in exploring issues surrounding *how* group members are interacting and developing opinions, which are of core interest to the methodology.

Galloway (2020) argues that focus groups generally require more complex transcription protocols in order to analyse not only what is said but how it is said. With suitable transcripts that can capture interaction in terms of intonation, stress, turn-taking and overlapping speech, conversation analysis techniques can be applied to focus group data to facilitate a more fine-grained examination of interaction within the data. This can generate knowledge of how the group develops knowledge and opinions as a social unit and how participants react to ideas raised by others in the group. Thus, for applied linguistics researchers, this fine-grained analysis of focus group data can be used to provide further evidence of group thinking.

Analysing visual data

Another usual additive to an analytical framework for focus group data includes multimodal analysis to capture non-verbal communication. Multimodal analysis can further capture interaction, agreement and dissention via analysis of visual cues, ideally captured via videoed records. If visual data can be added into the transcripts for analysis alongside verbal data, this can be useful to show evidence of engagement and reaction to ideas of dominant members or to extract the opinions of quiet members. In other words, while content analysis can analyse the volume of ideas yielded, and conversation analysis can measure the quality of these ideas, multimodal analysis can interpret reaction to these ideas via exploration of members' body language and other visual cues. Such analysis can thus further a researcher's understanding of the shared construction of meaning of the group.

New technology has introduced innovations in focus group methodology in recent years. Traditionally, focus groups were conducted in face-to-face settings, but technological developments have seen the emergence of 'virtual focus groups'. Focus groups can now be conducted via Voice over Internet Protocols (e.g. Skype) and other similar software, which now allow researchers to bring geographically distant groups of participants together for moderated discussion. Such protocols also allow sessions to be audio- and video-recorded with clearly captured facial images provided for all participants, which may enhance the quality of data for multimodal analysis.

Improving reliability and validity

Choosing and training a good moderator

Krueger and Casey (2014) suggest when conducting focus groups in international and culturally bounded contexts, it is often essential to hire a moderator from the same cultural group and with characteristics which are similar to the focus group members. This is especially important in contexts where a social or cultural distance between the participants and the moderator is seen to affect the comfort level for participants to voice their opinions. Rossman and Rallis (2016) note that power imbalance between the moderator and the focus group members can influence the data, resulting in the concealment of opinions. In such cases, hiring and training a peer moderator is essential, so group members see the moderator as an insider and equal, rather than someone who is evaluating their opinions or experiences.

In many contexts, there may be local traditions which may also affect the way in which people interact; thus, using a local moderator, who uses the local language and follows local customs, is essential for valid data collection. Local or peer moderators need adequate training for their roles, including good questioning techniques to encourage participation from all members and to avoid contaminating the data with their own opinions. In some cases, a moderator 'team' is necessary, especially when video recordings cannot be used. When a team is used, the lead moderator can facilitate the discussion while an assistant moderator can record the focus group session and take notes on group interaction and non-verbal communication during the session.

Multiple focus groups needed to draw meaningful conclusions

To improve the reliability of the data, multiple focus groups are an essential (i.e. not conditional) feature of the methodology. In the research literature on focus groups, the term *saturation* is used to refer to the point where a researcher has conducted enough focus groups that they are confident no new ideas are emerging from the addition of subsequent groups. The number of groups needed to reach saturation will vary depending on the diversity of the population and the complexity of the research topic. As a crude guideline, Krueger and Casey (2014) advise researchers to initially plan three or four groups for each participant variable predicted to influence opinion and then evaluate whether saturation has been reached with the addition of each new group. If important ideas are evident in the last group conducted, which were not yielded from a previous group, the researcher should then evaluate how many additional groups appear to be needed to reach saturation: the larger the number of new ideas present, the greater the number of additional focus groups will be needed. Of course, just like any data collection method, the study will have pragmatic limitations of time and human resources, as well as participant availability, so saturation may not be met in many studies. In such cases, the researcher should be transparent in the write-up of the research in terms of how close the data appeared to get to saturation.

Dealing with silent and dominant voices

Silent and dominant participants in a focus group can affect the validity of the data, in that the data may not represent all opinions of the group. Silent members' opinions may be masked by dominant speech, and dominant opinions may appear to be more greatly supported by the group. Various techniques can be employed to engage silent members, such as gently probing them to join in the discussion by asking open-ended or indirect questions. In the absence of voiced opinions, the researcher could try to evaluate opinions by more deeply analysing silent members' non-verbal cues for signs of agreement and disagreement.

Dealing with dominant or overly talkative participants can be challenging for a moderator. While talkative members can be very useful to generate ideas for discussion, they can also unduly detract from opportunities for a diversity of voices to be heard. It is important that a moderator does not silence a talkative member in a way that could be seen as reprimanding them for their input, as their enthusiasm is, after all, an asset in terms of data generation. If a member is judged to be so dominant that they are affecting the validity of the data by reducing opportunities for others to speak, the moderator must be sure to directly ask other members for their opinions and take a more-than-usual active role in questioning. At the turn of topics, the moderator might ask silent members for their thoughts first, in case they are reluctant to disagree with the dominant member. At the end of the focus group, if it is clear that a dominant member has injected bias in the data, additional focus groups with additional participants may be needed to reach saturation so that all other opinions can be elicited.

Case studies in applied linguistics research

Galloway (2020) notes a relative absence of focus group methodology in applied linguistics research, stating that in her review of abstracts in the journal *Applied Linguistics* from 2007 to 2017, only one study made mention

Table 9.2 Examples of focus groups in applied linguistics research

Researchers	Topic	Participants	Research design	Data collection method
Galloway (2017a)	Global Englishes	EFL students in Japan (*n* = 120)	Quasi-experimental	Focus groups, interviews, questionnaires
Galloway, Kriukow and Numajiri (2017)	English medium instruction	EMI students in Japan and China (*n* = 579)	Survey	Focus groups, interviews, questionnaires
Santello (2015)	Attitudes to language selection in advertising	Italian English Bilinguals (*n* = 8 + 103)	Experimental	Focus group data used to create constructs for experiment
Sato (2017)	L2 learners' peer interaction	Grade 10 English as a foreign language classes in Chile (*n* = 53)	Classroom research (field research)	Pre-task interviews; L2 development data; interaction data from focus groups
Razfar and Simon (2011)	Course-Taking Patterns of ESL Students	Latino ESL students' data (*n* = 1,479); plus focus group (*n* = 10);	Mixed methods: analysis of existing data plus Ethnographic research	Academic records; focus groups
Lanvers (2018)	Uptake of foreign language education	Language students (*n* = 99); teachers (*n* = 7); management (*n* = 4) in UK schools	Survey	Focus groups; interviews

of focus groups. In this section, we explore six empirical studies in wider applied linguistics literature to illustrate the use of this data collection method in the field. These six examples are outlined in Table 9.2. After a brief overview of each of these, two of the studies (Galloway, 2017a; Lanvers, 2018) are discussed in further detail in relation to the main issues raised in this chapter.

An overview of the studies

Of the studies outlined in Table 9.2, Galloway (2017a) and Lanvers (2018) adhere most closely to focus group conventions in terms of sampling, data collection to point of saturation and analysis. Galloway, Kriukow and Numajiri (2017) and Santello (2015) are also highly aware of focus group conventions. In Galloway, Kriukow and Numajiri (2017), eight focus groups are conducted, four with teachers and four with students in an English medium instruction setting. The focus groups are homogeneous in that they include students studying within the same university. This study is also highly cognizant of the fact that focus groups are used to explore interaction and incorporates this knowledge into its analysis of the data, thereby extracting insight beyond that which is typical in interviews. Santello (2015) uses focus group to explore issues surrounding attitudes to language in order to better establish the experiment in the study's main stage. Even though only one focus group is conducted, Santello is highly aware of focus group methodology as an exploratory method, utilizing research-informed techniques to moderate the groups, provide freedom for the bilingual participants to switch between languages and to create an informal atmosphere to put participants at ease.

The study by Sato (2017) is quite removed from typical focus group methodology, in that in this study, 'focus group' refers to a bounded unit of students within a class of students who are engaging in a research task. In fact, interviews are individually conducted with the focus group participants to elicit direct data from them; the 'focus groups' are instead used to explore interaction among members during completion of the task. While this method does not fit the traditional methodological procedure of a focus group, it is included here because its focus on analysis of interaction among members indicates how focus group data lend themselves to research questions that value interaction in the data yielded. All in all it is a rather innovative interpretation of the methodology.

The study by Razfar and Simon (2011) is highly typical of how focus groups are used in most applied linguistics research. Here, the researchers use focus groups as a qualitative add-on to a predominantly quantitative study. The data are analysed thematically with little attention to interaction or group thinking. There is also little transparency or consideration of group size or constitution and no attempt at saturation of data. The appendix to the study confirms interview questions have been used, rather than prompts. The methodology for this study would perhaps have better been described as 'group interviews' rather than focus groups, as there is little in this study, apart from collecting data from groups of participants, that suggests a focus group method has been applied during data collection. We choose this study not to criticize it, as we believe it is methodologically excellent in its application of procedures for its main data collection method, but we showcase this study as representative of the bulk of good studies in applied linguistics that have conducted group interviews under the banner of focus group methodology.

Galloway (2017): A simple and methodologically sound use of focus groups

The study presented in Galloway (2017a) is discussed in greater depth in this chapter as we consider it to be a good example of focus group methodology, as the use of groups in data collection is considered in all elements of the study: design, sampling, data collection and analysis. In this study, the researcher explored attitudes towards the explicit teaching of Global Englishes content to groups of Japanese students who were majoring in English at a university in Japan. Four focus groups are conducted within pre-existing classes taking part in a quasi-experimental study, thus the focus groups are deemed to be representative of their targeted population. In her study, she created homogeneous groups based on extant classes with two focus groups representing each of the two classes in the study. As Galloway was also in the position of a teacher to the students in the focus groups, the power distance between her and her students meant that she would be an unsuitable moderator for the groups. To counter this, she hired a peer moderator who was also a student in the university but not enrolled in the class and gave them detailed training guidelines to ensure they could adequately deal with both dominant and passive participants without injecting their own voice into the discussions. This training involved pilot sessions with the moderator and groups of broadly similar students.

To counter possible language barriers that were thought to threaten data reliability, all prompts were translated into Japanese, and participants were given the choice of conversing in Japanese or English in the focus groups. This countered a scenario of less proficient or less linguistically confident students being reluctant to voice their opinions fully in English in front of more able peers. In terms of analysis, Galloway video-recorded all sessions and applied conversation analysis techniques to explore group member interaction, including agreement and disagreement. Within these transcripts, she also includes some non-verbal communication such as laughter, smiling, nodding and head shaking.

One of the issues Galloway found with conducting focus groups in the Japanese cultural context, even when using a peer moderator, was that participants were reluctant to give strong opinions during group discussions, which was unlike their individual interviews where participants were reported to be more honest. This finding reveals the importance of cultural traditions in certain contexts, which may influence the data. In Japanese culture, where norms may dictate that one softens their opinion in front of their peers, focus groups as a method may need special consideration. To counter this, Galloway gave participants a short time to read and note down their own responses, since turn-taking strategies and the avoidance of interrupting a conversation are commonly employed in the Japanese context. She also ensured all participants were directly invited to give their opinions rather than relying on them to voluntarily offer them.

Galloway's work on focus groups is very thorough and stands as a good model of methodologically grounded practice. She further discusses the methodology of her focus groups in greater detail in Galloway (2020), and she also discusses the real-world issues of conducting research with her own students in Galloway (2017b). The pilot study for this project appears in Galloway (2013).

Lanvers (2018): A model in saturation

The study by Lanvers is an excellent example of research design, where data from focus groups form a large proportion of the data. So much so that the sample could be argued to be representative of the target population due to efforts to reach a saturation of opinions at each research site. In this study, Lanvers explores the uptake of foreign language education in four schools in the UK, interviewing heads of school and teachers at each site and conducting focus groups with 17–28 students within each school. With 3–5 focus groups at each school (18 in total), the researchers make a good case for achieving a saturated sample of student opinions. The focus groups were heterogeneously sampled to achieve a mix of gender within each group.

Even though the researcher moderated the focus groups, there was a stated awareness of the need to reduce the gap between the researcher and the students and decreased inhibition by ensuring the teacher was not present during data collection. Unfortunately, not all methodological decisions in creating the focus groups were transparently described in the published paper, and the prompts read somewhat like an interview. However, the excerpts in the paper clearly indicated that students were speaking with each other, and the researcher role was minimized during data collection. All in all, the number of focus groups conducted and the overall sample achieved in this study were impressive, and the opportunities for further data analysis with the focus group transcripts are greater than that presented in the published paper, perhaps due to word-length limitations.

Implications for researchers

Despite the long history of focus groups as a means of data collection, they are yet to enter the mainstream of applied linguistics research. This is surprising considering much applied linguistics research is interested in exploring interaction and construction of meaning within social groups. This is also unfortunate considering applied linguistics researchers are well equipped to apply expertise in analysing interaction to explore meaning making within the transcribed data. Applied linguists, therefore, should be at the forefront of innovative analysis of focus group data, rather than trailing behind other disciplines, as it does currently. Despite the relatively slow uptake of focus groups in our field, some good work has been undertaken by researchers, as highlighted in the case study section of this chapter.

Nevertheless, much research conducted under the banner of focus group data fails to meet the methodological requirements for valid and reliable research. When searching the field for focus group studies we encountered numerous group interviews labelled as focus groups – something we see as problematic for developing future good practice in focus group methodology. It is vital that we end the conflation of focus groups with group interviews and communicate this via appropriate methodological practice in our research.

Researchers intending to conduct focus groups in their research should abide by the following tenets of good practice:

1 As a general rule, focus groups should include 4–12 participants, and if group size differs from this, justifications should be provided as to how the number is able to provide evidence of group thinking.
2 Focus group methodology should aim for saturation of ideas, generally achieved through a series of replicable focus groups of similar participants. One focus group for each participant variable is generally insufficient to show saturation. If only one is conducted, this must be justified or discussed as a limitation affecting generalizability of the results to the target population.
3 Focus groups should ideally be video-recorded. If this is not possible, attempts should be made to use a moderation team so that visual data can be recorded by an observer.
4 Focus groups should be moderated by a trained peer moderator. If the researcher is the moderator, discussion should be included in the write-up of the research to explain how any power gap between the researcher and the participant has been minimized.
5 Prompts, rather than questions, should be used to encourage group interaction surrounding a topic. The format should ideally be a discussion with participants talking to each other, rather than predominantly communicating via the moderator.
6 Focus group data should be subjected to analysis of group interaction to capture reactions to points raised by numerous members of the group. Analysis of content alone is insufficient to capture such interaction.

If these principles of good practice are followed by future researchers, the rigour with which focus groups are used within our field will improve. This will also help to decouple focus groups as a data collection technique from interviews and avoid the conflation of the two distinct methods.

With upward trends in methodological rigour, and with innovative ways to conduct and analyse focus group data, we are entering an exciting time for focus group methodology. They remain a powerful and yet underutilized tool for data collection of group opinions and group interaction. Applied linguistics research, with its focus on communication and meaning making, coupled with its home-grown methods for analysing interaction, is in a unique position to lead future methodological innovation and development of this area of research, rather than lagging behind other disciplines in the social sciences.

Post-reading activities

Reflect
This chapter suggests that focus groups are relatively new to applied linguistics, compared to other social sciences. Why do you think the uptake on this data collection method has been so delayed?

Expand
Individually or in small groups, choose one of the studies in Table 9.2 to read and critique. After reading, consider and discuss: (1) Did the researcher conduct enough focus groups to reach saturation? (2) Do you think the sampling and grouping decisions were appropriate? (3) Thinking of the moderator roles and the language used, were there any aspects of the methodology which could have been improved in design or implementation? (3) Did the use of focus groups in this study add any more value than a series of interviews could have provided?

Apply
Imagine you are going to conduct focus groups with Mandarin-Chinese-speaking migrant parents in Canada on their thoughts on bilingual child development. You are particularly interested in their beliefs about whether the L1 of the parents should be used at home, and if so, how the language should be used and maintained by their children. You also want to investigate sociological issues surrounding bilingual development of Chinese. You think that socio-economic status will be a factor that may influence the comfort level of participants, in that parents fall within groups of those engaged in blue-collar and white-collar employment. Consider how you will decide on group membership, what the group size will be, who will be used as a moderator, and how you will otherwise improve reliability and validity of your data.

Resources for further reading

Galloway, N. (2020). Focus groups. In J. McKinley & H. Rose (Eds.), *The Routledge handbook of research methods in applied linguistics*. Abingdon: Routledge.

This chapter explores the growing use of focus groups in applied linguistics research and advocates for its use in certain fields of study where group thinking is important. The chapter begins with an overview of focus group methods in the wider social sciences before then exploring their current use in our field. The chapter includes a useful overview of the benefits of the method for the applied linguistics researcher and draws on a range of methodological resources within the social sciences. The chapter also explores various methodological concerns for focus group research, which are highlighted with examples from Galloway's own study, used to showcase various data analysis techniques.

Krueger, R. A., & Casey, M. A. (2014). *Focus groups: A practical guide for applied research* (5th edn.). London, UK: Sage.

This book is the current gold standard resource for focus group methodology. Now in its 5th edition, it provides a comprehensive overview of the full range of methodological considerations associated with focus groups. The book includes all facets of focus group methodology, from various theoretical designs, sampling and grouping issues, moderator training considerations, data collection procedures and data analysis.

10

Document Data Collection

Introduction

The use of documents in applied linguistics research is pervasive and yet not clearly defined in the research methods literature. Most literature on the use of documents as a source of research jumps directly into analysis without due consideration of how documents should be collected and treated by the researcher. When reading about the use of documents in research, information is mostly found in general resources, mixing forms of the word such as *documents, documentation* or *documentary research*. Much of this literature is not specific to applied linguistics and therefore contains a certain amount of irrelevant subject matter for applied linguistic researchers. As a major data collection method in our field, it is too often undervalued as a sole data source, except perhaps for researchers interested in topics such as text or genre analysis or those working in the field of language policy. This chapter will look at the importance of document collection in a wide array of applied linguistics research and discuss how the collection of documents for research purposes is subject to the same criteria of rigour as other data collection methods.

Documents, often referred to as *written texts* in applied linguistics research, vary widely, but the general understanding is that they all have two qualities: they can be read, and they provide some kind of message. They can include documents *about* language, such as language policies or curriculum documents, or indeed any text that can be subjected to linguistic analysis, such as newspaper articles, letters, essays or emails. More recently, innovative approaches take advantage of a multimodal perspective, which has further expanded the parameters of what a document is by including visual images as documents for multimodal analysis. This includes documentation through photography of language or symbols on signs and other public spaces in linguistic landscape studies. These new directions are discussed in greater depth in the key concepts section of the chapter.

Documents as a primary data collection method of secondary sources

Despite their obvious strengths as a valuable source of data, document research does not share the same prominence in applied linguistics research as other methods and is often relegated to the role of supplementary data, serving as an effective additional method for triangulation. Many of the documents we use in applied linguistics are socially constructed, so pairing them with other data collection methods makes much sense in some research. However, as document data collection methodology is used for qualitative, quantitative and mixed methods applied linguistics research, it can form the sole or main data collection method for a study.

In this chapter, we urge applied linguists to consider the strengths of conducting document-based research as a primary source of data collection, due to the advantages it offers researchers. First, researchers in our field have the expertise to work with varieties of texts, creating a multitude of opportunities for creative research. Second, researching documents avoids the messiness of conducting research with people, as researchers can often work independently. Working with documents also avoids the associated biases and threats to credibility of indirect measures, as they exist as artefacts of their time of production. Certainly, document data collection has its own risks, discussed later in this chapter, but it is time researchers took advantage of what this method has to offer to the field of applied linguistics as a data collection method. According to Payne and Payne (2004: 60), document collection methodology is used to 'categorise, investigate, interpret and identify the limitations of physical sources'. This can be extremely valuable in providing clear, concrete parameters for a research inquiry.

Key concepts

In this section, we first highlight the most significant feature of documents in applied linguistics research – that they are socially constructed. We then offer a discussion of the different types of documents used in applied linguistics research and finally some suggestions on what can be investigated using document methodology.

The social nature of documents in applied linguistics

At a surface level, documents are positioned as a piece of one-way communication, from the creator of the message to the intended reader or audience. However, much applied linguistics research adopts a view of writing as a social activity. Thus, any socially constructed document entails more than just one-way communication as it involves the co-construction of knowledge (see e.g. McKinley, 2015, on a social constructivist approach to text analysis). As a result, most researchers consider the sociocultural context of documents to be paramount to understanding them.

Whether a language policy, a lesson plan, a student's essay, a personal written communication or even a posted notice – these documents are influenced and defined by social, cultural and historical factors. The meaning given to the document by the reader is co-constructed; that is, the message is incomplete until it is given meaning by the reader. The intended reader or audience involved in communication through documents should be easily identifiable if the message is clear and is often – but not always – explicitly marked by the writer. In theory, the context in which the message is communicated needs to be agreed sufficiently by both the creator and reader for the message to be fully complete. Therefore, the understanding of documents as socially constructed requires that researchers see documents as two-way communication, albeit unmonitored, and therefore not necessarily always understood by the receiver as the creator of the message intended.

Researchers must also consider the driving forces behind the creation of the message. There are very likely certain socio-historical, socio-economic and/or sociopolitical motivations in the creation of documents (e.g. language policies). In some research, these motivations may be difficult to uncover. For example, a study which analyses policies related to the internationalization of higher education must consider the fact that these policies have been developed to address the quickly expanding influence of globalization and that there are many stakeholders involved in shaping these policies within separate political and economic agendas. Policies might be intentionally vague in some areas so that they can be interpreted in different ways by various readers. An understanding of the wider context during data collection and analysis may reveal a great deal about the 'real' meanings behind policy changes. These influences can be found at all levels of policy documentation from national policies written by a range of stakeholders to classroom policies written by individual teachers found in course descriptions.

The social nature of documents at the classroom level may be more straightforward. In documenting student learning, students' written texts can make ideal documents for investigation. If we understand student writing to be socially constructed, embodying their sociocultural identities, we can inquire into the entire process of developing that writing. In most cases, student writing is a response to specific instruction – an exercise in working with certain ideas about writing. If we know the context in which the writing is done, we can better understand the writing as a document of a student's learning at a stage in an ongoing process. We can also investigate whole portfolios of writing, including drafts, written feedback and written reflection, to gain a deeper understanding of the phenomenon of developing a student writer.

Beyond the classroom, we find a broad range of possibilities to understand the social nature of various forms of documents from electronic correspondence to signage and more. Whatever the form of a document, the language used in it is aimed at the discourse community in which the message is intended to be communicated (lest the message be misunderstood). Such documents allow us to identify the use of language in certain communities – what words (or symbols or images) are used, how they are used, by whom, when and why?

What qualifies as a document?

There is considerable ambiguity of what documents are. If we take our broad definition that a document can be read, and carries a message, this can include a broad range of texts. Some documents are collected for analysis of their content *about* language, such as the following:

- Legal documents such as language policies and language acts
- Texts outlining language guidelines or expectations
- Educational documents such as national, state/province, local district, institution and classroom language curricula, as well as course descriptions and lesson plans
- Educational materials, such as language textbooks
- Various components of student writing including drafts and peer-or-teacher written feedback

These documents are often subject to some type of content or thematic analysis (discussed later in this chapter), as the researcher is often interested in what these documents say about language in terms of their content and meaning.

Other documents are collected *for* the language used within them. This can include a wide range of documents including texts such as the following:

- Media texts from newspapers or online news sources
- Electronic texts, such as online forum, blog or social media posts
- Personal correspondence, such as letters, emails or messages
- Any linguistically analysable text from poems to graffiti
- Students' writing to analyse for its linguistic properties

These documents are usually subjected to linguistic analysis, as researchers are usually more concerned with how language is used by the creator of the document, or within the genre of the text, or interpreted by the reader.

While the definition of a document is wide, they do not include texts such as transcripts (see Chapter 6), which have been transformed into documents for ease of analysis by the researcher rather than being collected by the researcher as pre-existing texts. Such transcripts are primary researcher-created documents, rather than secondary documents which have been collected for the purposes of primary research. However, document analysis can be conducted in much the same way with these transcripts as with the documents listed above. From a discourse perspective, documentation of email and other correspondence via social media and online forums provides convenient avenues for applied linguistics research.

Documents are pervasively used in translation studies, where they are almost always discussed in terms of 'document analysis' (for content or linguistic aspects). In this subfield, researchers analyse texts for meaning for the purposes of translating. This requires an understanding of the context surrounding a text and the 'deeper meaning' of that text. As we are more concerned with documents as a data collection method, we will not attempt to cover this aspect of document methodology; for an overview of document data collection in translation studies, please see Venuti (2012).

For applied linguistics research, the texts commonly used include official documents, such as national education language policy, at the broad end, and curriculum at the narrow end of the spectrum. In the realm of sociolinguistics, applied linguists analyse a range of documents within diverse social realms to understand language use across genres and communities of practice. Understanding documents as *written texts* allows us to also consider students' writing – a very common form of document used in applied linguistics research. Indeed, even written feedback on writing is used as documentation for research. In Gebhard's (2004: 249) study of education reform and L2 literacy practices in the United States, document collection at the school level included student and state records, school reports, media pieces, correspondence with parents, and at the student level included student work, teacher-created materials, textbooks and more correspondence with parents. These document types have been used extensively in applied linguistics research, leading researchers to delve further into innovative approaches to the method in search of more document types.

Systematic reviews and meta-analyses

Two specific types of document research in academia are systematic reviews and meta-analyses. Both approaches aim to synthesize a large body of research on a certain phenomenon to draw conclusions to their research questions. Document data collection involves the selection of published and unpublished studies to include in the study by applying systematic inclusion criteria, while vetting the documents according to their contribution and relevance to the topic being investigated. Systematic reviews aim to evaluate the findings of the studies via weighted criteria concerning each study's rigour and provision of evidence; meta-analyses aim to reanalyse the data from the studies to be able to draw more definitive conclusions across the larger data set. Systematic reviews, therefore, are qualitative in nature, requiring researcher interpretation and evaluation, while meta-analyses are generally quantitative in their approach to data analysis.

Both systematic reviews and meta-analyses are types of primary (i.e. original) research, as they involve the systematic collection of data in the form of documents and apply original approaches to analyse these documents. In this way, they differ from narrative reviews, which are a type of secondary research. The main difference is that systematic reviews and meta-analyses have a clear research methodology and transparent data collection method. Narrative reviews can be subject to bias and a general lack of systematicity: bias in terms of which published studies are selected for inclusion and lacking in systematicity regarding how the studies are analysed (Macaro, 2020). Systematic reviews and meta-analyses, in contrast, have a transparent methodology and offer original findings to their research questions.

Even though systematic reviews and meta-analyses have their own distinct methodology, the approaches they take to data collection, in terms of their rigour and transparency, may be relevant to other types of document data collection. For more on systematic reviews, applied linguistic researchers should read Macaro (2020), and for more on meta-analyses and research synthesis in general, readers should refer to Ortega (2015).

Innovation in document methodology

We are in an age where new text types for written communication are rapidly emerging, and in some domains, replacing common spoken modes. Examples which have emerged in recent decades include email, social media correspondence, online comments and online forums. Email has been firmly established as a legitimate form of documentation; take for example Hillary Clinton's emails sent from her private email account that were considered a major contribution to her losing the US presidential election in 2016. Qualitative content/text analysis of those emails was of great interest to voters, and corpus software was used to locate any key terms, such as 'Benghazi'. As for social media and online forums, these have been of interest to discourse analysts for most of this century. Today, computer algorithms are set to read our correspondence and provide us with related advertising, having done an automated content analysis. These forms of documentation capture a use of language that is much less restricted by the formal usage found in traditional, official documents. The language is often much more of a spoken nature, containing combinations of various registers of language, translanguaging and a range of uses of images and symbols, with entire messages communicated using only emoticons. This last type leads us to consider multimodal documentation.

From a multimodal perspective, documentation also includes signs or instructions that may not include actual words but still contain a message that is read, thus qualifying as documents for research purposes. Linguistic landscape studies are an example of a subfield of research that examines the use of text and graphic imagery to analyse language to draw conclusions about social uses of language in public spaces. Adjustments need to be made to analysis tools, but these are developing quickly as *visual research* proliferates.

What to investigate

Document methodology provides opportunities to explore the use of language in delivering messages from a number of different perspectives. We can use documents to investigate vocabulary, particular discourse features, different ways of approaching pragmatics, linguistic standardization, variation, gender and so on (Coxhead, 2020). Quantitatively, word frequency can be very useful for identifying common terms within certain communication contexts and with certain communicators. Qualitatively, researchers can explore these contexts to investigate how these terms are used. For example, we might investigate what words tend to be used in thesis acknowledgements (see e.g. Hyland, 2004). The documents in this example include only the acknowledgement pages of a set of theses (note: sampling is important here, discussed in the next section under 'Document selection').

As illustrated earlier, there is a wide range of items that qualify as documents in applied linguistics research. Gebhard's (2004) study covered a range of documents, including materials and textbooks. As a specific area of document inquiry, published educational materials provide a rich area for investigation. For example, the work of Gray (e.g. 2013), investigating heteronormativity in published English language education materials, offers a valuable sociolinguistic perspective. Such studies do not require large samples. Weninger and Kiss's (2013) semiotic study of culture in EFL textbooks had a sample size of two and used no other sources of data collection.

Quantitative approaches to researching documents sometimes borrow methods from corpus research, even if the documents collected do not constitute a representative corpus. These tools allow researchers to analyse large-scale data within a relatively short time (see Chapter 11). Corpus research makes use of software to explore word frequencies, lexical properties and create concordances, usually concentrated on common or key words or phrases. Corpus linguistics is the name given to this area of research, which has been in practice since the 1960s with most credit given to Sinclair's (1987) COBUILD lexicography project for bringing it to prominence. The intention of this project was to use texts to locate the usage of words beyond their traditional dictionary definitions – by developing software that could locate these words and collate them to allow researchers to read around the words to gain an understanding of the words in use depending on the source of the text. This is a significant point about a quantitative approach in document methods – they ultimately require the addition of qualitative analysis for the data to have meaning.

Ultimately, document data collection in applied linguistics research is broad, so it is crucial to clarify specifically what in the data are being identified as 'documents' (whether or not the word 'document' is even used, as 'text' is much more common in applied linguistics) and how the use of these documents best responds to the research question(s).

Procedures and practicalities

In this section, we now address how to conduct document data collection. First, we discuss the selection of documents including a discussion on sampling, followed by some important points about how to ensure the quality of those documents. We then move to the main considerations for document data collection in qualitative research including coding, followed by a discussion of mixed methods research.

Document selection

When selecting the documents for applied linguistics research, researchers might consider the four criteria of authenticity, representativeness, meaning and credibility (Scott, 2006). That is, documents are socially constructed, reflecting aspects of their sociocultural context, and a research must justify how they are appropriate for answering the study's research questions. Both authenticity and credibility of documents in applied linguistics research are fairly straightforward. As the selection should be directly applicable to the immediate context under investigation, it will usually include documents generated for that context. For example, in classroom research, documents such as the course (or module or unit) outline and syllabus, lesson plans and text generated in or for use in the classroom might be collected for analysis. Problems with authenticity and credibility can arise where texts are generated outside of usual course content, such as asking students to write something only for a study. In this case, these documents are best viewed as primary data generated by the researcher for a project via data elicitation techniques (see Chapter 2) rather than an example of secondary document collection for primary research purposes. Beyond the classroom level, authenticity and credibility of documents should be considered regarding their ultimate influence on the context. For example, national or state-level curriculum that has not been taken into account by the school or instructor in setting up or delivering a course should be used with caution if the investigation is aimed at the classroom level.

In contrast, meaning in documents is somewhat more evasive, as a researcher's interpretation of meaning is subjective and dependent on the research inquiry. Here, the sociocultural context needs to be understood and reflected in understanding the document. Researchers need to consider specifically what is the message, who is communicating it and who is meant to be reading it. The rhetorical situation plays a powerful role, as the social construction of the text will have weighed on the register and tone used in the document. The genre should be discerned within the social context in which the document was created so we can hold our interpretation of it to the expected constructs of that genre. Documents that do not fit clearly into a category (see coding below) may have to be removed from the data set.

Representativeness is where researchers need to address issues of sampling, as it may be hard to achieve if little is known of the research context. The sampling of documents should be clarified and justified. While technically random sampling could be used, documents left out could be significant (causing the data set to fail to be representative). This is where a variety of sources can be useful, as they can help to discern overall patterns and help shape the direction of the study. However, more systematic sampling procedures are advised for rigorous research, such as those found in systematic reviews, which require a team of researchers to apply inclusion and exclusion criteria to form the sample (Macaro et al., 2018). Ultimately, the sample needs to be sufficient for investigation of 'the bigger picture' of the research phenomenon, which needs to be understood before selecting specific documents. For example, in a study of journal language guidelines, McKinley and Rose (2018) decided to look at journals from all twenty-seven discipline categories provided by an external ranking website to draw conclusions about the publishing industry. While this may seem to have created somewhat of a mixed data set, it is much more representative of what they set out to achieve, which was the ability to comment on issues of conceptualizations of language errors, standards, norms and nativeness in academic journals.

Finally, securing access to official documents that are not in the public domain, such as institutional curricula or meeting minutes, or anything that includes sensitive or confidential data, may require special permissions that may be beyond the scope of a study. These limitations need to be carefully considered in the planning stages. Only those documents that are accessible, that ensure confidentiality (when not in the public domain) and that answer the research questions should be selected and compiled for analysis.

Ensuring document quality

Having compiled documents according to set criteria, the next step is to remove any that does not meet quality standards. The accuracy of the documents can be determined by comparing them to similar documents or with other data collected. Finally, a data collection form with a summary of the data can be generated that includes the source information, such as the document type, citation information and specific document content that answers the evaluation questions. If a researcher needs to know how and why documents were produced in a certain way they sometimes can engage in some additional investigation, such as talking directly with the creators of the documents, if this is possible. Other researchers prefer not to do this if they prefer to analyse how the documents stand on their own. This is often justified as more authentic in situations where typical readers of the documents do not have access to the creators and thus need to interpret them in their own right. In systematic reviews, the quality of the documents is usually evaluated according to weighted criteria.

Document analysis: Qualitative research and coding

A particular point of confusion about qualitative document analysis is what to call it. Ultimately, this depends greatly on the specificity of the approach. There are several terms used to describe document analysis in qualitative applied linguistics research, mainly *qualitative text analysis* (Kuckartz, 2014), which is located within the tradition of *qualitative content analysis* (Mayring, 2000). Through qualitative text analysis, data can be analysed using *thematic text analysis* (Kuckartz, 2014), which combines concept-driven and data-driven categories (Schreier, 2014). Using a typical methodology of qualitative text/content analysis (see Schreier, 2014), a coding frame can be established based around central themes. These themes should be trialled in the data, evaluated and modified where new themes emerge.

We offer the following clarification of the differences between these key terms: *qualitative content analysis* is the umbrella term containing *qualitative text analysis* (which is not always differentiated) when the intention is to analyse written documents applying an existing theme for content relevant to that theme. Alternatively, within the tradition of qualitative text analysis, we find *thematic text analysis*, which functions in the opposite direction, where the researcher approaches the documents without a predetermined theme, instead searching for patterns, allowing themes to emerge.

When texts are analysed for their linguistic properties, this is often referred to as *discourse analysis*. Discourse analysis 'examines patterns of language across texts and considers the relationship between language and the social and cultural contexts in which it is used' (Paltridge, 2012: 2). When discourse analysis methods are used to analyse written texts, applied linguists often refer to this as *text analysis*. It is important to note that this is very different from the term *qualitative text analysis* as used by Kuckartz (2014), which is part of content analysis methodology. Text analysis, as part of discourse analysis, focuses on the linguistic patterns in the text, whereas qualitative text analysis focuses on the content of what is written. More detail on text analysis can be found in different frameworks, depending on what elements of the text researchers are interested in. Many are related to each other such as various levels of genre analysis (see Bhatia, 2014), as well as those found in systemic functional linguistics, rhetorical genre studies and corpus linguistics, among others. See Wang (2020) for an overview.

Document analysis: Mixed methods research and corpus studies

In mixed methods document analysis, there are several approaches in applied linguistics research to integrate quantitative approaches with qualitative elements to draw meaningful conclusions. The most common quantitative approaches are found in corpus studies, using software to analyse text, usually concentrated on keywords or phrases with concordances then generated for further qualitative investigation. To add a qualitative element to this type of corpus research, the researcher can, for example, explore further the words that 'stand out'. Martinez (2018), for example, ran statistical tests to first compare texts written by nonnative academic writers with those written by native writers to look for evidence of emergent English as a lingua franca forms in academic papers. He writes, 'Here "stood out" is essentially operationalized as a content word (i.e. not a grammatical or function word, such as an article or particle) (Schmitt, 2010: 54) or lexical bundle.' He then qualitatively explored concordance outputs surrounding the words to better understand how they were used in context. While corpus software can be fairly quick to use in the analysis stage, this is only an effective approach when there are solid research questions that warrant such an approach.

Word frequency is probably the most common quantitative component in document analysis. Coxhead (2020), well known for her development of the Academic Word List 20 years earlier which made use of corpus analysis (Coxhead, 2000), explains that frequency research helps us to identify words that learners are more likely to need to know in various contexts and to understand how words collocate. Using corpus analysis software such as AntConc (Anthony, 2014), texts can be entered into a programme and can provide a list of most frequent words. For more detailed information on this approach, see Chapter 11 in this volume.

Improving reliability and validity

As with interviews and observations, when documents are used as a qualitative data collection method, documents are perhaps better considered in terms of credibility, rather than reliability and validity. Whatever terms we use, documents need to be scrutinized just as much as any other data collection method, as there are some important limitations to consider, as well as ways of dealing with limitations.

As mentioned earlier in the chapter, researching documents avoids the inherent messiness involved in researching people. Document methodology is unobtrusive, as documents are authentic and naturally occurring, not produced for the study, and hold a position that is relatively concrete providing information about the social world of the creator(s) of the document (Payne & Payne, 2004). But it is important to understand the nature of the document, as the creator may have been produced them for very different purposes than how researchers position them in their research. These differences will impact on a researcher's ability to use them for their own research purposes. While documents seem in their nature to have lesser chance of lacking credibility, there are several threats that need to be addressed, mostly in consideration of how and why the documents were created. Document analysis raises several potential threats, as researcher bias weighs heavily on interpretation of document content, and quantitative measures of documents can involve words being misinterpreted and mistakenly categorized, due to the nuanced way language is used.

The first major drawback to document data collection is how time-consuming it can be to collect, review and analyse many documents. This usually results in researchers taking a narrower focus to their research, using documents available to them and shaping the study around that. For example, in Rose and McKinley's (2018) study of Japanese universities' plans for using education ministry funding as part of a recent higher education initiative, the study was limited to the information that was publicly available via the university websites. It was further limited to the information that was provided in English. Although the researchers justify their sample as analysis of information available to an international audience, nevertheless, these limitations challenge the reliability of the study, as it remains uncertain whether the English language documents are accurate reflections of their Japanese language counterparts. It also challenges validity, in that while documents state a university's intention, document analysis alone may yield an invalid picture of actual policy implementation.

Next, one of the greatest threats of the use of documents is irrelevance. As Cohen, Manion and Morrison (2018) explain, document types vary regarding information and accuracy. While some documents may be opinionated or subjective, others could be more factual and descriptive. Researchers, therefore, need to understand the nature of the document in relation to the research questions. The information provided in documents may be inapplicable. A document that is very poorly organized, incomplete or outdated may also be considered irrelevant. As mentioned, sifting through a great number of documents can be very difficult, so ensuring documents are relevant to the inquiry can be very helpful: applying relevance criteria (i.e. a sampling strategy) can help to reduce the number of documents. Of course, while this can be effective for narrowing the data set down to a manageable size, it is also reliant on a certain selective survival of documents and information. To overcome this point, researchers must be very clear about their relevance criteria, justifying their decisions to argue that what is considered a manageable size will differ according to the length of text and the research questions.

Finally, documents are also reliant on a researcher's own understanding of the context in which they were produced. When analysing documents on their own within a context of familiarity to the researcher, researchers are subject to their own biases; when analysing documents outside a researcher's own contexts, they are essentially working in the dark. This is where further data collection may be needed, such as interviewing the creator of the document or readers of the documents. However, it is indeed possible to conduct a study using documents as the sole data collection method, but a limitation should usually be acknowledged that the researcher is analysing the text as it stands, which may be different from the creator's intentions. It can usually be justified that documents are not produced with the idea that the creators will be given the opportunity to explain them. Indeed, in many cases, we do not have the ability to interview the creators of the documents collected for our research, so the point should be made that these documents were not intended to generate the discussions that we develop by investigating them.

Case studies in applied linguistics research

The use of documents in applied linguistics research is so varied. Table 10.1 provides examples of studies using mostly different data that qualify as documents – from students' writing to research articles, from author guidelines to university web pages and from technical documents to textbooks. Certainly, there are many more examples that could have been included here, but this list provides at least a starting point from which we can attempt to create parameters for this otherwise vast data collection method, specifically for applied linguistics research.

In addition to the range of types of documents and types of analysis, this list also shows a range of sample sizes from one into the hundreds. In document data collection for applied linguistics research, sample size depends on the intention of the study, and a large sample does not always indicate comprehensive coverage. For example, Weninger and Kiss's (2013) study of EFL textbooks adopts a case study design in its selection of two textbooks and does not require a large sample for its close-up analysis. Also, McKinley and Rose's (2018) study of 210 author guidelines used narrow sampling criteria (from the position of the highest impact journals) to investigate their research topic phenomenon. Although the sample size is large, it is certainly not representative. Hyland's (2004) study similarly provides a non-representative sample of the phenomenon being researched, despite its sample size of 240. However, a systematic approach such as the one applied by Macaro et al. (2018) provides a comprehensive of the phenomenon under investigation, with a final sample size of 83, and could be considered more representative.

Taking an in-depth look at two of these studies, we start first with Rose and McKinley (2018), as this provides a traditional qualitative approach to document research in applied linguistics and is a good example of a study that used documents as a stand-alone data collection method. The study sought to examine the stated implementation of a new higher education initiative at thirty-seven participating universities across Japan.

Table 10.1 Examples of document data collection in applied linguistics research

Researchers	Topic	Data collected	Research design	Data collection method
Hyland (2004)	Structure of dissertation acknowledgements	PhD and MA dissertation acknowledgements in Hong Kong; student and supervisor interviews ($n = 240$)	Move structure analysis	Corpus of a larger study of post-graduate research writing in Hong Kong
Macaro et al. (2018)	English medium instruction in higher education	Research publications on EMI in HE ($n = 83$)	Systematic review	Academic journals, applying inclusion/ exclusion criteria
Martinez (2018)	Nonnative English forms in international journals	Academic articles on food science written by English L2 scholars ($n = 192$)	Corpus analysis	Academic journals, identifying scholars' L1 by name
McKinley and Rose (2018)	Native standards in journal language policy	Journal submission guidelines ($n = 210$)	Interpretive qualitative text analysis	Journal web pages
Rose and McKinley (2018)	English policy in Japanese higher education	Ministry policy + university policy documents ($n = 37$)	Thematic text analysis	Ministry website + university websites
Ross (2005)	Impact of assessment on Japanese university students' L2 proficiency growth	8 years of student records and curriculum documents ($n = 2,215$) + statistical analysis	Mixed methods	School and instructor provided documents
Viburg and Grönlund (2017)	Mobile technology use in distance L2 education	Institutional + technical docs; interviews and observations ($n = 25$)	Mixed methods	Institution rules, user manuals, white papers, observations, interviews
Weninger and Kiss (2013)	Culture in EFL textbooks	EFL textbooks ($n = 2$)	Interpretive semiotic text analysis	Two EFL textbooks based on different language teaching principles

Documents were collected in the form of text extracted from thirty-seven publicly available university websites, which detailed policy implementation strategies. These were found by searching for each participating university's required publication of such a documentation in English for international readership (according to the policy document produced by Japan's education ministry). A thematic text analysis was employed by first reading all the documents and employing open coding as themes emerged. In the first round there were fourteen categories, but this was reduced to eleven due to a lack of coverage of three categories across documents. These categories, or 'nodes', were grouped by similarity and qualitatively analysed, although some quantitative procedures were also applied, including a cluster analysis of coding similarities across documents. This systematic analysis allowed the researchers to draw important conclusions regarding these universities' interpretations of the ministry initiative to develop 'global universities' in Japan. The authors state several limitations of the study (as discussed earlier in the chapter), including a need for future studies to explore Japanese language versions of the texts and to explore how the creators of the texts (i.e. the universities themselves) put these stated plans into action.

On a very different scale, the mixed methods study conducted by Ross (2005) presents a valuable opportunity afforded by using document data collection to generate a large data set. In his study on the impact of changes in assessment criteria on Japanese university students' L2 proficiency growth, Ross collected course curriculum documents and student records for all 2,215 students in the same programme over a period of 8 years. With this large data set, the researcher generated statistical values for assessment criteria that could then be analysed for comparative reliability.

Implications for researchers

Document data collection in applied linguistics research has not previously been defined to the extent we have offered in this chapter. With the understanding that documents in this specific field can include anything that can be read, and provide a message, the possibilities for research are almost endless. We maintain that documents are forms of concrete data that present messages that are socially, culturally and historically contextualized. This is important, as an analysis of language policy documents or students' writing from 30 years ago would require a socio-historic lens that embraces the social, cultural, economic and political influences at the time. With this understanding, we see that document data collection in applied linguistics will forever provide opportunities for fresh perspectives and will go through regular periods of change as influencing factors go through their own stages of evolution.

Establishing definitive parameters of document methods in applied linguistics research requires some clarity about the field itself. In much of this chapter, we have mostly discussed documents related to language education; this is because the more narrowly focused areas of translation and discourse analysis have been discussed in greater depth within the literature specific to these fields of study (see, e.g., Paltridge, 2012; Wang, 2020 for research methods related to discourse). We have intended this chapter to extend the discussion of the use of documents in applied linguistics research in an effort to promote the strengths of the data collection method specific to the field.

We also see document data collection as an opportunity to generate various sizes of data sets with larger data sets having the potential to raise the profile of applied linguistics research. While most qualitative data collection can be time-consuming, as in-depth investigation and 'thick description' require going into the details of the research phenomenon, analysing large data sets of documents can be relatively quick with, for example, the help of corpus software. If documents are the sole data collected, different perspectives can be achieved by applying multiple data analysis techniques to them. We therefore encourage researchers to consider ways of increasing sample sizes by using various selection criteria for documents and exploring mixed methods approaches to analysis.

Post-reading activities

Reflect
Setting aside discourse analysis and corpus research, this chapter suggests that documents are relatively underutilized as a primary method of data collection in applied linguistics research *about language*. Why do you think this is so?

Expand
Individually or in small groups, choose one of the studies in Table 10.1 to read and critique. After reading, consider and discuss: (1) Did the researcher(s) sufficiently justify the use of documents for the study?

(2) Do you think the relevance criteria were appropriate? (3) Thinking of the type of analysis used, were there any aspects of the methodology which could have been improved in design or implementation?

Apply

Imagine you are going to investigate classroom language policy regarding use of the target language alongside other languages in an immersion setting, taking an entire school as a case study. What documents could you use? How could these documents alone serve sufficiently as the sole source of data collection? If other methods were added to triangulate the research, what other data would be collected?

Resources for further reading

Aside from work within discourse analysis (which focuses on analysis, rather than data collection) few publications exist on document data collection methods which are specific to the field of applied linguistics. We therefore present the following two resources that provide useful, comprehensive discussions about approaches to the method.

Denscombe, M. (2014). *The good research guide: For small-scale social research projects* (5th edn.). Ch. 14: Documents. Maidenhead: Open University Press.

This overview of document research, not specific to applied linguistics research, provides a good introduction to various ways the data collection method can be used, most of which have been covered in this chapter. From the more general perspective taken by Denscombe in his comprehensive book, the chapter on documents specifies the basics, such as what qualifies as a document, how to access them, how to ensure validity and credibility, evaluation of online documents, and the use of images – both 'created' and 'found' – for document research. The chapter closes with a discussion of some advantages and disadvantages of the method, along with a checklist for using documents in social research.

Macaro, E. (2020). Systematic reviews in applied linguistics research. In J. McKinley & H. Rose (Eds.), *The Routledge handbook of research methods in applied linguistics*. Abingdon: Routledge.

This handbook chapter provides clear, to-the-point instructions for the use of research articles as documents in a systematic review. The focus is on aiming to reduce the potential bias that is inherent in other types of reviews – what we often refer to as 'narrative' reviews of the literature. Macaro has rigorously interrogated the method to draw out fundamental guidelines that any researcher embarking on a systematic review in applied linguistics research should follow, such as to always work in a team, establish a clear understanding of the purpose of the review, confirm credible inclusion and exclusion criteria, and follow the review process including working with the first trawl, doing the systematic mapping activity, conducting an in-depth review and writing up the in-depth analysis. Macaro admits that total avoidance of bias is impossible, but by following these procedures, a systematic review can overcome serious challenges to the method.

11

Constructing and Using Corpora

Pre-reading activities

Think

Before reading this chapter, think about your answers to the following questions: How would you define a corpus? Is there a difference between a text archive and a corpus? Between the Web and a corpus? If so, what is the difference? What different types of corpora can you think of? What different purposes do different types of corpora serve?

Discuss

In small groups, or as a class, discuss the following: what kinds of research questions will a corpus help to answer? What kinds of questions will a corpus not be able to answer? What type(s) of information could be added to corpus data to facilitate its analysis? What features of a corpus might make the results of its analysis more or less reliable and valid?

Imagine

Imagine you are conducting a study on the use of anaphoric, cataphoric and exophoric reference in written academic English (cohesive links in writing to something stated previously, later or external to the text). Search the Web for existing corpora that might usefully serve as the basis for your research and think about the following questions in relation to each: what target discourse domain (i.e. type of language) is represented by the corpus? What types of texts are included in the corpus? Can the corpus be subdivided in any way? What is the size of the corpus and its subdivisions, and how might you determine whether the size of the corpus is appropriate for your intended research aim?

Introduction

A *corpus* – literally meaning 'body' in Latin – is a collection of texts that meets three specific criteria: the texts included are (1) authentic (i.e. naturally occurring), (2) representative (i.e. sampled in a principled manner from a larger population of texts) and (3) machine-readable (i.e. can be analysed using software). This final feature indicates the strong relationship between corpus linguistics and technology. Indeed, a lack of suitable technology initially withheld corpus research from fulfilling its potential as a primary contributor to the body of knowledge about language use. In tandem with technological advances, however, in recent decades corpus linguistic research in applied linguistics has flourished. Corpus linguistic work has informed, inter alia, lexicography, lexical studies, grammatical studies, research into language variation and change; language teaching and learning; contrastive analysis; computational linguistics; and translation and interpretation studies.

The use of the term *text* in corpus research may be initially misleading: 'texts' refers to both written and spoken language, ranging from academic journal articles to text messages, from political speeches to football chants. Corpora differ from text archives (mentioned in the previous chapter), because although both are a collection of texts, archives are often developed merely for reasons of posterity and contain texts selected at random, whereas corpora are always compiled systematically and for a pre-specified purpose. Likewise, therefore, the internet is not a corpus because the texts it includes are undefined and not compiled for linguistic purposes.

Corpora facilitate a range of different analyses – both qualitative and quantitative – from purely linguistic endeavours to research focusing on discourse from a social and cultural perspective. They are a vital resource for applied linguistics research because they provide examples of authentic language use in context; allow for objective analysis of linguistic data; and can store, recall and reorganize information on an unmatched scale. What they cannot do is explain the phenomena they exemplify: to find out why a particular linguistic feature is used in a certain way, complementary methodologies must be employed. Furthermore, corpora do not provide *negative evidence*: they are a repository of what is possible in a language but not what is impossible and (sometimes) not what is atypical or peripheral. Finally, the extent to which generalizations can be made from corpus linguistic research is inextricably linked to the features of the corpus analysed.

That is, if a corpus is not truly representative of the target discourse domain (i.e. the language, variety, genre or register it was designed to exemplify), then findings yielded from its analysis may only apply as far as the sample included in the corpus.

This chapter lays the theoretical groundwork for constructing and using corpora in applied linguistics research, outlining key concepts and issues before showcasing examples of sound use of corpora in the literature.

Key concepts

In this section, we explore key concepts underpinning the construction and use of corpora. These include discussion of the different types and models of corpora and of representativeness, balance and size.

Types of corpora

There is a plethora of types of corpora. *General corpora* are intended to yield a picture of a language (or language variety) as a whole, whereas *specialized corpora* focus on language use in a particular genre (e.g. advertising text) or domain (e.g. law). *National corpora*, such as the British National Corpus (BNC), are a type of general corpus designed to represent use of the national language in a particular country. They aim to include a balanced range of data such that generalizations about national language usage can be drawn. For example, the BNC includes written and spoken data, data from different 'domains' (e.g. arts, commerce/finance, world affairs), data from different time periods and data from a range of sources (e.g. books; speeches). Spoken BNC data are further categorized by features such as formality of the discourse context (e.g. leisure, business), region (e.g. north, south), age of speakers and interaction type (e.g. monologic, dialogic).

National corpora tend to adopt a *static sample model*, whereby data are collected cross-sectionally to provide a 'snapshot' of language use within a given time period (with, in some cases, the same sampling frame applied at subsequent time points as a means of keeping the corpus in line with contemporary language usage). *Dynamic models*, on the other hand, refer to the practice of constantly adding to a corpus such that it grows exponentially over time and nuanced language changes can be tracked. New texts are sampled that maintain the particular proportion of text types overall, meaning that newer versions of the corpus are held comparable to former versions. Corpora which adopt a dynamic model are referred to as *monitor corpora* – a well-known example being the Corpus of Contemporary American English (COCA). Because they are constantly being added to, monitor corpora are commonly much larger than static corpora (e.g. COCA is (at the time of writing) approximately 5–6 times larger than the BNC).

Specialized corpora are intended to yield a picture of a specific domain (e.g. law), genre (e.g. children's fiction), register (e.g. academic discourse), time point/period and/or context. While general corpora always follow a sample model, specialized corpora can in some cases be complete (e.g. the complete works of Sylvia Plath) and in others may take a sample. One example of a static sample specialized corpus is the Michigan Corpus of Academic Spoken English (MICASE), which sampled contemporary academic speech events at the University of Michigan. *Diachronic corpora* are samples of texts from different historical time points compiled to analyse language change and variation. For example, the ARCHER (A Representative Corpus of Historical English Registers) corpus was designed to probe change and variation in written and spoken British and American English between 1600 and 1999. *Learner corpora* are collections of texts produced by second/additional users of the language in question, such as the International Corpus of Learner English (ICLE). As learner language is likely to deviate from L1 user norms, the transcription, annotation and analysis of learner corpora can be more complex than when dealing with 'standard' language varieties. However, learner corpora are particularly useful for engendering comparison between L1 and L2 users and within groups of L2 users (e.g. by proficiency level, by L1 background).

Comparable corpora are two (or more) corpora constructed using the same (or very similar) sampling frame yet sample texts from different languages (or language varieties), such as the CorTec Corpus of technical discourse in Portuguese and English. *Parallel corpora* (e.g. the Arabic English Parallel News Corpus) contain exactly the same texts yet in one of the corpora the texts have been translated into another language. Parallel corpora are linguistically aligned (e.g. at the sentence level) such that translation equivalents in one language will be yielded when a linguistic feature is searched for in the other language. Parallel corpora are thus particularly useful for studies using contrastive analysis and for researchers in translation and interpreting. *Multilingual corpora* function in the same way as parallel corpora and align three or more languages. Whereas most corpora are text-based and monomodal, in recent years a number of *multimodal corpora* have been developed, which align different data modalities such as video and audio. For example, the Nottingham Multimodal Corpus (NMMC: Knight et al., 2009) is a 250,000-token corpus of monologic and dialogic academic discourse in which video, audio and text-based transcriptions are aligned such that patterns in the relationships between verbal and non-verbal behaviour can be analysed.

Representativeness

Other chapters in this volume have discussed in detail the importance of sampling participants from a research population in such a way that the study's findings are generalizable to the population (see Chapter 8 on questionnaires). The notion of *generalizability* also holds in corpus linguistic research. According to Leech (1991: 27), a corpus is representative 'if the findings based on its contents can be generalized to the said language variety'. In order for a corpus to have *representativeness*, therefore, the sample (of texts) must mirror the extent and range of variability that exists in the wider population (the language (or language variety/genre/domain) as a whole) (e.g. Biber, 1993). Representativeness is a key construct in corpus linguistic research because it determines the appropriateness of using certain corpora to address specific research questions: for example, a corpus of newspaper articles is not representative of academic language use and would therefore not be a representative corpus for questions relating to academic discourse. Similarly, representativeness informs the extent to which broader claims about language use can be made.

Balance

The notion of balance in corpus linguistic research is strongly allied to that of representativeness. *Balance* refers to the range and proportion of different types of texts in a corpus with the ideal range and proportion of text types corresponding to informed, logical judgements about the range and proportion of text types in the wider population of language use. For example, an informed and logical judgement about general language use is that on balance people are likely to be exposed to more spoken than written language. Therefore, to achieve good balance a general corpus should include at least as many if not more spoken texts than written texts. However, a good balance in this regard is rarely achieved in general corpora because spoken language is so much more complex to sample (for this reason, the BNC contains disproportionately more written than spoken language). Thus, while balance is a principal tenet guiding corpus construction, it is not always achieved in practice. The notion of using informed, logical judgement to achieve balance denotes that there is an element of subjectivity in the process: for this reason, the decisions taken as regards balance in corpus construction are usefully taken in collaboration with (other) experts in the target discourse domain and should be documented and justified in detail in any write-up of the research.

Size

In terms of *corpus size*, generally speaking, the bigger, the better. To ascertain the minimum size for a corpus the main consideration is that of frequency. That is, the object of the research (i.e. the linguistic unit(s) of interest) must occur sufficiently frequently in the corpus to enable detailed analysis of it. If, for example, the object is a particular grammatical class of a certain word form (e.g. 'drink' as a verb), then the corpus must be large enough that any patterns in its use can be detected. Sinclair (2004a) posits a bare minimum of twenty occurrences for a specific word form, rising to at least fifty for a lemma (headword) in English. Target objects that are more complex than a single word (e.g. lexical sequences, subordinate clauses) will require a larger corpus than single-item objects because the odds of the component features occurring together may be lower than the odds of one of the individual components occurring alone. Another consideration as regards corpus size is the type of methodology that will be employed: if the researcher intends on including further tiers of analysis after an initial frequency search (e.g. if they search for verb + noun collocations initially and then group the collocations by mutual information score (see 'Data analysis' section) to perform group-level analyses), then the corpus must provide sufficient frequency of the object at every analytical tier. Thus, corpus size should be determined a priori based on the object and methods of the intended research.

Procedures and practicalities

Whether a researcher constructs a corpus or uses an existing corpus, there are a number of key procedures and practicalities to be observed. These include accessing corpora, how texts are collected or sampled, how texts are transcribed and processed and how corpora can be tagged and analysed. We cover each of these considerations in this section.

Accessing corpora

If a corpus already exists that represents well the discourse domain a researcher is interested in examining, then the first step is to find and access those data. Most corpora are catalogued by a corpus archive/distribution site, such as the Linguistic Data Consortium (LDC) or the Oxford Text Archive (OTA), so a good starting place is to visit their websites and search the holdings for corpus descriptions and user agreements and to download request information. Accessing the data itself can be more complex: while some corpora are openly available for download in their entirety (e.g. the British Academic Spoken and Written corpora), many are at least partially restricted due to copyright issues or funding body stipulations. Lee (2010) provides a detailed discussion of locating and accessing corpora, covering the accessibility of many of the major English language resources. When a corpus is not available for download or purchase, one option is to contact the corpus developer to enquire as to whether they are willing to share their data. If this possibility is available, we recommend establishing with the developer whether and to what extent they will also share their mark-up of the data: if the annotation already applied is reliable, well-documented and pertinent to the types of analyses intended to be carried out, then obtaining ready-marked-up texts will save a lot of time.

Collecting and sampling texts

Corpora can be constructed via sampling of existing texts (e.g. newspaper articles), via collecting newly generated data (see Chapter 2 for a detailed discussion of data elicitation techniques) or via a combination of the two. Regardless of the source of texts, the researcher must first decide what constitutes a 'text' for the purpose of the corpus. It is advisable to define 'text' at the smallest unit of analysis possible (e.g. 'individual essay' rather than 'Year 9 cohort essays'), such that data do not need to be subdivided at the analysis phase. Furthermore, Sinclair (2004a) recommends that, where possible, complete texts are used (i.e. sampling complete learner essays, entire speech events) so that each individual text is a comprehensive example of the target discourse domain and the corpus is not skewed towards language characteristic of one or more specific parts of the domain (e.g. greetings, conclusions).

For a spoken corpus, collecting texts involves recording participants' speech. Recording spoken data should be done in such a way that the quality and clarity of the recording is maximized. Where individual (or pairs or small groups of) speakers are recorded, it is recommended that the recording takes places in a quiet (ideally soundproofed) room. If, however, classroom or naturalistic discourse is to be recorded, then the adequacy of the recording devices and microphones to pick up speech in the target environment needs to be thoroughly piloted in advance of the main data collection. If a participant is likely to be moving during the recording, such as a teacher in class, then a lapel or headset microphone should be used in tandem with one or more digital recording devices. Thompson (2004) advises keeping written notes about the context and environment of an audio recording (e.g. the relationship between the speakers) to help situate the discourse for the transcriber. A video recording would also serve this purpose. Likewise, detailed field notes should be taken about the equipment used and any issues with it that might be useful for future recordings. Video recording is a prerequisite for studies that require transcribing and coding of paralinguistic information and are a primary data source in multimodal corpora. In such cases, the question of where to position video cameras requires consideration of perspective: in order to best address the aims of the study, whose perspective (researcher or participants) matters most?

Ethical considerations are another important component of the process of collecting and sampling texts. In corpus construction, dissimilarly to many other types of empirical data collection procedures, it is vital that *a priori consent* is obtained not only to record, transcribe, analyse and write about the data but also to preserve and distribute the data. That is, participant contributors need to give specific consent for their data (in raw or transcribed form) to be made available to specified end users, who may include future researchers exploring similar phenomena. In the case of a corpus constructed for open-access use, this means that contributors must permit their data to be included in the corpus and to understand the manner in which and to whom the corpus will be available. Anonymity is another primary ethical concern: any potentially identifying information should either be modified or omitted from the data. As discussed by Wray et al. (1998), this practice may extend beyond modification or removal of individuals' names to the treatment of certain words, phrases or topics that, if traced to a particular participant, may cause him or her harm.

Transcription

Transcription refers to the transformation of spoken data to written form. Transcription is a very time-consuming process, so if a researcher intends on personally transcribing spoken data, this will likely have implications for the size of the corpus. Transcribing spoken text is also an interpretative process in that the transcriber must make a number of decisions about what exactly to transcribe and how. First, *what* to transcribe and not transcribe? What to include should be a decision derived from careful operationalization of the object of interest: if, for example, the focus is purely on the vocabulary the speakers use, then detailed prosodic information will unlikely be necessary. If the analysis will look at, say, turn-taking, however, then the transcriber will need to transcribe overlaps between speakers and likely also prosodic and possibly paralinguistic features of the discourse. Second, *how* to transcribe the elements chosen for inclusion? There are many existing transcription conventions available to download from the Web that can be applied to or adapted for use with other spoken corpora. These include the conventions developed for transcription of the spoken component of the BNC (http://corpora.lancs.ac.uk/bnc2014/doc/BNC2014manual.pdf) and those used for the British Academic Spoken English (BASE) corpus (http://www2.warwick.ac.uk/fac/soc/celte/research/base/conventions.doc). Key decisions to be taken include the treatment of contractions (e.g. 'innit'), incomplete words (e.g. 'shou–'), marginal words (e.g. 'mmhmm') and non-words (e.g. laughing). It is important that whatever transcription conventions are applied to the raw data, they are applied consistently and documented in detail with a full version of the transcription scheme available as an appendix to the paper, dissertation or thesis.

Processing texts

Once raw data have been collected and transcribed, they must be processed and formatted into the corpus. Sinclair (2004b) proffers a useful five-point checklist for the processing of corpus texts:

1 Save a copy of each text in its original format.
2 Create a copy of each text in plain text (.txt) format. This is because most corpus software will only read texts in plain text.
3 Label each text with a reference or serial number that allows for details about the text (e.g. source, date procured) that are stored in an offline

document to be linked to the text itself. This can be done by adding a header to the text in mark-up format (e.g. inside angle brackets < >) so that when the text is read by corpus software, the added information is not included as part of the text.

4 Consult the user manual for the software you intend to use and carry out any specified preprocessing on the data that the programme requires in order to run its analyses.

5 Make a security copy of the complete processed corpus (e.g. on an external hard drive) so that if the working copy becomes corrupted in any way during your analyses, you are able to revert to its original form.

Software

There are a seemingly infinite number of technological tools available for corpus building and analysis. A fairly comprehensive list is available at https://corpus-analysis.com/. Which one a researcher chooses to use will depend on a number of factors, such as the operating system used, the types of mark-up and analyses intended and the price of the software. Many corpus builders contain built-in tools for annotation and analysis, which are detailed on the website or in the user manual for the builder. However, if a researcher does not require automated mark-up, then they may not need to use a builder: depending on size, a corpus can be simply saved into a computer (or cloud) folder and then uploaded to an analytical tool when needed.

Mark-up

Once the texts for a corpus have been collected and processed, then *mark-up* (additional information to help the researcher analyse the corpus) can be added to them. Existing corpora have differing extents of mark-up: to determine what kind and how much mark-up has been added, researchers should consult the most up-to-date user manual for the corpus, which is usually available to view online or as an open access download. Mark-up can be added either at the level of the document (document mark-up) or at the linguistic level (annotation). The term *tagging* is also used interchangeably in the literature to refer to the addition of metadata to a corpus. Document mark-up may include adding codes to specify text features (e.g. to indicate where headings, sentences, paragraphs and chapters begin and end) so that when a linguistic object is searched for, the researcher can also see where in a document it most and least commonly occurs. Codes can also be added to the beginning of each text (e.g. as a header) in order to indicate, for example, the text source and author. Sometimes this kind of metadata is not included in the header but rather implanted within the text to indicate, for example, the gender, age or L1 background of each speaker in a dialogic spoken text.

Annotation can be carried out manually, semi-automatically (i.e. first annotated by a computer programme and then hand-checked) or completely automatically. While each approach carries with it a lessening burden of time, some types of annotation cannot reliably be carried out completely automatically, such as the annotation of phonological features of a text. There are many different forms of annotation that can be added. *Part-of-speech (POS)* tagging involves adding metadata to each token in a corpus to indicate its grammatical part of speech and is therefore useful for examining, inter alia, the occurrence of different forms of the same token (e.g. 'bear' as a noun and as a verb). For example:

```
The/DT owl/NN and/CC the/DT pussycat/NN went/VBD
to/TO sea/NN

CC:   coordinating conjunction
DT:   determiner
NN:   noun, singular or mass
TO:   'to', preposition or infinitival marker
VBD:  verb, past tense
```

There are a number of different POS tagsets (i.e. tagging schemes) available, which are more or less detailed and can be selected based on the level of POS detail required to answer the research questions, such as the Penn Treebank POS tagset (45 tags), the Brown tagset (87 tags) and the CLAWS tagset (137 tags). Many POS taggers can be freely downloaded from the internet, and corpus building programmes (e.g. Wmatrix, Sketch Engine) commonly include built-in POS taggers for a variety of languages. Other POS taggers offer a limited online version (restricted by token count) and can be obtained in their full version via purchase of a license. Many POS tagging programmes have been shown to be reliable to around the 97 per cent mark (Manning, 2011), meaning that manual checking of the analysis can be limited to smaller random samples.

Another form of annotation is *syntactic parsing*, whereby mark-up indicating phrase structure is added, facilitating analyses of syntactic relationships. For example:

```
(S
  (NP
    (NP (DT The)  (NN owl))
    (CC and)
    (NP (DT the)  (NN pussycat)))
  (VP (VBD went)
    (PP (TO to)
      (NP (NN sea))))))
```

```
S:    sentence
NP:   noun phrase
VP:   verb phrase
PP:   prepositional phrase
```

Because parsing programmes are generally less accurate than automated POS taggers, syntactic parsing is usually carried out semi-automatically (i.e. first parsed by a computer programme and then hand-checked) or manually. However, there are often ambiguities in syntactic parsing that are difficult to resolve: to address this issue, manual parsing should be guided by detailed, predetermined guidelines, and where hand-checking is carried out by more than one person, an index of *inter-rater reliability* should be calculated and reported (see Chapter 4 for a detailed discussion of inter-rater reliability). Pre-parsed corpora are commonly referred to as *treebanks* (e.g. the Penn Treebank) and are used to train automatic parsers.

Other common forms of annotation include *semantic tagging*, whereby the semantic properties of tokens are marked up (e.g. tagging the intended meaning of a polysemous word, such as 'pupil'); *lexical annotation*, in which each word is tagged with its lemma, as per in a dictionary entry (e.g. 'owlet' tagged with the lemma OWL); *pragmatic annotation*, whereby text units are tagged with the speech or discourse act they represent (e.g. apology, request); *phonetic/prosodic annotation*, in which phonological features of the text are tagged; and *discourse tagging*, whereby, for example, anaphoric, cataphoric and exophoric references are tagged. *Learner corpora* may further be *error tagged*, allowing for the proportion of erroneous language use to be calculated and to determine the proportions of types of errors made (e.g. L1 transfer; over-generalization of L2 rule). Whatever type of annotation is applied to a corpus, the annotation should be heavily documented. That is, a detailed report of how, when, why and by whom the annotations were made must be provided in the write-up of the research, including details of coding and annotation schemes (such as the specific POS tagset used) and a judgement on the quality of the mark-up.

Data analysis

Corpus analysis engenders reorganization of the data in two main ways. First, wordlists can be generated that help characterize the data. Wordlists can be yielded on a frequency basis (i.e. from most to least frequently occurring), can list alphabetically all words containing a particular feature (e.g. ending in a particular suffix) and can identify *keyness* (i.e. words unusually frequent in one corpus when compared with their frequency of occurrence in a usually larger reference corpus). If a word occurs, say, 30 per cent of the time in the main corpus yet only 7 per cent of the time in the reference corpus, then it has a strong level of keyness. Corpus analysis can also yield concordances. *Concordances* allow the researcher to see how a search term has been used in context in the corpus (also termed *Key Word in Context* or KWIC) and are thus very useful for investigating collocations and patterns of language use. The search term can be a single word (e.g. 'owl'), a sequence of words (e.g. 'night owl') or a part of a word or sequence (e.g. 'owl*' to yield occurrences of 'owl', 'owlet', 'owlery', 'owls', 'owling' and 'owler'). Corpus software allows researchers to sort concordance output in various ways, such as alphabetical sorting of the word immediately to the left or right of the search term.

Descriptive statistics are widely reported in corpus analysis. Common descriptives specific to corpus-based research include *raw frequency* (i.e. the arithmetic count of occurrences of an object in the corpus), *proportional frequency* or 'coverage' (i.e. the percentage of the corpus made up by the object) and *normalized frequency* (i.e. the expected number of occurrences of the object per, for example, one thousand or million words). Normalized frequency, also termed 'relative frequency', is particularly useful when a researcher would like to describe the frequency of an object in two or more corpora of different sizes. It should be noted that the base of normalization needs to be proportionate to the size of the corpus (e.g. a base of one million words is appropriate for analyses of the BNC, which contains over 100 million words). If the base is groundlessly inflated or diminished, then the normalized frequencies yielded will be distorted.

Another common descriptive analysis is the *type–token ratio* (TTR), which is a measure of the diversity or range of vocabulary in a corpus. To calculate TTR, the number of different word *types* (different words) in a corpus is divided by the number *tokens* (running words). For example, 'The owl and the pussycat went to sea' has seven types (because the type 'the' occurs twice) and eight tokens, yielding a raw TTR of 0.875. TTR is a value between 0 and 1 whereby the closer the value is to 1, the greater the range of vocabulary the corpus includes (for ease of interpretation raw TTRs are also commonly multiplied by 100). However, TTR is text-length sensitive and thus cannot be used to compare lexical diversity across corpora of different token counts. To facilitate a valid comparison, a normalized (or standardized TTR) can be calculated, for example via WordSmith Tools or other widely used analysis software. Various other indices of lexical diversity have been designed in attempts to circumvent the issue of differing token counts across corpora, such as VOCD-D (Malvern & Richards, 1997; McKee, Malvern & Richards, 2000) and MTLD (McCarthy & Jarvis, 2010).

Inferential approaches to corpus data analysis are tests for the statistical significance of features of texts, for example to determine whether the difference in the frequency of an object across two corpora is statistically significant. Three common analyses for testing differences are the *chi-square test*, the *log-likelihood test* and *Fisher's exact test*. The chi-square test and the log-likelihood test both test the difference between an observed (raw) frequency and an expected frequency. Both analyses yield a test score: if the score is 3.84 or greater, then the odds of the score occurring by chance are less than 5 per cent. In other words, a test score of >3.84 equals a significance value of $p < 0.05$. The log-likelihood test does not assume that the values analysed are normally distributed and is thus arguably a more robust test than chi-square, yet neither of these tests is a reliable method where frequencies are very low. Fisher's exact test is a more reliable option where there are expected values of <5. There are also specific indices for collocations in corpus linguistic research, such as the *mutual information* (MI) *score*, the *t score* and the *z score*. For example, MI indicates the strength of a collocation with an MI score of 3 or higher indicating a significant collocational relationship, a score of 0 indicating that any co-occurrence is by chance and a negative MI score indicating that the words tend to occur apart from one another. There are a number of online significance test calculators (e.g. the University of Lancaster's Stats Tools Online, http://corpora.lancs.ac.uk/stats/toolbox.php)

that will run some or all of these inferential analyses on data inputted by the user. Where a significant finding is yielded, it is imperative to report an *effect size* along with the significance value to indicate the practical significance of the finding (for a detailed discussion of statistics including effect sizes in corpus linguistic research, see Brezina, 2018).

Improving reliability and validity

Now that we have explored the types and purposes of corpora and addressed the procedures and practicalities inherent in their development, use and analysis, we turn to a discussion of how corpus linguistic research can be enhanced in terms of its reliability and validity.

At the outset of this chapter we discussed the concept of *representativeness*, which refers to the extent to which findings from the analysis of a corpus can be generalized to the wider target discourse domain it was constructed to represent. In other words, representativeness is a form of *generalizability* or *external validity*. But how can the *internal validity* of corpus linguistic research (i.e. the extent to which a corpus engenders reliable representations of the target linguistic domain) be determined? Miller and Biber (2015) argue that if a corpus is internally valid, then any replication of that corpus (i.e. using the original sampling frame) would yield similar linguistic representations of the target discourse domain. That is, replication should reveal stable internal representations. However, for many scholars, particularly postgraduate students and postdoctoral researchers on a time-limited project, constructing two comparable corpora for the purposes of testing internal validity is not feasible. Besides replication, Miller and Biber (2015) focus on issues of size in relation to internal validity, which is a factor that can be addressed regardless of time constraints. They argue for greater size on the whole-corpus level because the larger the corpus, the more stable the identification of its key linguistic features will be. Also, greater size on the text level is needed (i.e. longer individual texts and a greater number of texts overall) because in addition to the impact on overall corpus size, text number and size are related to the extent and type of linguistic variation sampled. Furthermore, they suggest that if a finding holds stable across multiple random samples of a corpus (i.e. if the corpus is divided into subcorpora and the same analysis is run on each subcorpus to yield similar findings), then the argument for internal reliability of the corpus is strengthened. Therefore, via consideration and exploration of the concepts of representativeness and stability, estimations can be made as regards the external and internal validity of corpus linguistic research.

Case studies in applied linguistics research

There have been numerous studies which have used a corpus linguistic approach to address key questions relevant to applied linguistics. Table 11.1 showcases a section of these, some of which used existing corpora to address their research aims with others detailing the construction of an original corpus.

John, Brooks and Schriever's (2017) study is an example of researcher-developed learner corpora in applied linguistics research. The researchers investigated the 'structural idiosyncrasy' of communication in a branch of English for specific purposes, maritime English, by comparing it with non-nautical English communication. To do this, they constructed a spoken learner corpus of 'bridge team communication' training exercises carried out in English over a period of 2 years by L1-German undergraduate students of Nautical Science in Germany. Six hundred minutes of exercises were transcribed by the researchers and analysed for (1) lexical diversity (using TTR), (2) lexical frequency (via frequency-based wordlists), (3) lexical density (via analysis of the ratio of content words per utterance), (4) distribution of discipline-specific lexis (words derived from a document containing standard marine communication phrases) and (5) syntactic diversity (operationalized as a ratio using POS tagging, whereby the number of grammatical word classes in an utterance is divided by the token count of the utterance). The same analyses were run on reference (i.e. comparison) corpora in the form of the Brown corpus (an L1-English corpus of standard written American English) and the Vienna-Oxford International Corpus of English (a corpus of spoken L2-English in English as a lingua franca interactions). Significance testing was employed to determine whether maritime English as represented by the constructed corpus differed significantly from the language in the non-nautical reference corpora.

Durrant (2017) and Dang and Webb (2014) are examples of research in which existing corpora of academic discourse were lexically analysed.

Table 11.1 Examples of corpus studies in applied linguistics research

Researchers	Topic	Participants	Research design	Data collection method
Dang and Webb (2014)	Lexical profiling of academic spoken English	Speakers in academic lectures and seminars at UK universities (n not stated)	Cross-sectional; within-corpus comparison; lexical analysis; quantitative	Use of the British Academic Spoken English (BASE) corpus
Demjén (2016)	Cancer patients' written use of humour to cope with illness	Cancer patients on an online discussion forum (n = 68)	Cross-sectional; between-(sub)corpus comparison; semantic analysis; mixed methods	Use of subsets of the Metaphor in End-of-Life Care (MELC) corpus
Durrant (2017)	Disciplinary variation in the use of lexical bundles in academic writing	Students of various subjects at UK universities (n = 285)	Cross-sectional; within-corpus comparison; lexical analysis; mixed methods	Use of the British Academic Written English (BAWE) corpus
John, Brooks and Schriever (2017)	Linguistic profiling of spoken L2 maritime English	L1-German undergraduate students of Nautical Science in Germany (n = 23)	Cross-sectional; between-corpus comparison; lexical and syntactic analysis; quantitative	Construction of corpus of maritime spoken bridge team communication
Laufer and Waldman (2011)	Verb-noun collocation use in L2-English writing	L1-Hebrew/L1-Arabic L2 learners of English (n = 759)	Cross-sectional; between-corpus comparison; lexical and error analysis; quantitative	Construction of the Israeli Learner Corpus of Written English (ILCoWE)
Vyatkina (2012)	Linguistic complexity development in beginner L2-German learners' writing	Beginner L2 learners of German enrolled at a US university (n not stated)	Longitudinal; within-corpus comparison; syntactic and lexical analysis; mixed methods	Construction of longitudinal learner corpus of written L2-German

Durrant (2017) analysed the British Academic Written English (BAWE) corpus, which is a corpus of summative coursework from students attending UK universities to determine whether use of four-word lexical bundles would reflect disciplinary variation. Particularly interesting in this study was the selection of the individual writer as the unit of analysis: rather than dividing students (and therefore texts) into disciplinary groups a priori and then analysing for group differences, Durrant sought to identify lexical bundle patterns within individual writers' texts and use these patterns to characterize groups of writers to then see if the bottom-up grouping aligned with subject disciplinary categories. Dang and Webb (2014) analysed the sister corpus of the BAWE, the British Academic Spoken English (BASE) corpus, to determine how many word families an L2 listener would need to know to attain 95 per cent and 98 per cent coverage (i.e. to be able to 'know' 95–98 per cent of the word families used) of the texts included. BASE is a corpus of seminars and lectures recorded at UK universities comprising texts from four disciplinary categories: Arts and Humanities, Life and Medical Sciences, Physical Sciences and Social Sciences. Using the RANGE programme (Nation & Heatley, 1994; Heatley, Nation & Coxhead, 2002), Dang and Webb (2014) estimated word knowledge estimates for 95 per cent and 98 per cent lexical coverage for the BASE as a whole (i.e. combining the four discipline-specific subcorpora) and then for each subcorpus individually in order to yield vocabulary knowledge targets for L2-English academic listeners in general and by broad subject discipline.

While the above-described studies focused on lexical analysis of corpora, we now detail two studies that utilized sematic and syntactic analyses. Demjén (2016) employed subsets of the Metaphor in End-of-Life Care (MELC) corpus, which is a 1.5 million-token corpus comprised of interviews with and contributions to online fora of cancer patients, medics and carers, to explore how patients use conversational humour to help them cope psychologically with their illness. She analysed a 530,055-token discussion thread called 'Warped', on which sixty-eight colorectal cancer patients shared humorous stories and anecdotes over a period of 13 months. To facilitate this analysis, Demjén selected a 950,000-token comparison thread of patient-carer interaction from the same online forum: that is, the research investigated whether humour was used differently among patients alone compared with between patients and carers. She used Wmatrix (Rayson, 2009) to annotate the corpora with POS and semantic tagging and then applied significance testing to determine features that had statistically significantly ($p < 0.001$) more keyness in Warped than the comparison corpus. The significant categories that occurred in humorous exchanges specifically related to cancer were retained for qualitative analysis.

Vyatkina (2012) researched the development of linguistic complexity, operationalized as sentence length, clausal complexity, the use of coordinating and subordinating conjunctions, and lexicogrammatical variety, among beginner learners of German enrolled on a four-semester-long L2-German course at a US university. Nineteen written tasks were collected from each participant and were automatically tagged for POS and sentence length. The POS tagging allowed for subsequent automatic analysis of finite verb units (the unit of analysis for clausal complexity) and co/subordination. Standardized TRR was calculated as a measure of lexicogrammatical variety, and concordances were generated using WordSmith Tools to facilitate qualitative analyses of coordinating and subordinating conjunctions. At the data analysis phase these measures of linguistic complexity were correlated with each other and with the variable of time (i.e. the nineteen data collection time points).

We choose now to showcase one study to highlight the principled use and construction of corpora in applied linguistics research.

Laufer and Waldman (2011): Constructing a learner corpus of L2 English writing

Laufer and Waldman (2011) constructed the Israeli Learner Corpus of Written English (ILCoWE) – an L2-English learner corpus comprising approximately 300,00 tokens of 759 descriptive and argumentative essays written by L1-Hebrew young adults. The authors note (presumably with reference to the representativeness of their corpus) that although the ILCoWE is small compared to general corpora, its size is generous when compared to other learner corpora. Focusing on the frequency and accuracy of verb + noun collocations, the authors compared the ILCoWE with a reference corpus of writing samples from L1-English young adults (the Louvain Corpus of Native English Essays, or LOCNESS) and made within-ILCoWE comparisons by dividing their learner corpus into three subcorpora based on the contributors' English proficiency level (advanced, intermediate and basic). As the three subcorpora were of differing lengths and token counts, they were standardized prior to the analyses (i.e. brought to the same token count while retaining the original proportions of verb + noun collocations).

The analyses began with the reference (L1-English) corpus: the 220 most frequent nouns were extracted via WordSmith Tools, using the arbitrary cut-off point of inclusion of any noun with twenty or more occurrences. Then, concordances for these nouns were generated to find the verbs with which they co-occurred. The initial verb + noun collocations were then checked against two collocation dictionaries: if a verb + noun collocation was listed in either dictionary, then it was deemed to be a 'true' collocation. Next, the learner corpus was analysed: all verb + noun collocations were extracted from the learner corpus (overall and by proficiency level). Then, all 'deviant' (i.e. non-target-like) verb + noun collocations were extracted from this list and appraised by two L1-Hebrew English teachers, who determined which erroneous collocations showed evidence of L1 influence (with high inter-rater reliability). Finally, the two corpora were compared on their use of collocations that included one of the 220 most common nouns as first identified in LOCNESS. A series of chi-square tests was run on an online calculator (using the raw values) to compare the frequency of verb + noun collocations across both corpora and the frequency of deviant collocations across the three proficiency levels in the ILCoWE.

Implications for researchers

Hunston (2002: 1) stated, 'It is no exaggeration to say that corpora, and the study of corpora, have revolutionised the study of language, over the last few decades.' As a discipline we have benefitted hugely from corpus linguistic research, and its potential for impactful contribution will only increase as technological advances enable more and more sophisticated analysis of corpora. Technological development drives forwards corpus linguistic research in two main ways: it facilitates the storage, processing and retrieval of datasets on a scale formerly unimaginable, and it engenders an increasing variety of ever more complex (quantitative) analytical procedures. Therefore, while it is fair to say that corpus linguistic research is highly methodologically distinct from other empirical approaches in the field of applied linguistics, it is also the case that within corpus linguistic research there is an increasingly high level of methodological eclecticism.

The multiplicity of possible approaches in corpus linguistic research is both an opportunity and a threat to the novice researcher: the sheer range of existing corpus linguistic aims, tools, procedures and applications, coupled with the adjacent potential for ever more ground-breaking technological advances, allows for blue skies thinking at the project development stage. Yet the diversity, dispersion and complexity of many key stages in and approaches to corpus building and analysis present a challenge to the uninitiated. The challenges are, however, a justifiable trade-off for what is indubitably the most objective approach to the study of language use available to us as a field. As per Leech (1997), corpus-based research has the potential to enlighten every single branch of language learning and linguistics.

Post-reading activities

Reflect

This chapter has suggested that for corpus linguistic research to be valid, the corpus analysed must be a balanced and comprehensive representation of the target discourse domain. To what extent do you think that representativeness and balance are *absolute* constructs? In other words, what (if any) kinds of caveats might be applied to these constructs without significant loss of validity to the research?

Expand

Individually or in small groups, choose one of the studies in Table 11.1 to read and critique. After reading, consider and discuss: (1) What target discourse domain is represented by the corpus? What conclusions are you able to draw about the representativeness of the corpus, and on what do you base your conclusions? (2) What type(s) of mark-up were added to the texts, and why? To what extent was the annotation applied automatically or manually? (3) Were there any aspects of the study design or corpus analysis which could have been improved? If so, what, and how?

Apply

Design a study which aims to determine whether and how task topic influences the lexical profile of responses to the spoken component of a high-stakes English language test (e.g., IELTS, TOEIC). You are particularly interested in determining whether certain topics are significantly associated with a higher level of lexical diversity among test-takers' responses. Plan a methodological approach that will facilitate the construction of a corpus of L2-English learners' speaking test responses, and pay particular attention to the following decisions: how will you collect/sample your data? What level of detail will you require in your transcription protocol? What kind(s) of mark-up will you add to the data to facilitate the analyses? What software programmes might you use for annotation and analysis? How might the corpus be subdivided in the analysis phase? What descriptive and inferential statistics will be calculated and reported? How will you address and evaluate the reliability and validity of the findings?

Resources for further reading

O'Keeffe, A., & McCarthy, M. (Eds.) (2010). *The Routledge handbook of corpus linguistics*. London: Routledge.

Aimed at undergraduate and graduate students, this handbook brings together a wide range of experts to provide a comprehensive overview of issues and approaches in corpus linguistic research. The volume covers the historical and theoretical background to corpus-based approaches; key considerations in designing, building and analysing corpora; and the application of corpus linguistic methods to a variety of research aims (e.g. L2 pedagogy, materials development). Of particular note are the chapters which emphasize the applications of corpus linguistic research: these sections address the main research aims of corpus linguistic research in different domains and discuss the types and characteristics of the corpora and the analytical approaches best suited to address them. The inclusion of detailed descriptions of a broad array of empirical corpus-based studies gives the reader a keen insight into both the findings yielded and methodologies adopted by corpus linguists at large.

Wynne, M. (Ed.) (2005). *Developing linguistic corpora: A guide to good practice*. Oxford: Oxbow Books. Retrieved from http://ota.ox.ac.uk/documents/creating/dlc/ [Last accessed 13 December 2018].

This online edited volume is an excellent resource for anyone involved in the process of constructing a linguistic corpus. The book contains six substantive chapters on key considerations in corpus development, such as corpus building and annotation, from a range of experts in corpus linguistic research. Useful checklists for various aspects of the design and processing are proffered, and links to a range of further useful resources are provided.

The volume covers issues that go beyond written English language corpora to discuss, for example, character encoding of logographic languages and the compilation of spoken corpora. The volume closes by detailing the considerations inherent in archiving, distributing and preserving a corpus – an important topic in light of the growing movement towards the requirement for open-access datasets by academic journals and funding bodies.

12

Strengthening Data Collection: Triangulation, Replication and Realities

Where does data collection in applied linguistics go from here?

Now that the book has explored various types of data collection, we turn to issues that cut across the spectrum of applied linguistic research to take a macro-perspective of research methodology. The key concepts discussed in this chapter are triangulation, replication, realities of data collection, transparency and innovation in research.

As applied linguistics as a research discipline has matured, we have entered an era of methodological innovation, where many researchers are challenging traditional data collection methods. The parameters of the field have expanded, and applied linguists have carved out new domains of study – many of which draw connections with research in the broader disciplines of education, linguistics, sociology, psychology, law, information technology and even medicine. These new domains bring exposure to different approaches to research and at times the creation of new methodological approaches to data collection.

As outlined in Chapter 1, applied linguists also recognize the strengths of blended and mixed methods approaches to research and rely heavily on triangulating data collection to improve reliability, validity and credibility. This has led to the need for more reflection on methods and clearer definitions of data collection procedures. Clarity of methods used in research is essential if future researchers are to build on the findings of previous studies or to methodologically innovate them.

Replication has been a mainstay of research in the hard sciences but has been significantly underutilized in social research, especially in applied linguistics. Replication gives the researcher the chance to confirm existing theory generated from previous studies by conducting the same study in a similar context, applying the same data collection procedures. In this chapter, we will discuss the potential replication has of contributing greatly to knowledge in the field, while still being mindful of the limitations of this practice.

The realities of social research reveal significant limitations regarding what we can reliably do with, and say about, the data we collect. Applied linguistics research often demands that researchers be flexible with their data collection, adjusting as needed along the way, as we deal with the emergence of unexpected findings or methodological obstacles. In reality, applied linguistics researchers often need to deal with problems in situ during data collection, such as participants dropping from the study, getting insufficient questionnaire responses, or managing the different expectations of the participants. In this chapter, we will argue for a need to embrace these challenges and report honestly about potential threats to the validity, reliability and credibility of our research, rather than attempting to divert them.

Embracing these realities raises the issue of transparency in applied linguistics research, as we too often feel that it is best not to mention incidents in the data collection process that were problematic or 'messy'. We might even try to hide our biases, rather than acknowledge and deal with them through reflexive practices. If we agree that transparency is important, then we agree that revealing the problems experienced in the data collection process are potentially valuable to the field, as it could, for example, inform others of a common mistake that could be addressed to improve the method in future research. Honest and transparent reporting, therefore, leads to a more credible (and replicable) study.

Applied linguistics continues to be an evolving field with plenty of emerging opportunities to engage in original research that will contribute to knowledge. We encourage applied linguistics researchers to place more emphasis on ways data collection methods can contribute this knowledge and consider ways in which triangulation, replication, honesty, transparency and innovation can continue to drive the field forward.

Triangulation in data collection

Each chapter in this book has discussed data collection methods in isolation, but in practice, we regularly use multiple methods in a single study as different research questions require variant and multiple methods. The use of multiple methods helps to improve the credibility of our research through a process known as triangulation, which has been mentioned briefly in previous chapters. Triangulation is defined as a practice of supporting validation of data by using two or more sources for cross verification. This practice gives us a more comprehensive understanding of social phenomena. Prominent scholars in sociology such as Denzin (2017) and Patton (2015), among others, have put forward various types of triangulation, as it can be applied at all stages and levels of research, targeting both macro and micro issues. Regarding applied linguistics research methods, a recent book on triangulation edited by Baker and Egbert (2016) focuses on corpus-based research, but many of the same principles apply.

In Chapter 1, we explored the three levels of quantitative and qualitative methods, and it is at these three levels where triangulation can also occur:

1 Triangulation of research designs – where multiple designs are used to explore a research question. For example, a researcher conducting an experiment with two groups of students on an intervention might also decide to choose some participants as case studies to explore the findings in further depth. This approach would mix an experimental design with a case study design.

2 Triangulation of data collection methods – where multiple instruments are used to collect data on the same phenomenon. For example, a researcher conducting research into attitudes towards language use in multilingual workplaces might decide to collect data from participants using questionnaires, post-observation interviews and focus groups.

3 Triangulation of data analysis – where multiple techniques are applied to the same data to compare the results. For example, different statistical tests could be run to ensure significance is maintained across types of analysis. Likewise, the same corpora could be subjected to both quantitative and qualitative analysis to add breadth and depth to the findings.

Other types of triangulation could include the use of multiple researchers at various stages of the research (i.e. data collection or data analysis).

One of these types, 'triangulation of data collection methods' – sometimes referred to as methodological triangulation – directly addresses the main focus of this book. This type of triangulation can be done in two different ways. One way is to use two or more applications of a data collection method in a study, such as using multiple questionnaires to measure the same problem. The other way is to use two or more data collection methods in a study, such as possibly mixing qualitative data collection methods (such as interviews and documents) and quantitative (such as corpus analysis) methods. However, triangulation does not necessarily mean a study must adopt a mixed methods design, as two types of quantitative or two types of qualitative methods can be used. If this is the case, the term *multiple-method* (rather than *mixed-method*) is more appropriate to describe the approach.

Triangulation targets the understanding that the use of multiple data collection methods or applications helps to balance strengths and weakness of those tools. Bringing together procedures or techniques allows researchers to exploit the strengths of each, and in the process, overcoming their flaws (Denzin, 2017). It is important to note that triangulation does not necessarily mean that the data should be combined. While there are advantages to comparing the results across methods, each procedure of data collection will provide its own results and thus can generate its own discussion. Triangulation then serves as a 'next step' for treating the data and discussing why similarities and differences between the two findings have been observed. Triangulation can also lead to researcher reflection, as a practice of improving reliability, validity and credibility.

Replication in applied linguistics

Replication in applied linguistics research is the practice of repeating the data collection procedures of a previous study with different participants and circumstances. Replication helps to confirm that the results of the original study can be applied to other contexts and that their findings are maintained. Despite historical calls for more replication (e.g. Polio and Gass, 1997), scholars have observed an overall lack of replication studies in applied linguistics (Marsden et al., 2018a). This lack may be attributed to a misunderstanding of the practice – that it is only for quantitative research or that it amounts to research that is unoriginal. But applied linguistics scholars have been drawing our attention to the positive contribution of replication for decades, as a practice that is 'necessary to advance the field' (Santos, 1989: 700). More recently, we have seen great developments in conceptualizing replication in both quantitative and qualitative applied linguistics research (see e.g. Mackey, 2012) that takes us well beyond the concerns about originality. Based on this body of theoretical work, we can confidently confirm that replication research is original research: it applies well-developed and vetted methods to new research contexts, eliciting original data and generating original findings and insight. We draw especially on the recent work of Porte and McManus (2019); Marsden et al. (2018a); and Marsden, Mackey and Plonsky (2016) and their instruments for research into second languages (IRIS) database.

In their book on the practicalities of how to carry out replication studies in applied linguistics research, Porte and McManus (2019) explain the process of identifying an appropriate study for replication with thorough consideration given to the most advantageous replication approach, carrying it out, discussing it and writing it up. In the introduction, they describe the status of replication research in applied linguistics as changing. They raise the issue that much of the discussion of replication in the field is spent on the feasibility or need of replication, seeing it as a practice characteristically scientific – a practice useful for testing hypotheses.

A systematic review of replication studies in applied linguistics (discussed in greater depth in the 'Case studies in applied linguistics' section of this chapter) highlighted the value of replication research (Marsden et al., 2018a). The review found that replication research tended to be high impact, as measured by a high number of citations for the original research and a larger-than-average number of citations for the replication study. Despite the clear interest in these studies, the review also found that replication research in applied linguistics was infrequent, and exact replication research was non-existent. That is, in most replication studies, researchers tended to adapt the research design or data collection instruments – an issue the authors partly attribute to a general lack of transparency or availability of the data collection procedures and instruments in research. Such research is perhaps better referred to, and explicitly labelled as, *partial replication*.

It is clear that there is a need for replication in applied linguistics research to move the field forward, and therefore a need for open sharing of data collection instruments. We recommend consulting online repositories of research instruments, like IRIS (https://www.iris-database.org/). Here, researchers can find deposited instruments, which have been used in previous research projects, and include links to their published articles. In many cases the published articles provide information on the development of the measure, including any validation processes (if conducted). The published papers often also include contact information for the authors, so researchers can contact the developers directly to ask for further information regarding the use of the measure for research purposes.

At the time of writing over 4,200 materials were in the IRIS database – many of these could be used for replication research. The site had facilitated 29,894 downloads of these materials, which included grammaticality judgement tasks (1,814 downloads), interview protocols (1,121 downloads), questionnaires (1,382) and observation protocols (498 downloads), among numerous other types of data collection methods covered in this book. Due to the recent calls for replication research in applied linguistics, and the increased availability of research instruments used in published studies, researchers who are venturing into new data collection methods for the first time are very much encouraged to explore the resources available through IRIS.

Realities in data collection processes

Collecting data in applied linguistics research is often described in the literature as a process that, if meticulously planned, will go smoothly. In this literature (e.g. Mackey & Gass, 2005), research methods, data collection instruments and analytical tools are presented with their accompanying threats to validity and reliability if researchers fail to follow the exact plan. For example, the risk of getting a low response rate for a questionnaire is covered frequently in research methods books, usually paired with project-rescuing advice for improving response rates. What is not mentioned in these otherwise well-intended instructions is the reality that an applied linguistics study with a low response rate is common and that where that rate cannot be increased, it can still be a potentially valuable contribution to knowledge in the field.

Instead, many researchers (particularly novice ones) continue to blame themselves for insufficient planning when things inevitably go wrong. They must have failed to recognize the possibility of the misstep, or failed to make a contingency plan, or failed to avert the problem when they faced it. This thinking completely ignores the reality of data collection processes in applied linguistics, which can sometimes be inherently messy. As Dörnyei (2007: 309) notes, 'Making compromises is part and parcel of being a researcher.'

This is not an idea that is widely debated, especially not in research methods literature. When the idea is raised that doing applied linguistics research is not as straightforward as it is so often depicted, it is sometimes to make the point that we are denying ourselves the opportunity to advance the field by embracing the realities. Three applied linguists in Finland created a reading circle focused on McKinley and Rose's (2017) book *Doing research in applied linguistics: Realities, dilemmas and solutions.* They wrote an insightful, reflective piece to share their experience, raising the question: 'Could the things that some authors seem to view as "missteps", "messiness", "sidetracks", or something else in need of "cure", instead be seen as integral parts of the actual real-life research process?' (Ennser-Kananen, Saarinen & Sivunen, 2018: 72). Indeed, if these are inherent qualities of data collection processes in applied linguistics research, then why are they targeted as problems to be overcome?

Bias in data collection is another major threat to the credibility, validity and reliability of the research that must be dealt with and somehow overcome so applied linguistics researchers can have unbiased results and make unbiased claims. Researchers of philosophy and reason, however, discuss the idea that everyone is inherently biased (see e.g. Earle, 2018). So if we are all biased, why is it suggested that for research to be credible, bias needs to be overcome, or indeed, that it even can be? It seems that facing the realities of applied linguistics research, acknowledging and addressing them, rather than averting them, or 'curing' them, offers much more opportunity for development of the field.

When reading applied linguistics research, we do not usually know when things went wrong in the data collection process, as it is common for researchers to hide such details in publications. For example, a researcher may have been denied access to the first-choice research site, but the paper does not mention the fact that the data were instead collected in the second-choice site. Typically, the new site is described using altered criteria so that the site appears to have always been the ideal, first choice. Such practices obscure the realities of research and perpetuate the myth that research remains methodologically pristine. Embracing the obstacles faced during the data collection process requires an element of honesty and transparency in the write-up of the study – two issues discussed next.

Transparency in research

Leading on from both replication and realities is the need to be transparent and honest in reporting research, because (1) it allows the reader to more fully understand the research process and (2) it is important in replication that readers have an honest and thick description of the research. In the methodological literature, journal articles are described as 'pristine and logical' (Marshall & Rossman, 2010: 55), where researchers inadvertently obscure methodological problems by participating in 'highly standardized reporting practices' (Bargar & Duncan, 1982: 2). Data collection procedures that have been sanitized and idealized for publication ignore all of the real work and effort of the researchers in bringing the study to fruition. As Prior (2017: 172) observes, what is left unsaid 'in neatly packaged (and deliberately sanitized) publications' is 'any discussion of the behind-the-scenes dilemmas that had a hand in shaping the analysis, the final product, and even the researcher'. It also denies the readers the opportunity to learn about the difficulties of implementing certain procedures in certain contexts or under certain conditions or how they might be inherently problematic, which may in fact make a study impossible to replicate.

There is also an ethical point to the need for transparency in research, in that an honest record of data collection processes should be seen as less of a choice and more of a researcher's obligation. If real methods and intentions are obscured in much of the research we read, theories within the field could be interpreted as having being informed by somewhat dishonest accounts of evidence. One way to increase transparency is to ensure gatekeepers of research (i.e. examiners, reviewers and editors) place explicit value on honest portrayals of research, even if by traditional views they could be seen to threaten the reliability of the study. Trustworthiness, often used in place of reliability and validity in qualitative research, should in fact be applied to *all* types of research. Even the most scientific quantitative study is subject to some bias at the write-up stage – that is, writing up research is inherently a qualitative and interpretive endeavour undertaken by an author. Thus, trustworthiness should be maintained throughout the write-up via the transparent and honest reporting of the research and its procedures.

Another way in which transparency in research can be achieved is through *registered reports*, which refers to the pre-registering of research so that researchers are held accountable to the planned procedures of a project before collecting data. This initiative is occurring across research disciplines and is part of a push for *Open Science*, which aims at 'enhancing transparency in research methods, observation, data collection, data access, and communication of findings, provid[ing] important mechanisms for enhancing the validity, credibility, and reliability of scientific endeavors' (Marsden et al., 2018b: 1). Pre-registering projects in a publicly accessible domain ensures greater transparency of the intentions of research and is particularly important in experimental research to avoid questionable practices (Chambers, 2017). These practices can include HARKing (hypothesizing after results are known), where the null hypothesis is obscured or changed based on a study's findings. Some journals in applied linguistics, such as *Language Learning*, are leading the initiative of providing avenues for researchers to pre-register their studies and aim to make the practice inclusive of a range of methodological approaches (i.e. not only laboratory or experimental research). This high-profile initiative will likely raise awareness of the practice of registering research in future applied linguistics research.

Innovative research

A final concept to address – and one that has been raised several times throughout the book – is the challenge to 'be original' in conducting applied linguistics research. Originality is a feature of all research that is linked to facilitating a researcher's contribution to knowledge in the field. Originality is often believed to be best achieved through innovation – in filling gaps in both topic and theoretical knowledge. In applied linguistics research, innovation is positioned as a valuable endeavour in all areas, from translation studies to discourse analysis to speech therapy. It is also discussed in reference to new ideas and approaches to language pedagogy such as developments in curriculum, assessment, materials and classroom practices. While indeed there is a need for innovation in research within these domains, the methods used to study them are less commonly referred to as innovative themselves.

Despite ongoing challenges to the 'norms' in academia and attention drawn to innovation in research, applied linguistics continues to adhere largely to the methodological catalogue of social science research. The norms in applied linguistics research are defined by traditional approaches to research such as experiments, surveys and ethnographic research, often drawing on widely used data collection methods. These norms can be problematized as barriers to cultivating more creative, generative approaches to data collection, sometimes labelled 'non-traditional' or 'alternative' research methods. In the context of globalization, multilingualism and developing technologies, questions surrounding relationships among language and other semiotic resources (e.g. image, film/video, sound) and the social contexts of their use are increasingly foregrounded.

Thus, the field of applied linguistics is at a pivotal moment in considering how best to investigate this explosion of domains and dimensions of the resources used to make meaning. Larsen-Freeman (2018: 64) raises some examples of innovative research designs in SLA that could prove to effectively advance the field, including 'design studies, social network analysis, and process tracing'. Looking more broadly across the field, certainly there are many opportunities for innovation. Major theoretical shifts, such as those occurring within the social turn (see Ortega, 2011) and the multilingual turn (see May, 2014; Ortega, 2013), have challenged the way many applied linguists have historically approached research. This disrupts the foundations upon which much current research is based, including the methods used to generate this evidence.

Other emergent theories, such as complex dynamic systems theory, have challenged notions of viewing (and therefore measuring) non-linear constructs like language development or learner psychology as linear (see Lowie & Verspoor, 2018). Other groups of researchers, such as those in the Douglas Fir Group (2016), have emphasized a need to embrace and explore more fully the social and contextual realms, alongside the cognitive and psychological, when researching second language learning. These new perspectives challenge existing ways researchers engage in data collection and data analysis and provide innovative avenues for future research.

Case studies in applied linguistics research

Pfenninger and Singleton's (2019) study is an excellent example of data triangulation in applied linguistics research. The study reports on a 5-year longitudinal study of 636 bilingual and monolingual EFL students in Switzerland – half of whom had studied English in primary school and half of whom had not. By taking thirteen different sociolinguistic contextual measures of parents, siblings and home life, and seven different types of proficiency measures, the researchers were able to explore the effects of early age of onset of English learning on their language development. Although not explicitly labelled as such, the methodology could be considered to adopt a complex dynamic systems theory approach to data collection, while also highly valuing socio-contextual factors in second language learning.

Seals and Kreeft Peyton (2017) and Hedgcock and Lee (2017a) are both examples of honesty in the reporting of research but also in reflexivity during data collection. Both studies involved major changes to data collection due to the methodological issues encountered when collecting their data. They describe their experience of needing to adopt alternative data collection methods and research strategies to maintain their desired research focus. Both studies are accompanied by separately published narratives that expand on behind-the-scene data collection challenges, which are presented in Seals (2017) and Hedgcock and Lee (2017b). Seals and Kreeft Peyton (2017) is discussed in greater depth below.

Handley (2018) and Coxhead (2018) are provided here as examples of published papers that outline a need for replication of research into

Table 12.1 Example studies in research replication, transparency and triangulation

Researchers	Topic	Participants/data	Research design	Data collection method
Coxhead (2018)	Replication of formulaic sequences	N/A	N/A	N/A
Handley (2018)	CALL replication	N/A	N/A	N/A
Hedgcock and Lee (2017a)	Teacher learning in language teacher education	Language teacher candidates ($n = 2$)	Action research	Questionnaire; focus groups
Marsden et al. (2018a)	Replication in L2 research	L2 replication studies ($n = 67$)	Systematic review	Document collection
Pfenninger and Singleton (2019)	Age effects in L2 acquisition	Secondary school students in Switzerland ($n = 636$)	Longitudinal survey	Questionnaire of 13 sociolinguistic context measures; 7 proficiency measures
Seals and Kreeft Peyton (2017)	Heritage language learning	Russian-Ukrainian language learners ($n = 2$)	Ethnography; case study	Observations, audio/video recordings, interviews, document collection

language teaching and learning. Handley (2018) calls for replication of experimental research in the field of computer assisted language learning to increase evidence for good-quality software and activity design. She singles out two studies (Neri et al., 2008; Satar & Özdener, 2008) in need of replication and outlines appropriate methods and considerations for future studies. Coxhead (2018) calls for more replication research into formulaic sequences, especially in terms of their use alongside appropriate teaching methodologies and within language teaching materials. She recommends replication of two studies (Alali & Schmitt, 2012; Jones & Hayward, 2004). Finally, Marsden et al.'s (2018a) is a systematic review which investigates replication research as a whole. Due to its clear relevance to issues raised in this chapter, it is discussed further below.

Seals and Kreeft Peyton (2017) and Seals (2017)

The study reports on the lead author's longitudinal ethnographic investigation of participants within a heritage language programme at a case study school in the United States. Her data collection included school observations, audio and video classroom recordings, audio home recordings, interviews with students, parents, administrators, and teachers, and classroom and community document collection. During her data collection, the school dismantled the programme she was researching, so she needed to work around severe changes and uncertainty within her planned research site, including the attrition of her participants as they departed from the school. The write-up of the study is honest and transparent, and the authors provide a thick description of the research process and the changes that took place during data collection.

In a related publication, Seals (2017) writes in further depth on this experience, focusing on the methodological processes she applied to manoeuvre through her data collection challenges, deciding to reposition her study to embrace the dynamic changes to her research site. In this narrative, it becomes clear that additional data collection research methods were added to her project to deal with changes; thus, the study is also a good example of triangulation at the data collection level. Even though the final study included fewer participants than the researcher had planned, the addition of in-depth data collection methods such as having the participants wear audio-recording wristwatches to record language interactions in the playground and at home provided the researcher with a much richer dataset. With this additional method, she could triangulate data on language use derived from other methods such as observations and interviews.

Marsden et al. (2018a)

This study reports on a systematic review of replication studies extracted from twenty-six journals within the broad field of second language research. The researchers coded the articles for 136 characteristics, which were used for comparison and further analysis. The study found that replication tended to only be carried out on highly cited articles. The researchers noted a lack of frequency in replication in second language research, calculating that one replication study occurred for every 400 published studies, often with long periods between the original study and replication of it with a mean length of time of 6.64 years. They also found that when replication studies were carried out by the original researchers, or when materials from the original studies were available, the likelihood of the replication supporting the findings of the original study was greater. The researchers also found no exact replication studies, in that replications often made changes to the initial studies 'which likely obscured, if not undermined, the interpretability of replication studies' (Marsden et al., 2018a: 322).

In the conclusion of the study, the researchers make sixteen suggestions to improve the quality of replication research within applied linguistics, of which some are of direct relevance to the topic of data collection. These include recommendations to

1 increase open availability of materials, including proficiency measures;
2 make more research fully transparent and open for replication by making data available; and
3 encourage more journals to give more and stronger incentives to their authors for systematically making materials and data openly available (Marsden et al., 2018a: 369–370).

Through the open sharing of both data collection instruments, and the data yielded from them, the authors argue that replication research could be more easily facilitated and their results more readily comparable. Thus, a key finding of the study is the need for greater availability of data collection measures and greater transparency of the procedures by which these instruments are applied in research – two issues that resonate with the points raised in this chapter.

Implications for researchers

Originality can be achieved in multiple forms, which extend beyond simply addressing a gap in knowledge. Originality can be found in new forms of triangulation by bringing together two methods of data collection that may not commonly be paired in the area of inquiry. It can also be achieved via replication research by applying data collection procedures from an existing study to research in a similar, but not the same, context. Without replication it is difficult to achieve a large enough body of evidence to drive theory forward. Originality can also be accomplished by applying a new theoretical construct or a new analytical lens to examine previously explored constructs. A number of concepts have been raised in this book such as furthering applications for abductive reasoning in research or working within new theories such as complex dynamic systems theory – both of which have direct implications for the ways research questions are formulated, and data are collected and analysed.

Researchers can also achieve originality by seeking innovative forms of data collection methods, including those raised in this book. We are constantly seeing the emergence of new instruments that enhance the quality of data collection, such as online questionnaires, keylogging software, eye-tracking hardware, and corpus and document collection tools. Also, as tasks, tests, measures, questionnaires, protocols and schemes are developed, shared and reported, our awareness of how to apply these instruments to our research grows. We encourage applied linguistics researchers to place more emphasis on ways data collection methods can contribute to the quality of knowledge in our field.

While the field of applied linguistics may offer plenty of opportunities to engage in original and innovative research, we want to emphasize that innovation alone does not take precedence over conducting good, well-informed research. A study should always be carried out according to the procedures that the research questions point to and via the most appropriate data collection research methods to answer these questions. When good research practices are followed, procedures are transparently reported via a chain of evidence (or thick description), and data collection instruments (and data collected from them) are made available, a project vastly increases its contribution to the field.

Post-reading activities

Reflect
This chapter has suggested that as researchers we need to be honest in our write-up of research procedures, including any problems we encountered. Reflect on how a researcher could balance a need for honesty with a need to present their study as rigorous.

Expand
Individually or in small groups, choose one of the replication-focused articles in Table 12.1 (i.e. Coxhead, 2018 or Handley, 2018) or find another in an issue of *Language Teaching*. Explore the elements of the original study that the authors focus on to show that the study is worthy of replication. Devise some criteria that researchers could use to assess other studies in terms of their replicability.

Apply
Choose a study related to your field of research that you believe warrants replication. Write up a case for replication, noting the strengths of the study, and how replication should be best achieved.

Resources for further reading

Ellis, N. C., Trofimovich, P., Marsden, E., Morgan-Short, K., & Crossley, S. (Eds.). (2018). *Language Learning, 68*(2), 305–585.

This issue of *Language Learning* contains three articles related to replication, transparency and the registering of research. The opening editorial is titled *Introducing registered reports at language learning: Promoting transparency, replication, and a synthetic ethic in the language sciences* (Marsden et al., 2018b) and discusses the importance of registered reports for the field of applied linguistics as one way to increase methodological transparency. The issue also includes a systematic review of replication in second language research (Marsden et al., 2018a), titled *Replication in second language research: Narrative and systematic reviews and recommendations for the field*. The issue contains a further article on multisite replication.

McKinley, J., & Rose, H. (Eds.). (2017). *Doing research in applied linguistics: Realities, dilemmas and solutions*. Abingdon: Routledge.

This edited book explores issues surrounding honestly and transparency in applied linguistics research. Each chapter showcases a behind-the-scenes look at a published study in applied linguistics, outlining methodological obstacles that researchers faced during different stages of a study. Part Two of the five-part book focuses on problems during data collection, although other parts of the book, which range from problems in research planning to reporting research, also have implications for data collection. The book contains a number of chapters highlighted in reference to transparency and addressing problems during data collection, including Prior (2017), Seals (2017), Hedgcock and Lee (2017b) and the introductory chapter by Rose and McKinley (2017).

Glossary

Abductive reasoning: The use of an unclear premise based on observations, pursuing theories to try to explain it. See also *deductive reasoning* and *inductive reasoning*.

Action research: A type of research conducted by practitioners in their own classrooms to trial innovations in teaching practice to improve learning and teaching practices or to solve problems.

Autoethnography: A type of research which combines features of autobiography and ethnography, allowing the researcher to report on their own lived experiences of the phenomenon being studied.

Buffer trial: A series of psycholinguistic task items that appear to the participant as true experimental trials yet are included solely to acclimatize the sample to the task type(s) and are excluded from the data analysis.

Case study: A research design that involves the in-depth and contextualized study of a specific object or set of objects (e.g. a person, a class, a community) to understand its particularity and complexity.

Coding: A process of grouping or categorizing qualitative data.

Concordancing: A method of corpus analysis that yields a list of all occurrences of a search term accompanied by the linguistic content before and after each occurrence (also termed Key Word in Context or KWIC).

Construct validity: The extent to which a test or measure is a true and comprehensive measure of the construct it is intended to probe.

Content analysis: A systematic approach of evaluating texts for their topics (content) to count them in quantitative studies or to code them for interpretation in qualitative studies. See also *discourse analysis, qualitative content analysis* and *thematic text analysis*.

Continuous data: Variables comprised of values on a continuum within a (potentially infinite) range (e.g. age in years).

Conversation analysis: A data analysis technique used to facilitate a fine-grained examination of interaction between speakers.

Corpus: A collection of authentic, machine-readable written and/or spoken texts that have been sampled in a principled manner from a larger population of texts.

Counterbalancing: A technique used to mitigate order effects in research design, whereby participants are divided into groups and all possible task presentation orders are rotated equally between groups.

Criterion-referenced scoring: A test score reported as an indication that the test-taker has achieved a given level in the ability being tested against a set of benchmarked criteria.

Critical discourse analysis: A type of analysis that explores the power relationship between people or communities of people represented in the language used by and about them.

Critical ethnography: A type of research that challenges the beliefs and practices observed within ethnographic research to explore what these beliefs and practices should be.

Deductive reasoning: The use of a premise as a hypothesis, testing it to show whether it is true. See also *inductive reasoning* and *abductive reasoning*.

Delayed post-test: A measure used in experimental research to ascertain whether the effects of an intervention are long-lasting.

Descriptive statistics: A range of statistical analyses that yield values which serve to describe and characterize a given dataset.

Detached (unobtrusive) observation: An observation where the researcher is, or attempts to be, unnoticed by those being observed. The researcher role is sometimes identified as a 'detached observer' or 'complete observer'. See also *observer as participant* and *participant observer.*

Diary: A self-opinionated journal, which can contain one's thoughts, reflections, moods and emotions, and is written in the author's own time and usually by their own volition. See also *journals* and *logs.*

Direct test: A test in which respondents are required to engage directly in the behaviour that is being tested.

Discourse analysis: The analysis of texts for their linguistic properties. See also *content analysis, qualitative content analysis* and *thematic text analysis.*

Discourse completion task: An elicitation task commonly used to measure pragmatic competence that presents respondents with a situation and/ or prompt to which they respond in oral, written or cloze form.

Document research: A category of research which involves the exploration of content within a collection of texts (written, spoken or multimodal).

Documents: Data sources often referred to as 'written texts'; they must have two qualities: they can be read and they provide a message. See also *text.*

Duoethnography: The study of two or more contrasting lived experiences of author-researchers on a shared phenomenon.

Ecological validity: The extent to which the control a researcher exerts over a data collection methodology reflects the real-world relevance of the data.

Edumetric measure: A test designed to measure changes in knowledge, skills or ability, usually as a result of some form of intervention.

Emic approach: A perspective positioned inside the social group being investigated.

Ethnography: A research design that positions the participants (and its communities and cultures) as the primary focus of investigation, involving descriptive and analytical explanations of the participants' behaviours, values, beliefs and practices.

Etic approach: A perspective positioned outside the social group being investigated.

Event contingent journal: A type of journal design that requires participants enter information after they experience or complete the event being researched. They are useful to measure participant reaction to, or completion of, a task. See also *signal-contingent journal* and *interval-contingent journal.*

Experiment: A research design that attempts to isolate cause and effect of a 'thing' being manipulated (referred to as the independent variable) and the effects of the manipulation on the 'thing' being measured (referred to as the dependent variable).

External variables: Any construct external to a study that could affect the observed results.

Eye-tracking: Technology used to monitor eye movements and gaze when completing a task. Eye-tracking measures an eye's movements (saccades) and stops (fixations), as well as movements back in a text when reading (regressions).

Factor analysis: A statistical procedure that seeks to identify patterns in responses to questionnaire items on a given construct via intercorrelation.

Field notes: Data collected through observations as notes taken in the field or of recordings that can be used to respond to research questions. See also *observation.*

Field research: A research design that aims to research a phenomenon in its natural setting.

Filler: A task item designed to distract respondents from developing a (subliminal) understanding of the distribution of stimuli in a psycholinguistic experiment.

Focus group: A type of data collection technique that involves having groups of participants engaged in a moderated discussion that focuses on a particular topic, situation or phenomenon to elicit their thoughts, experiences or opinions.

Grammaticality judgment task: A psycholinguistic task in which sentences are presented to respondents, who judge (usually under timed conditions) whether each is grammatical or ungrammatical.

Group interview: Interviewing a group of participants at the same time; not to be confused with *focus group*.

Hawthorne Effect: Sometimes called the 'observer effect'; it is when observed participants modify their behaviour due to an awareness of being observed.

Heterogeneous groups: A strategy in focus group methodology, where groups are organized so that diverse groups of people of differing perspectives are placed within the same group.

Homogeneous groups: A strategy in focus group methodology, where groups are organized so that members sharing a key characteristic are placed within the same group.

Indirect test: A test in which competence is assessed via a task(s) that does not require the respondent to engage directly in the skill or behaviour that is being tested.

Inductive reasoning: The use of a premise as the basis for an investigation for which there is no hypothesized conclusion but rather leads to a non-predetermined probable conclusion. See also *deductive reasoning* and *abductive reasoning*.

Inferential statistics: A range of statistical tests that yield significance values which enable generalization to the population and/or the testing of hypotheses.

Internal consistency: A form of reliability estimated via the extent to which responses to items pertaining to the same construct are correlated and thus engender similar scores.

Inter-rater reliability: The degree to which different raters'/observers' scores converge.

Interval contingent journal: A type of journal design that requires participants to enter information at set intervals in time. They are useful for systematic study of the topic being researched. See also *signal-contingent journal* and *variable-scheduled journal*.

Interview schedule: A list of predetermined questions asked in a structured or semi-structured interview.

Introspective protocols: Tasks that require participants to look inward at their own behaviours, thoughts and beliefs and verbalize these actions and processes to a researcher.

Item analysis: Statistical scrutiny of individual test items to ascertain their relative difficulty and their ability to discriminate between test-takers who perform well and less well on the test overall.

Joint autoethnography: See *duoethnography*.

Journal: A data collection instrument usually produced by participants, which records are kept of activities, accounts or thoughts surrounding the constructs or behaviours being investigated. See also *diaries* and *logs*.

Keyness: The extent to which the frequency of a linguistic feature is idiosyncratic to one corpus as compared to another corpus.

Keystroke logging: Online tracking software for recording writing on a computer by logging keystrokes, pauses and editing, allowing a researcher to explore text production processes.

Latent construct: An unobservable phenomenon, such as motivation or aptitude, that cannot be directly measured.

Lexical decision task: A type of yes/no identification task used in psycholinguistic research to probe how lexical items are organized and processed in the mind.

Likert scale: A questionnaire response format which requires the participant to read a statement and choose one of (usually) five options from 'Strongly disagree' to 'Strongly agree'.

Log: A highly constrained version of journal, which often collects specific information usually in the form of numbers or words in predefined categories. See also *journals* and *diaries*.

Log-likelihood test: A significance test commonly used in corpus-based research to compare the difference in the observed (raw) frequency of a given linguistic object between two corpora.

Mark-up: Extra annotated information that is added to corpus data to facilitate its analysis.

Member-checking: Presenting data coding and findings to participants to ensure they agree with the manner in with the data have been interpreted by the researcher(s).

Meta-analysis: An approach to document evaluation involving mostly quantitative reanalysis of data from a set of existing studies identified using inclusion and exclusion criteria.

Mindfulness: The practice of suspending evaluation by first observing, describing and interpreting phenomena.

Mixed methods research: The combination of qualitative and quantitative approaches at the design, data collection or data analysis level. See also *multiple method research*.

Moderator: A person in focus group methodology, who introduces the topics to the group, steers discussion on the topic and monitors group participation.

Multimodal analysis: A data analysis method used to interpret a range of verbal, non-verbal and visual communication for meaning.

Multimodal interview: An interview involving various modes of either questioning or responding with either the interviewer or interviewee using at least some writing to communicate.

Multiple method research: A study using (at least) two types of quantitative or (at least) two types of qualitative methods. See also *mixed methods research*.

Naturalistic research: See *field research*.

Nominal data: Variables comprised of categories that cannot be meaningfully ordered or ranked which are arbitrarily assigned numerical values (e.g. 0 = 'Male'; 1 = 'Female').

Non-verbal cue: An intentional or unintentional communication through unspoken behaviour, gesture, facial expression, body language, pacing or emotion.

Normalized frequency: A calculation of the expected frequency of a given linguistic object in a corpus per a set number of tokens (e.g. per one thousand, per one million).

Norm-referenced scoring: A test score expressed as the rank of a particular test-taker against that of all other takers of the test.

Null hypothesis: An assumption that there is no significant difference between researched populations. This is (usually) the hypothesis a researcher hopes to reject (disprove) during data analysis.

Observation: The act of watching, recording and, in qualitative approaches, interpreting and reflecting on human activity and behaviour. See also *field notes*.

Observation scheme: A system of using checklists or predetermined categories in structured observations, keeping track of the number of instances activities occur and in some cases the length of time spent on them.

Observer as participant: An observation where the observer role involves participating naturally in observed activities without directing or steering them. This facilitates more natural behaviour of those being observed, especially in smaller spaces. See also *detached observation* and *participant observation*.

Online interview: An interview conducted online via videoconferencing software or apps. Some scholars also claim that open-ended questionnaires conducted online can be called online interviews.

Online observation: The systematic observation of online activities, such as those on social media websites.

Oral proficiency interview: A standardized measure of L2-speaking proficiency in the form of a guided conversation between test-taker and interviewer.

Ordinal data: Variables comprised of a fixed number of ordered/ranked categories which have been assigned correspondingly ordered numerical values (e.g. a frequency scale from 0 = 'Never' to 5 = 'Always').

Participant (obtrusive) observation: An observation where observer roles can range from participant (engaging in activities but still taking notes) to complete participant (fully engaged with all notes taken after the observed phenomena). See also *detached observation* and *observer as participant.*

Part-of-speech (POS) tagging: A form of corpus annotation whereby metadata are added to each token to indicate its grammatical part of speech (e.g. verb, preposition).

Priming: The notion that exposure to one stimulus affects the cognitive processing of a subsequent stimulus.

Probability-based sampling: A family of sampling procedures that involve random selection of individuals from the population to the sample.

Psychometric measure: A test designed to measure the extent to which an individual exhibits a particular characteristic—such as foreign language aptitude or anxiety—to distinguish individual differences among a sample.

Purposive sampling: A sampling procedure whereby the researcher deliberately selects certain individuals to include in the sample via predetermined inclusion and exclusion criteria relevant to the focus of the study.

Qualitative content analysis: A data analysis method used to capture the content of verbal, visual or written data in the form of key topics, which are organized within emergent themes. See also *content analysis* and *thematic text analysis.*

Qualitative data: Data in the form of words or that which can be interpreted into words.

Qualitative data analysis: The analysis of linguistic or thematic content within a data set.

Qualitative research: A research paradigm involving the investigation of a phenomenon based on building a contextualized, holistic picture, conducted in a natural setting.

Quantitative data: Data in the form of numbers.

Quantitative data analysis: The investigation of variables via statistical procedures.

Quantitative research: A research paradigm involving theory testing, composed of variables.

Quasi-experiments: A type of experimental design that does not meet the two conditions of a true experiment, which are random assignment and full experimenter control, but tries to meet these conditions as much as possible.

Quota sampling technique: A sampling strategy where the target population is divided into categories according to key characteristics, and then the participants are sampled in representative numbers within each category.

Reflexivity: The act of referring to the self and social influences in investigatory research – an act designed to affect the researcher and inform the research.

Registered reports: The act of preregistering research so that researchers are held accountable to the planned procedures of a project before collecting data.

Replication research: The practice of repeating the data collection procedures of a previous study with different participants and circumstances to confirm that the results of the original study can be applied to other contexts and that their findings are maintained.

Representativeness: The extent to which the findings from corpus analysis can be generalized to the linguistic domain that the corpus was compiled to represent (akin to generalizability in other forms of quantitative research).

Research design: The methodological framework or blueprint of a study, which informs other methodological decisions.

Retrospective protocols: A type of introspection requiring participants to look inward at their own behaviours, thoughts and beliefs regarding a recently completed past activity and verbalize these actions and processes to a researcher.

Retrospective think aloud: An introspective technique which requires a participant to verbalize their thoughts or explain their actions immediately after completing a task.

Same-subject design: A type of experimental research design where the same groups receive all treatments.

Self-observation: The act of observing one's own activity and behaviour either introspectively or retrospectively.

Semantic categorization task: A psycholinguistic task in which respondents are required to indicate whether target words (often accompanied by non-target lexical primes) belong to a predetermined semantic category.

Semi-structured interview: A systematic approach using an interview schedule to ask participants a series of predetermined questions with the flexibility of asking additional probing or follow-up questions and recording their responses.

Semi-structured observation: A systematic approach of using predetermined categories for observed phenomena with flexibility to record additional phenomena that do not fit into those categories.

Signal contingent journal: A type of journal design that requires participants to enter information only when signalled to do so. They are useful if temporal factors have impact on the topic being researched. See also *variable-scheduled journal*.

Stimulated recall: A type of retrospective protocol that uses stimulus to help improve the accuracy of a participant's recollections of their thoughts and behaviours when carrying out a previously completed task.

Stratified random sampling: A sampling strategy where the target population is divided into key characteristics or strata, and then the participants are randomly sampled within each category.

Structured interview: A systematic approach using an interview schedule to ask participants a series of predetermined questions and record their responses.

Structured observation: A systematic approach of using predetermined categories for observed phenomena.

Surveys: Survey research involves the widespread exploration of a topic within a target population, aiming for representativeness in its findings and also to cross-sectionally explore differences in segments of the sample.

Syntactic parsing: A form of corpus annotation in which basic morphosyntactic categories (e.g. parts of speech) are combined into higher order phrase structures to facilitate the analysis of syntactic relationships within a body of texts.

Systematic review: A qualitative approach to document evaluation involving inclusion and exclusion criteria to identify documents fitting the criteria for analysis and then using criteria to evaluate the document's contribution to answering a research question.

Text: A term used in applied linguistics research to refer to existing written data but also widely used to include spoken discourse, symbols and images. See also *document*.

Text analysis: A wider category of analysis that can include both quantitative and qualitative analysis for their linguistic and/or thematic content. See *content analysis* when texts are analysed for words, *thematic text analysis* when texts are analysed for themes, *qualitative content analysis* when the content of texts are organized by theme or *discourse analysis* for analysis of linguistic properties/features.

Thematic text analysis: A qualitative approach of evaluating texts for their themes and coding them for interpretation. See also *content analysis, discourse analysis* and *quantitative content analysis.*

Thick description: A description of data in which details of behaviours, activities and context are provided, usually along with some researcher interpretation so those outside the context can better understand the phenomena.

Think aloud: An introspective technique which requires a participant to verbalize their thoughts or explain their actions while simultaneously completing a task.

Transparency in research: The practice of reporting research honestly and openly using thick description, allowing others to more easily understand the real processes undertaken in the research.

Triangulation: The practice of supporting validation of data by using two or more sources for cross verification.

Type–token ratio (TTR): A measure of lexical diversity in which the number of different word types in a text or corpus is divided by the total number of words.

Unstructured interview: A conversational approach to interviewing with possibly just one or a few predetermined questions or topics, often prompting longer narrative responses.

Unstructured observation: An approach in which there are no predetermined categories for observed phenomena, in which the researcher takes field notes.

Variable-scheduled journal: A type of journal design that requires participants to enter information at predetermined variable intervals in time. They are useful if temporal factors have impact on the topic being researched. See also *signal-contingent journal.*

References

Adair, J. G. (1984). The Hawthorne effect: A reconsideration of the methodological artifact. *Journal of Applied Psychology, 69*(2), 334–345.

Adamson, J., & Muller, T. (2018). Joint autoethnography of teacher experience in the academy: Exploring methods for collaborative inquiry. *International Journal of Research & Method in Education, 41*(2), 207–219.

Alali, F., & Schmitt, N. (2012). Teaching formulaic sequences: The same as or different from teaching single words? *TESOL Journal, 3*(2), 153–180.

Alderson, J. C., & Banerjee, J. (2002). Language testing and assessment (Part 2). *Language Teaching, 35*(2), 79–113.

Androutsopoulos, J. (2014). Computer mediated communication and linguistic landscapes. In J. Holmes & K. Hazen (Eds.), *Research methods in sociolinguistics: A practical guide, vol. 5* (pp. 74–90). Hoboken, NJ: John Wiley & Sons.

Androutsopoulos, J. (2015). Networked multilingualism: Some language practices on Facebook and their implications. *International Journal of Bilingualism, 19*(2), 185–205.

Anthony, L. (2014). *AntConc computer software [version 3.4.3].* Tokyo: Waseda University.

Appleby, R. (2017). Dealing with controversial findings. In J. McKinley & H. Rose (Eds.), *Doing research in applied linguistics realities, dilemmas, and solutions* (pp. 203–213). Abingdon: Routledge.

Aubrey, S. (2017a). Measuring flow in the EFL classroom: Learners' perceptions of inter and intra-cultural task-based interactions. *TESOL Quarterly, 51*(3), 661–692.

Aubrey, S. (2017b). Inter-cultural contact and flow in a task-based Japanese EFL classroom. *Language Teaching Research, 21*(6), 717–734.

Azaz, M. (2017). Metalinguistic knowledge of salient vs. unsalient features: Evidence from the Arabic construct state. *Foreign Language Annals, 50*(1), 214–236.

Azaz, M., & Frank, J. (2017). The role of perceptual salience in the L2 acquisition sequence of the Arabic construct state. *International Journal of Applied Linguistics, 27*, 621–635.

Bachman, L. F. (1990). *Fundamental considerations in language testing.* Oxford: Oxford University Press.

Bachman, L. F., & Palmer, A. S. (1996). *Language testing in practice.* Oxford: Oxford University Press.

Bailey, K. M. (1983). Competitiveness and anxiety in adult second language learning: Looking at and through the diary studies. In H. W. Seliger & M. H. Long (Eds.), *Classroom-oriented research in second language acquisition* (pp. 67–102). Rowley, MA: Newbury House.

Bailey, K. M. (1990). The use of diary studies in teacher education programmes. In J. C. Richards & D. Nunan (Eds.), *Second language teacher education* (pp. 215–226). New York: Cambridge University Press.

Baker, P., & Egbert, J. (Eds.) (2016). *Triangulating methodological approaches in corpus linguistic research.* New York: Routledge.

Banegas, D. L., & Busleimán, G. I. M. (2014). Motivating factors in online language teacher education in southern Argentina. *Computers & Education, 76,* 131–142.

Banegas, D. L., & Consoli, S. (2020). Action research in language education. In J. McKinley & H. Rose (Eds.), *Handbook of research methods in applied linguistics* (in press). Routledge.

Bargar, R. R., & Duncan, J. K. (1982). Cultivating creative endeavor in doctoral research. *The Journal of Higher Education, 53*(1), 1–31.

Barkhuizen, G. (2006). Immigrant parents' perceptions of their children's language practices: Afrikaans speakers living in New Zealand. *Language Awareness, 15*(2), 63–79.

Barkhuizen, G. (2014). Narrative research in language teaching and learning. *Language Teaching, 47*(4), 450–466.

Bartlett, R., & Milligan, C. (2015). *What is diary method?.* London: Bloomsbury Publishing.

Bhatia, V. K. (2014). *Analysing genre.* London: Routledge.

Biber, D. (1993). Representativeness in corpus design. *Literary and Linguistic Computing, 8*(4), 243–257.

Block, D. (2000). Problematizing interview data: Voices in the mind's machine? *TESOL Quarterly, 34,* 757–763.

Block, D. (2017). Positioning theory and life-story interviews: Discursive fields, gaze and resistance. In S. Bagga-Gupta, A. L. Hansen, & J. Feilberg (Eds.), *Identity revisited and reimagined* (pp. 25–39). Cham: Springer.

Bolger, N., Davis, A., & Rafaeli, E. (2003). Diary methods: Capturing life as it is lived. *Annual Review of Psychology, 54,* 579–616.

Borg, S. (2015). *Teacher cognition and language education: Research and practice.* London: Bloomsbury.

Bowles, M. A. (2010). *The think-aloud controversy in second language research.* New York: Routledge.

Brezina, V. (2018). *Statistics in corpus linguistics: A practical guide.* Cambridge: Cambridge University Press.

Briggs Baffoe-Djan, J., & Smith, S. A. (2020). Descriptive statistics in data analysis. In H. Rose & J. McKinley (Eds.), *The Routledge handbook of research methods in applied linguistics* (in press). London: Routledge.

Briggs, J. G. (2015). Out-of-class language contact and vocabulary gain in a study abroad context. *System, 53*, 129–140.

Briggs, J. G., Dearden, J., & Macaro, E. (2018). English medium instruction: Comparing teacher beliefs in secondary and tertiary education. *Studies in Second Language Learning & Teaching, 8*(3), 675–698.

Brinkmann, S. (2014). Interview. In *Encyclopedia of critical psychology* (pp. 1008–1010). New York: Springer.

Brinkmann, S., & Kvale, S. (2014). *InterViews: Learning the craft of qualitative research Interviewing* (3rd edn.). Thousand Oaks, CA: Sage.

Brown, J. D. (2001). *Using surveys in language programs.* Cambridge, England: Cambridge University Press.

Brown, J. D. (2014). Classical theory reliability. In A. J. Kunnan (Ed.), *The companion to language assessment* (pp. 1165–1181). Oxford, UK: Wiley-Blackwell.

Brown, P., & Levinson, S. C. (1987). *Politeness: Some universals in language usage.* Cambridge: Cambridge University Press.

Bryman, A. (2016). *Social research methods* (5th edn.). Oxford: Oxford University Press.

Carson, J. G., & Longhini, A. (2002). Focusing on learning styles and strategies: A diary study in and immersion setting. *Language Learning, 52*, 401–438.

Casanave, C. P. (2012). Diary of a dabbler: Ecological influences on an EFL teacher's efforts to study Japanese informally. *TESOL Quarterly, 46*(4), 642–670.

Casanave, C. P. (2015). Case studies. In B. Paltridge & A. Phakiti (Eds.), *Research methods in applied linguistics: A practical resource* (pp. 119–136). New York: Bloomsbury.

Casanave, C. P. (2017). Representing the self honestly in published research. In J. McKinley & H. Rose (Eds.), *Doing research in applied linguistics: Realities, dilemmas, and solutions* (pp. 235–243), Abingdon: Routledge.

Chambers, C. (2017). *The seven deadly sins of psychology: A manifesto for reforming the culture of scientific practice.* Princeton, NJ: Princeton University Press.

Chaudron, C. (2003). Data collections methods in SLA research. In C. J. Doughty & M. H. Long (Eds.), *The handbook of second language acquisition* (pp. 762–828). Oxford: Blackwell.

Cohen, A. (1984). Studying second-language learning strategies: How do we get the information? *Applied Linguistics, 5*(2), 101–112.

Cohen, A. D. (2004). Assessing speech acts in a second language. In D. Boxer & A. D. Cohen (Eds.), *Studying speaking to inform second language learning* (pp. 302–337). Clevedon: Multilingual Matters.

Cohen, A. D. (2010). Strategies for learning and performing speech acts. In N. Ishihara & A. D. Cohen (Eds.), *Teaching and learning pragmatics* (pp. 227–243). Harlow, UK: Longman/Pearson.

Cohen, L., Manion, L., & Morrison, K. (2018). *Research methods in education* (8th edn.). London: Routledge.

Conklin, K., & Pellicer-Sánchez, A. (2016). Using eye-tracking in applied linguistics and second language research. *Second Language Research, 32*(3), 453–467.

Cook, T. (2009). The purpose of mess in action research: Building rigour though a messy turn. *Educational Action Research, 17*(2), 277–291.

Corder, S. P. (1974). Error analysis. In J. P. B. Allen & S. P. Corder (Eds.), *Techniques in applied linguistics* (The Edinburgh Course in Applied Linguistics). Oxford: Oxford University Press.

Coxhead, A. (2000). A new academic word list. *TESOL Quarterly, 34*(2), 213–238.

Coxhead, A. (2018). Replication research in pedagogical approaches to formulaic sequences: Jones & Haywood (2004) and Alali & Schmitt (2012). *Language Teaching, 51*(1), 113–123.

Coxhead, A. (2020). Analysis of corpora. In J. McKinley & H. Rose (Eds.), *The Routledge handbook of research methods in applied linguistics* (in press). Abingdon: Routledge.

Creswell, J. W. (1994). *Research design: Qualitative and quantitative approaches.* Thousand Oaks, CA: Sage.

Creswell, J. W., & Plano Clark, V. L. (2011). *Designing and conducting mixed method research.* Thousand Oaks, CA: Sage.

Curdt-Christiansen, X. L. (2016). Conflicting language ideologies and contradictory language practices in Singaporean multilingual families. *Journal of Multilingual and Multicultural Development, 37*(7), 694–709.

Dang, T. N., & Webb, S. (2014). The lexical profile of academic spoken English. *English for Specific Purposes, 33*, 66–76.

Declerck, M., & Kormos, J. (2012). The effect of dual task demands and proficiency on second language speech production. *Bilingualism: Language and Cognition, 15*(4), 782–796.

Demjén, Z. (2016). Laughing at cancer: Humour, empowerment, solidarity and coping online. *Journal of Pragmatics, 101*, 18–30.

Denzin, N. K. (2017). *The research act: A theoretical introduction to sociological methods.* New York: Routledge.

Derrick, D. J. (2016). Instrument reporting practices in second language research. *TESOL Quarterly, 50*(1), 132–153.

Derwing, T. M., Rossiter, M. J., Munro, M. J., & Thomson, R. I. (2004). Second language fluency: Judgments on different tasks. *Language Learning, 54*, 655–679.

Diependaele, K., Brysbaert, M., & Neri, P. (2012). How noisy is lexical decision? *Frontiers in Psychology, 3*, 348.

Dörnyei, Z. (2003). *Questionnaires in second language research.* Mahwah, NJ: Lawrence Erlbaum.

Dörnyei, Z. (2007). *Research methods in applied linguistics*. Oxford: Oxford University Press.

Dörnyei, Z. (with Taguchi, T.) (2010). *Questionnaires in second language research: Construction, administration, and processing* (2nd edn.). London: Routledge.

Dörnyei, Z., & Csizér, K. (2012). How to design and analyze surveys in SLA research? In A. Mackey & S. Gass (Eds.), *Research methods in second language acquisition: A practical guide* (pp. 74–94). Malden, MA: Wiley-Blackwell.

Doughty, C., & Long, M. H. (2000). Eliciting second language speech data. In L. Menn & N. Bernstein Ratner (Eds.), *Methods for studying language production* (pp. 149–177). Mahwah, NJ: Lawrence Erlbaum Associates.

Downe-Wamboldt, B. (1992). Content analysis: method, applications, and issues. *Health care for women international, 13*(3), 313–321.

Dulay, H., & Burt, M. (1974). Natural sequences in child second language acquisition. *Language Learning, 24*, 37–53.

Durrant, P. (2017). Lexical bundles and disciplinary variation in university students' writing: Mapping the territories. *Applied Linguistics, 38*, 165–193.

Earle, W. J. (2018). Recent work on rationality. *The Philosophical Forum, 49*(1), 105–129.

Egi, T. (2008). Investigating stimulated recall as a cognitive measure: Reactivity and verbal reports in SLA research methodology. *Language Awareness, 17*, 212–217.

Ellis, C., & Bochner, A. P. (2000). Autoethnography, personal narrative, reflexivity: Researcher as subject. In N. K. Denzin & Y. S. (Eds.), *The Sage handbook of qualitative research* (pp. 733–768). Thousand Oaks, CA: Sage.

Ellis, R. (2009). Measuring implicit and explicit knowledge of a second language. In R. Ellis, S. Loewen, C. Elder, R. Erlam, J. Philp & H. Reinders (Eds.), *Implicit and explicit knowledge in second language learning, testing and teaching* (pp. 1–30). Tonawanda, NY: Multilingual Matters.

Ennser-Kananen, J., Saarinen, T., & Sivunen, N. (2018). It's not messy but it's not clean either: Reviewing and discussing an applied linguistics textbook through a research ethics lens. *Apples: Journal of Applied Language Studies, 12*(1), 71–76.

Fang, F. G., & Ren, W. (2018). Developing students' awareness of global Englishes. *ELT Journal, 72*(4), 384–394.

Farrell, T. S., & Ives, J. (2015). Exploring teacher beliefs and classroom practices through reflective practice: A case study. *Language Teaching Research, 19*(5), 594–610.

Fitzpatrick, T., & Izura, C. (2011). Word association in L1 and L2: An exploratory study of response types, response times and inter-language mediation. *Studies in Second Language Acquisition, 33*, 373–398.

Freed, B. F., Dewey, D., Segalowitz, N., & Halter, R. (2004). The language contact profile. *Studies in Second Language Acquisition, 26*(2), 349–356.

Fröhlich, M., Spada, N., & Allen, P. (1985). Differences in the communicative orientation of L2 classrooms. *TESOL Quarterly, 19*(1), 27–57.

Fulcher, G., & Davidson, F. (2007). *Language testing and assessment: An advanced resource book.* Abingdon: Routledge.

Gage, N. L. (1989). The paradigm wars and their aftermath: A 'historical' sketch of research on teaching since 1989. *Educational Researcher, 18*(7), 4–10.

Galante, A., & Thomson, R. I. (2017). The effectiveness of drama as an instructional approach for the development of second language oral fluency, comprehensibility, and accentedness. *TESOL Quarterly, 51*(1), 115–142.

Galloway, N. (2013). Global Englishes and English Language Teaching (ELT)– Bridging the gap between theory and practice in a Japanese context. *System, 41*(3), 786–803.

Galloway, N. (2017a). *Global Englishes and change in English language teaching: Attitudes and impact.* Abingdon: Routledge.

Galloway, N. (2017b). Researching your own students: negotiating the dual teacher-researcher role. In J. McKinley & H. Rose, (Eds.), *Doing Research in Applied Linguistics Realities, Dilemmas, and Solutions* (pp. 146–156). Abingdon: Routledge.

Galloway, N. (2020). Focus groups. In J. McKinley & H. Rose (Eds.), *The Routledge handbook of research methods in applied linguistics.* Abingdon: Routledge.

Galloway, N., & Rose, H. (2014). Using listening journals to raise awareness of global Englishes in ELT. *ELT Journal, 68*(4), 386–396.

Galloway, N., & Rose, H. (2018). Raising awareness of global Englishes in the ELT classroom. *ELT Journal, 72*(1), 3–14.

Galloway, N., Kriukow, J., & Numajiri, T. (2017). Internationalisation, higher education and the growing demand for English: an investigation into the English medium of instruction (EMI) movement in China and Japan. *ELT Research Papers, 17*(02). British Council.

Gass, S. (2015). Experimental research. In B. Paltridge & A. Phakiti (Eds.), *Research methods in applied linguistics: A practical resource* (pp. 100–118). New York: Bloomsbury.

Gass, S. M., & Mackey, A. (2000). *Stimulated recall methodology in second language research* (2nd edn.). Mahwah, NJ: Lawrence Erlbaum.

Gass, S. M., & Mackey, A. (2017). *Stimulated recall methodology in applied linguistics and L2 research.* New York: Routledge.

Gass, S., Mackey, A., Alvarez-Torres, M. J., & Fernández-García, M. (1999). The effects of task repetition on linguistic output. *Language Learning, 49*, 549–581.

Gebhard, M. (2004). Fast capitalism, school reform, and second language literacy practices. *The Modern Language Journal, 88*(2), 245–265.

Goh, C. C. (1997). Metacognitive awareness and second language listeners. *ELT Journal, 51*(4), 361–369.

Golafshani, N. (2003). Understanding reliability and validity in qualitative research. *The Qualitative Report, 8*(4), 597–606.

Goodwin, L. D., Sands, D. J., & Kozleski, E. B. (1991). Estimating interviewer reliability for interview schedules used in special education research. *The Journal of Special Education, 25*(1), 73–89.

Gorsuch, R. L. (1983). *Factor analysis* (2nd edn.). Hillsdale, NJ: Erlbaum.

Gray, J. (2013). LGBT invisibility and heteronormativity in ELT materials. In J. Gray (Ed.), *Critical perspectives on language teaching materials* (pp. 40–63). London: Palgrave Macmillan.

Grey, S., Cox, J. G., Serafini, E. J., & Sanz, C. (2015). The role of individual differences in the study abroad context: Cognitive capacity and language development during short-term intensive language exposure. *The Modern Language Journal, 99*, 137–157.

Gu, Y. (2014). To code or not to code: Dilemmas in analysing think-aloud protocols in learning strategies research. *System, 43*, 74–81.

Guilloteaux, M. J., & Dörnyei, Z. (2008). Motivating language learners: A classroom-oriented investigation of the effects of motivational strategies on student motivation. *TESOL Quarterly, 42*(1), 55–77.

Hall, G. (2008). An ethnographic diary study. *ELT journal, 62*(2), 113–122.

Hambleton, R., & Zenisky, A. (2011). Translating and adapting tests for cross-cultural assessment. In D. Matsumoto & F. van de Vijver (Eds.), *Cross-cultural research methods in psychology* (pp. 46–73). Cambridge: Cambridge University Press.

Handley, Z. (2018). Replication research in computer-assisted language learning: Replication of Neri et al. (2008) and Satar & Özdener (2008). *Language Teaching, 51*(3), 417–429.

Hashemi, M. R., & Babaii, E. (2013). Mixed methods research: Toward new research designs in applied linguistics. *The Modern Language Journal, 97*(4), 828–852.

Hatch, E., & Lazaraton, A. (1991). *The research manual.* New York: Newbury House.

Heatley, A., Nation, I. S. P., & Coxhead, A. (2002). *Range* [Computer software]. Retrieved from http://www.victoria.ac.nz/lals/staff/paul-nation/nation.aspx [Last accessed 14 July 2019].

Hedgcock, J. S., & Lee, H. (2017a). An exploratory study of academic literacy socialization: Building genre awareness in a teacher education program. *Journal of English for Academic Purposes, 26*, 17–28.

Hedgcock, J. S., & Lee, H. (2017b). Adjusting to contextual constraints: Methodological shifts in local research projects. In J. McKinley & H. Rose (Eds.), *Doing research in applied linguistics* (pp. 61–71). New York: Routledge.

Henning, G. (1987). *A guide to language testing: Development, evaluation, research.* London: Newbury House.

Hessel, G. (2017). A new take on individual differences in L2 proficiency gain during study abroad. *System*, *66*, 39–55.

Hinds, P. J., Neeley, T. B., & Cramton, C. D. (2014). Language as a lightning rod: Power contests, emotion regulation, and subgroup dynamics in global teams. *Journal of International Business Studies*, *45*(5), 536–561.

Hofer, B., & Jessner, U. (2019). Multilingualism at the primary level in South Tyrol: How does multilingual education affect young learners' metalinguistic awareness and proficiency in L1, L2 and L3? *The Language Learning Journal*, *47*(1), 76–87.

Holt, A. (2010). Using the telephone for narrative interviewing: A research note. *Qualitative Research*, *10*(1), 113–121.

Howell-Richardson, C., & Parkinson, B. (1988). Learner diaries: Possibilities and pitfalls. In P. Grunwell (Ed.), *Applied linguistics in society: Papers from the annual meeting of the British Association for Applied Linguistics* (pp. 74–79). Nottingham, UK: British Studies in Applied Linguistics.

Hudson, T., Detmer, E., & Brown, J. D. (1995). *Developing prototypic measures of cross-cultural pragmatics* (Technical Report #7). Honolulu: University of Hawai'i, Second Language Teaching and Curriculum Center.

Hunston, S. (2002). *Corpora in applied linguistics*. Cambridge: Cambridge University Press.

Hyland, K. (2004). Graduates' gratitude: The generic structure of dissertation acknowledgements. *English for Specific purposes*, *23*(3), 303–324.

Hyland, K. (2016). Methods and methodologies in second language writing research. *System*, *59*, 116–125.

Iwaniec, J. (2014). Motivation of pupils from southern Poland to learn English. *System*, *45*, 67–78.

Jackson, D., & Cho, M. (2018). Language teacher noticing: A socio-cognitive window on classroom realities. *Language Teaching Research*, *22*(1), 29–46.

Jarvis, J. (1992). Using diaries for teacher reflection on in-service courses about teacher-training. *ELT Journal*, *46*(2), 133–142.

Jiang, N. (2012). *Conducting reaction time research in second language studies*. New York: Routledge.

Jin, Y. X., & Dewaele, J.-M. (2018). Positive orientation and foreign language classroom anxiety. *System*, *74*, 149–157.

John, P., Brooks, B., & Schriever, U. (2017). Profiling maritime communication by non-native speakers: A quantitative comparison between the baseline and standard marine communication phraseology. *English for Specific Purposes*, *47*, 1–14.

Johnson, R. B., Onwuegbuzie, A. J., & Turner, L. A. (2007). Toward a definition of mixed methods research. *Journal of Mixed Methods Research*, *1*(2), 112–133.

Jones, L. L., & Estes, Z. (2012). Lexical priming: Associative, semantic, and thematic influences on word recognition. In J. S. Adelman (Ed.), *Visual word recognition, vol. 2: Meaning and context: Individuals and development* (pp. 44–72). Hove, UK: Psychology Press.

Jones, M., & Haywood, S. (2004). Facilitating the acquisition of formulaic sequences: An exploratory study in an EAP context. In N. Schmitt (Ed.), *Formulaic sequences* (pp. 269–291). Amsterdam: John Benjamins.

Kang, O. (2015). Learners' perceptions toward pronunciation instruction in three circles of world Englishes. *TESOL Journal, 6*(1), 59–80.

Kang, O., Rubin, D., & Lindemann, S. (2015). Mitigating US undergraduates' attitudes toward international teaching assistants. *TESOL Quarterly, 49*(4), 681–706.

Keenan, J., & MacWhinney, B. (1987). Understanding the relation between comprehension and production. In H. W. Dechert & M. Raupach (Eds.), *Psycholinguistic models of production* (pp. 149–155). Norwood, NJ: Ablex.

Kemmis, S., & McTaggart, R. (1988). *The action research planner.* Geelong: Deakin University.

Khabbazbashi, N. (2017). Topic and background knowledge effects on performance in speaking assessment. *Language Testing, 34*(1), 23–48.

Kim, Y., & Taguchi, N. (2015). Promoting task-based pragmatics instruction in EFL classroom contexts: The role of task complexity. *The Modern Language Journal, 99*(4), 656–677.

Kinsey, A., Pomeroy, W., & Martin, C. (1948). *Sexual behavior in the human male.* Philadelphia: W.B. Saunders.

Kinsey, A., Pomeroy, W., Martin, C., & Gebhard, P. (1953). *Sexual behavior in the human female.* Philadelphia: W.B. Saunders.

Kline, P. (1994). *An easy guide to factor analysis.* New York: Routledge.

Knight, D., Evans, D., Carter, R., & Adophs, S. (2009). HeadTalk, HandTalk and the corpus: Towards a framework for multi-modal, multi-media corpus development. *Corpora, 4*(1), 1–32.

Kormos, J. (1999). Monitoring and self-repair in L2. *Language Learning, 49*(2), 303–342.

Krishnamurty, P. (2008). Diary. In P. J. Lavrakas (Ed.), *Encyclopedia of survey research methods* (pp. 197–198). Thousand Oaks, CA: Sage.

Krueger, R. A. (1998). *Developing questions for focus groups. The focus group kit, 3.* Thousand Oaks, CA: Sage.

Krueger, R. A., & Casey, M. A. (2014). *Focus groups: A practical guide for applied research* (5th edn.). London, UK: Sage.

Kubota, R. (2017). Studying up, down, or across?: Selecting who to research. In J. McKinley & H. Rose (Eds.), *Doing research in applied linguistics: Realities, dilemmas and solutions* (pp. 35–44). Abingdon, UK: Routledge.

Kuchah, K., & Pinter, A. (2012). 'Was this an interview?' Breaking the power barrier in adult-child interviews in an African context. *Issues in Educational Research, 22*(3), 283–297.

Kuckartz, U. (2014). *Qualitative text analysis: A guide to methods, practice & using software*. London: Sage.

Kumaravadivelu, B. (1999). Theorising practice, practising theory: The role of critical classroom observation. In H. Trappes-Lomax & I. McGrath (Eds.), *Theory in language teacher education* (pp. 33–45). Harlow: Longman.

Kvale, S. (2007). *Doing interviews*. London: Sage.

Lachaud, C. M., & Renaud, O. (2011). A tutorial for analyzing human reaction times: How to filter data, manage missing values, and choose a statistical model. *Applied Psycholinguistics, 32*, 389–416.

Lanvers, U. (2018). 'If they are going to university, they are gonna need a language GCSE': Co-constructing the social divide in language learning in England. *System, 76*, 129–143.

Larsen-Freeman, D. (2018). Looking ahead: Future directions in, and future research into, second language acquisition. *Foreign Language Annals, 51*(1), 55–72.

Larsen-Freeman, D., & Long, M. H. (1991). *An introduction to research on second language acquisition*. London: Longman.

Laufer, B., & Nation, I. S. P. (1999). A vocabulary-size test of controlled productive ability. *Language Testing, 16*, 33–51.

Laufer, B., & Waldman, T. (2011). Verb-noun collocations in second-language writing: A corpus analysis of learners' English. *Language Learning, 61*(2), 647–672.

Lazaraton, A. (1996). Interlocutor support in oral proficiency interviews: The case of CASE. *Language Testing, 13*, 151–172.

Lee, D. Y. W. (2010). What corpora are available? In M. McCarthy & A. O'Keeffe (Eds.), *The Routledge handbook of corpus linguistics* (pp. 107–121). London: Routledge.

Leech, G. (1991). The state of the art in corpus linguistics. In K. Aijmer & B. Altenberg (Eds.), *English corpus linguistics: Linguistic studies in honour of Jan Svartvik* (pp. 8–29). London: Longman.

Leech, G. (1997). Teaching and language corpora: A convergence. In A. Wichmann, S. Fligelstone, T. McEnery & G. Knowles (Eds.), *Teaching and language corpora* (pp. 1–23). London: Longman.

Leijten, M., & Van Waes, L. (2013). Keystroke logging in writing research: Using Inputlog to analyze and visualize writing processes. *Written Communication, 30*(3), 358–392.

Leijten, M., Van Waes, L., & Janssen, D. (2010). Error correction strategies of professional speech recognition users: Three profiles. *Computers in Human Behaviour, 26*, 964–975.

Lennon, P. (1990). Investigating fluency in EFL: a quantitative approach. *Language Learning, 40*(3), 387–417.

Liamputtong, P. (2011). *Focus group methodology: Principles and practice*. Thousand Oaks, CA: Sage.

Loewen, S. (2009). Grammaticality judgment tests and the measurement of implicit and explicit L2 knowledge. In R. Ellis, S. Loewen, C. Elder, R. Erlam, J. Philp, & H. Reinders (Eds.), *Implicit and explicit knowledge in second language learning, testing and teaching* (pp. 94–112). Tonawanda, NY: Multilingual Matters.

Loewen, S., Lavolette, E., Spino, L. A., Papi, M., Schmidtke, J., Sterling, S., & Wolff, D. (2014). Statistical literacy among applied linguists and second language acquisition researchers. *TESOL Quarterly, 48,* 360–388.

Loschky, L., & Bley-Vroman, R. (1993). Creating structure-based communication tasks for second language development. In G. Crookes & S. Gass (Eds.), *Tasks and language learning: Integrating theory and practice* (pp. 123–167). Clevedon, England: Multilingual Matters.

Lott, D. (1983). Analysing and counteracting interference errors. *English Language Teaching Journal, 37*(3), 256–262.

Lowie, W., & Verspoor, M. (2018). Individual differences and the ergodicity problem. *Language Learning* (advanced online access).

Lupker, S. J., & Pexman, P. M. (2010). Making things difficult in lexical decision: The impact of pseudohomophones and transposed-letter nonwords on frequency and semantic priming effects. *Journal of Experimental Psychology: Learning, Memory, and Cognition, 36,* 1267–1289.

Luppescu, S., & Day, R. R. (1990). Examining attitude in teachers and students: The need to validate questionnaire data. *Second Language Research, 6,* 125–134.

Ma, R., & Oxford, R. L. (2014). A diary study focusing on listening and speaking: The evolving interaction of learning styles and learning strategies in a motivated, advanced ESL learner. *System, 43,* 101–113.

Macaro, E. (2020). Systematic reviews in applied linguistics research. In J. McKinley & H. Rose (Eds.), *The Routledge handbook of research methods in applied linguistics.* Abingdon: Routledge.

Macaro, E., Curle, S., Pun, J., An, J., & Dearden, J. (2018). A systematic review of English medium instruction in higher education, *Language Teaching, 5*(1), 36–76.

Mackey, A. (2012). Why (or why not), when and how to replicate research. In G. Porte (Ed.), *Replication research in applied linguistics* (pp. 21–46). Cambridge, UK: Cambridge University Press.

Mackey, A., & Gass, S. M. (2005). *Second language research: methodology and design.* London: Routledge.

Mackey, A., & Gass, S. M. (2013). *Stimulated recall methodology in second language research.* New York: Routledge.

Mackey, A., & Gass, S. M. (2016). *Second language research: Methodology and design* (2nd edn.). London: Routledge.

Macpherson, I., Brooker, R., & Ainsworth, P. (2000). Case study in the contemporary world of research: Using notions of purpose, place, process and product to develop some principles for practice. *International Journal of Social Research Methodology, 3*(1), 49–61.

Malvern, D. D., & Richards, B. J. (1997). A new measure of lexical diversity. In A. Ryan & A. Wray (Eds.), *Evolving models of language* (pp. 58–71). Clevedon, UK: Multilingual Matters.

Manning, C. D. (2011). Part-of-speech tagging from 97% to 100%: Is it time for some linguistics? *Proceedings of the 12th international Conference on Computational Linguistics and Intelligent Text Processing* (Vol. Part I) (pp. 171–189). Retrieved from https://nlp.stanford.edu/pubs/CICLing2011-manning-tagging.pdf [Last accessed 13 December 2018].

Marsden, E., Mackey A., & Plonsky, L. (2016). The IRIS repository: Advancing research practice and methodology. In A. Mackey & E. Marsden (Eds.), *Advancing methodology and practice: The IRIS repository of instruments for research into second languages* (pp. 1–21). New York: Routledge.

Marsden, E., Morgan-Short, K., Thompson, S., & Abugaber, D. (2018a). Replication in second language research: Narrative and systematic reviews and recommendations for the field. *Language Learning, 68*(2), 321–391.

Marsden, E., Morgan-Short, K., Trofimovich, P., & Ellis, N. (2018b). Introducing registered reports at *language learning*: Promoting transparency, replication, and a synthetic ethic in the language sciences [Editorial]. *Language Learning, 68*(2), 309–320.

Marshall, C., & Rossman, G. B. (2010). *Designing Qualitative Research* (5th edn). Thousand Oaks: Sage.

Martinez, R. (2018). "Specially in the last years…": Evidence of ELF and non-native English forms in international journals. *Journal of English for Academic Purposes, 33*, 40–52.

May, S. (2014). Introducing the 'multilingual turn'. In S. May (Ed.), *The multilingual turn. Implications for SLA, TESOL and bilingual education* (pp. 1–6). New York, NJ: Routledge.

Mayring, P. (2000). Qualitative content analysis. *Forum: Qualitative Social Research, 1*(2), 10. Retrieved from http://www.qualitative-research.net/index.php/fqs/article/view/1089 [Last accessed 1 January 2019].

McCarthy, P. M., & Jarvis, S. (2010). MTLD, vocd-D, and HD-D: A validation study of sophisticated approaches to lexical diversity assessment. *Behavior Research Methods, 42*, 381–392.

McCray, G., & Brunfaut, T. (2018). Investigating the construct measured by banked gap-fill items: Evidence from eye-tracking. *Language Testing, 35*(1), 51–73.

McDonough, K. (2006). Interaction and syntactic priming: English L2 speakers' production of dative constructions. *Studies in Second Language Acquisition, 28*, 179–207.

McKee, G., Malvern, D., & Richards, B. J. (2000). Measuring vocabulary diversity using dedicated software. *Literary and Linguistic Computing, 15*(3), 323–337.

McKinley, J. (2015). Critical argument and writer identity: Social constructivism as a theoretical framework for EFL academic writing. *Critical Inquiry in Language Studies, 12*(3), 184–207.

McKinley, J. (2017a). Identity construction in learning English academic writing in a Japanese university. *The Journal of Asia TEFL, 14*(2), 228–243.

McKinley, J. (2017b). Overcoming problematic positionality and researcher objectivity. In McKinley, J., & Rose, H. (Eds.), *Doing research in applied linguistics: Realities, dilemmas and solutions* (pp. 37–46). Abingdon, UK: Routledge.

McKinley, J. (2018). Integrating appraisal theory with possible selves in understanding university EFL writing. *System, 78*, 27–37.

McKinley, J. (2019). Developing contextual literacy EAP through CLIL. In T. Dobinson & K. Dunworth (Eds.), *Literacy unbound: Multilingual, multicultural, multimodal* (pp. 67–86). Cham, Switzerland: Springer.

McKinley, J., & Rose, H. (Eds.) (2017). *Doing research in applied linguistics: Realities, dilemmas, and solutions.* Abingdon: Routledge.

McKinley, J., & Rose, H. (2018). Conceptualizations of language errors, standards, norms and nativeness in English for research publication purposes: An analysis of journal submission guidelines. *Journal of Second Language Writing, 43*, 1–11.

Meara, P. (2005). *LLAMA language aptitude tests: The manual.* Swansea, UK: Lognostics.

Menold, N., & Bogner, K. (2016). Design of rating scales in questionnaires. In *GESIS survey guidelines.* Mannheim, Germany: GESIS – Leibniz Institute for the Social Sciences. doi: 10.15465/gesis-sg_en_015.

Merton, R. K., Fiske, M., & Kendall, P. L. (1990). *Focused interview* (2nd edn.). New York: The Free Press.

Meyer, D. E., & Schvaneveldt, R. W. (1971). Facilitation in recognizing pairs of words: Evidence of a dependence between retrieval operations. *Journal of Experimental Psychology, 90*, 227–234.

Miles, M. B. & Huberman, A. M. (1994). *Qualitative data analysis: An expanded sourcebook.* Thousand Oaks, CA: Sage.

Miller, D., & Biber, D. (2015). Evaluating reliability in quantitative vocabulary studies: The influence of corpus design and composition. *International Journal of Corpus Linguistics, 20*(1), 30–53.

Morgan, D. L. (1997). *Focus groups as qualitative research* (2nd edn.). Thousand Oaks, CA: Sage.

Murphy, L. (2008). Learning Logs and Strategy Development for Distance and Other Independent Language Learners. In S. Hurd & T. Lewis (Eds.), *Language Learning Strategies in Independent Settings* (pp. 199–217). Bristol: Multilingual Matters.

Murphy, V. A. (1997). The effect of modality on a grammaticality judgment task. *Second Language Research, 13*, 34–65.

Nassaji, H. (2017). The effectiveness of extensive versus intensive recasts for learning L2 grammar. *The Modern Language Journal, 101*(2), 353–368.

Nation, I. S. P. (1990). *Teaching and learning vocabulary.* New York: Newbury House.

Nation, I. S. P., & Heatley, A. (1994). Range: A program for the analysis of vocabulary in texts [software]. Retrieved from http://www.victoria.ac.nz/lals/staff/paul-nation/nation.aspx [Last accessed 13 December 2018].

Neri, A., O. Mich, M. Gerosa, & D. Giuliani (2008b). The effectiveness of computer assisted pronunciation training for foreign language learning by children. *Computer Assisted Language Learning, 21*(5), 393–408.

Norris, J. (2017). Duoethnography. In L. M. Given (Ed.), *The SAGE encyclopedia of qualitative research methods* (pp. 233–236). Thousand Oaks, CA: Sage.

Norris, J. M., Plonsky, L., Ross, S. J., & Schoonen, R. (2015). Guidelines for reporting quantitative methods and results in primary research. *Language Learning, 65*(2), 470–476.

Norris, W. E. (1970). *Teaching English as a second language: A survey of 1969, a projection for 1970.* Washington, DC: Center for Applied Linguistics.

Nunan, D. (1989). *Understanding language classrooms: A Guide for instructor initiated action.* New York: Prentice-Hall.

Nunnally, J. C., & Bernstein, I. H. (1994). The assessment of reliability. *Psychometric Theory, 3,* 248–292.

O'Brien, I., Segalowitz, N., Collentine, J., & Freed B. (2006). Phonological memory and lexical, narrative and grammatical skills in second language oral production by adult learners. *Applied Psycholinguistics, 27,* 377–402.

O'Keeffe, A., & McCarthy, M. (Eds.) (2010). *The Routledge handbook of corpus linguistics.* London: Routledge.

O'Reilly, K. (2009). *Key concepts in ethnography.* Los Angeles: Sage.

O'Sullivan, B. (Ed.) (2011). *Language testing: Theories and practices.* Basingstoke, UK: Palgrave Macmillan.

Onwuegbuzie, A. J., & Leech, N. L. (2005). On becoming a pragmatic researcher: The importance of combining quantitative and qualitative research methodologies. *International Journal of Social Research Methodology, 8*(5), 375–387.

Onwuegbuzie, A. J., Dickinson, W. B., Leech, N. L., & Zoran, A. G. (2009). A qualitative framework for collecting and analyzing data in focus group research. *International Journal of Qualitative Methods, 8*(3), 1–21.

Ortega, L. (2011). SLA after the social turn: Where cognitivism and its alternatives stand. In D. Atkinson (Ed.), *Alternative approaches to second language acquisition* (pp. 179–192). New York: Routledge.

Ortega, L. (2013). SLA for the 21st century: Disciplinary progress, transdisciplinary relevance, and the bi/multilingual turn. *Language Learning, 63* (suppl. 1), 1–24.

Ortega, L. (2015). Research synthesis. In B. Paltridge & A. Phakiti (Eds.), *Research methods in applied linguistics: A practical resource* (pp. 225–244). London: Bloomsbury Academic.

Oxford, R. L. (1990). *Language learning strategies. What every teacher should know.* Boston: Heinle.

Oxford, R. L., Lavine, R. Z., Hollaway, M. E., Felkins, G., & Saleh, A. (1996). Telling their stories: Language learners use diaries and recollective studies. In R. L. Oxford (Ed.), *Language learning strategies around the world: Cross-cultural perspectives* (pp. 19–34). Manoa: University of Hawaii Press.

Paltridge, B. (2012). *Discourse analysis: An introduction.* London: Bloomsbury Publishing.

Paltridge, B. (2014). What motivates applied linguistics research? *AILA Review, 27*(1), 98–104.

Paradis, J., & Genesee, F. (1996). Syntactic acquisition in bilingual children: Autonomous or interdependent? *Studies in Second Language Acquisition, 18,* 1–25.

Parkinson, B., & Howell-Richardson, C. (1990). Learner diaries. In C. Brumfit & R. Mitchell (Eds.), *Research in the language classroom.* ELT Documents, 133: 128–140. Oxford: Pergamon.

Patton, M. Q. (2015). *Qualitative research & evaluation methods: Integrating theory and practice* (4th edn.). London: Sage.

Payne, G., & Payne, J. (2004). *Key concepts in social research.* Thousand Oaks, CA: Sage.

Pellicer-Sánchez, A. (2016). Incidental L2 vocabulary acquisition from and while reading: An eye-tracking study. *Studies in Second Language Acquisition, 38*(1), 97–130.

Petrić, B., & Czárl, B. (2003). Validating a writing strategy questionnaire. *System, 31,* 187–215.

Pfenninger, S. E., & Singleton, D. (2019). Starting age overshadowed: The primacy of differential environmental and family support effects on L2 attainment in an instructional context. *Language Learning 69,* 207–234.

Phakiti, A. (2014). *Experimental research methods in language learning.* London: Bloomsbury Publishing.

Philp, J. J. (2003). Constraints on 'noticing the gap': Nonnative speakers' noticing of recasts in NS-NNS interaction. *Studies in Second Language Acquisition, 25,* 99–126.

Philp, J. J. (2016). Epilogue: New pathways in researching interaction. In M. Sato & S. Ballinger (Eds.), *Peer interaction and second language learning: Pedagogical potential and research agenda* (pp. 377–396). Amsterdam: John Benjamins.

Plonsky, L., & Derrick, D. J. (2016). A meta-analysis of reliability coefficients in second language research. *The Modern Language Journal, 100*(2), 538–553.

Plonsky, L., Marsden, E., Crowther, D., Gass, S., & Spinner, P. (2019). A methodological synthesis and meta-analysis of judgment tasks in second language research. *Second Language Research*. https://journals.sagepub.com/doi/10.1177/0267658319828413 [Last accessed 31 March 2019].

Polio, C., & Gass, S. (1997). Replication and reporting: A commentary. *Studies in Second Language Acquisition, 19*, 499–508.

Polio, C., Gass, S. M., & Chapin, L. (2006). Using stimulated recall to investigate native speaker perceptions in native-nonnative speaker interaction. *Studies in Second Language Acquisition, 28*, 237–267.

Poplack, S., Wheeler, S., & Westwood, A. (1989). Distinguishing language contact phenomena: Evidence from Finnish-English bilingualism. In K. Hyltenstam & L. K. Obler (Eds.), *Bilingualism across the lifespan: Aspects of acquisition, maturity, and loss* (pp. 132–154). Cambridge, UK: Cambridge University Press.

Porte, G., & McManus, K. (2019). *Doing replication research in applied linguistics*. New York: Routledge.

Porto, M. (2007). Learning diaries in the English as a Foreign Language classroom: A tool for accessing learners' perceptions of lessons and developing learner autonomy and reflection. *Foreign Language Annals 40*(4), 672–696.

Prior, M. T. (2011). Self-presentation in L2 interview talk: Narrative versions, accountability, and emotionality. *Applied Linguistics, 32*(1), 60–76.

Prior, M. T. (2017). Managing researcher dilemmas in narrative interview data and analysis. In J. McKinley & H. Rose (Eds.), *Doing research in applied linguistics: Realities, dilemmas, and solutions* (pp. 172–181). Abingdon: Routledge.

Rayson, P. (2009). Wmatrix: A web-based corpus processing environment. Computing Department, Lancaster University. Retrieved from https://ucrel-wmatrix4.lancaster.ac.uk/ [Last accessed 18 December 2018].

Razfar, A., & Simon, J. (2011). Course-taking patterns of Latino ESL students: Mobility and mainstreaming in urban community colleges in the United States. *TESOL Quarterly, 45*(4), 595–627.

Reid, J. M. (1990). The dirty laundry of ESL survey research. *TESOL Quarterly, 24*, 323–338.

Reis, H. T., & Gable, S. L. (2000). Event-sampling and other methods for studying everyday experience. In T. H. Reis & M. C. Judd (Eds.), *Handbook of research methods in social and personality psychology* (pp. 190–222). New York: Cambridge University Press.

Richards, J. C. (1971). A non-contrastive approach to error analysis. *English Language Teaching Journal, 25*, 204–219.

Richards, K. (2003). *Qualitative inquiry in TESOL*. New York: Palgrave Macmillan.

Richards, K. (2009). Trends in qualitative research in language teaching since 2000. *Language Teaching, 42*(2), 147–180.

Richards, K., Ross, S., & Seedhouse, P. (2012). *Research methods for applied language studies: An advanced resource book for students*. Abingdon: Routledge.

Robson, C. (2002). *Real world research*. Oxford: Blackwell.

Rose, H. (2013). L2 learners' attitudes toward, and use of, mnemonic strategies when learning Japanese kanji. *The Modern Language Journal, 97*(4), 981–992.

Rose, H. (2015). Researching language learner strategies. In B. Paltridge & A. Phakiti (Eds.), *Research methods in applied linguistics: A practical resource* (pp. 421–438). New York: Bloomsbury.

Rose, H., & Galloway, N. (2017). Debating standard language ideology in the classroom: Using the 'Speak Good English Movement' to raise awareness of global Englishes. *RELC Journal. 48*(3), 294–301.

Rose, H., & McKinley, J. (2017). Realities of doing research in applied linguistics. In J. McKinley & H. Rose (Eds.), *Doing research in applied linguistics: Realities, dilemmas and solutions* (pp. 3–14). Abingdon, UK: Routledge.

Rose, H., & McKinley, J. (2018). Japan's English-medium instruction initiatives and the globalization of higher education. *Higher Education, 75*(1), 111–129.

Rose, H., & Montakantiwong, A. (2018). A tale of two teachers: A duoethnography of the realistic and idealistic successes and failures of teaching English as an international language. *RELC Journal, 49*(1), 88–101.

Ross, S. J. (2005). The impact of assessment method on foreign language proficiency growth. *Applied linguistics, 26*(3), 317–342.

Rossman, G. B., & Rallis, S. F. (2016). *Learning in the field: An introduction to qualitative research* (4th edn.). London: Sage.

Saito, K., Suzukida, Y., & Sun, H. (2019). Aptitude, experience and second language pronunciation proficiency development in classroom settings: A longitudinal study. *Studies in Second Language Acquisition. 41*(1), 201–225.

Sanchez, H. S. & Grimshaw, T. (2020). Stimulated recall. In J. McKinley & H. Rose (Eds.), *The Routledge handbook of research methods in applied linguistics*. Abingdon: Routledge.

Santello, M. (2015). Advertising Italian English bilinguals in Australia: Attitudes and response to language selection. *Applied Linguistics, 36*(1), 95–120.

Santos, T. (1989). Replication in applied linguistics research. *TESOL Quarterly, 23*(4), 699–702.

Sasaki, M. (1998). Investigating EFL students' production of speech acts: A comparison of production questionnaires and role plays. *Journal of Pragmatics, 30*(4), 457–484.

Satar, H. M., & Özdener, N. (2008). The effects of synchronous CMC on speaking proficiency and anxiety: Text versus voice chat. *The Modern Language Journal, 92*(4), 595–613.

Sato, M. (2017). Interaction mindsets, interactional behaviors, and L2 development: An affective-social-cognitive model. *Language Learning, 67*(2), 249–283.

Schauer, G. A., & Adolphs, S. (2006). Expressions of gratitude in corpus and DCT data: Vocabulary, formulaic sequences and pedagogy. *System, 34,* 119–134.

Schon, D. (1983). *The reflective practitioner.* New York: Basic Books.

Schorn, A. (2000). The 'theme-centered interview'. A method to decode manifest and latent aspects of subjective realities. *Forum Qualitative Sozialforschung/Forum: Qualitative Social Research, 1*(2), 23.

Schreier, M. (2014). Qualitative content analysis. In U. Flick (Ed.), *The SAGE handbook of qualitative data analysis* (pp. 170–183). London: Sage.

Schrijver, I., Van Vaerenbergh, L., & Van Waes, L. (2012). An exploratory study of transediting in students' translation processes. *Hermes, Journal of Language and Communication in Business, 49,* 99–117.

Scott, J. P. (Ed.) (2006). *Documentary research.* Thousand Oaks, CA: Sage.

Seals, C. A. (2017). Dealing with participant attrition in longitudinal studies. In J. McKinley & H. Rose (Eds.), *Doing research in applied linguistics: Realities, dilemmas, and solutions* (pp. 72–80). London: Routledge.

Seals, C. A., & Kreeft Peyton, J. (2017). Heritage language education: Valuing the languages, literacies, and cultural competencies of immigrant youth. *Current Issues in Language Planning, 18*(1), 87–101.

Shiu, L.- J., Yalçın, Ş., & Spada, N. (2018). Exploring second language learners' grammaticality judgment performance in relation to task design features. *System, 72,* 215–225.

Shuy, R. W. (2003). In-person versus telephone interviewing. In J. A. Holstein & J. F. Gubrium (Eds.), *Inside interviewing: New lenses, new concerns* (pp. 175–193). Thousand Oaks, CA: Sage.

Sinclair, J. (2004a). Corpus and text: Basic principles. In M. Wynne (Ed.), *Developing linguistic corpora: A guide to good practice.* Oxford: Oxbow Books.

Sinclair, J. (2004b). Appendix: How to build a corpus. In M. Wynne (Ed.), *Developing linguistic corpora: A guide to good practice.* Oxford: Oxbow Books.

Sinclair, J. M. (Ed.) (1987). *Looking up: An account of the COBUILD project in lexical computing and the development of the Collins COBUILD English language dictionary.* London: HarperCollins.

Singleton, D., & Pfenninger, S. E. (2017). Reporting on politically sensitive issues. In J. McKinley & H. Rose (Eds.), *Doing research in applied linguistics: Realities, dilemmas, and solutions* (pp. 214–224). Abingdon: Routledge.

Skehan, P. (2016). Foreign language aptitude, acquisitional sequences, and psycholinguistic processes. In G. Granena, D. Jackson, & Y. Yilmaz (Eds.), *Cognitive individual differences in L2 processing and acquisition* (pp. 15–38). Amsterdam, The Netherlands: John Benjamins.

Smith, S. A., Briggs, J. G., Pothier, H., & Garcia, J. (2019). "Mental workouts for couch potatoes": executive function variation among Spanish-English bilingual young adults. *Applied Linguistics, 40*(3), 413–431.

Spada, N. (1994). Classroom interaction analysis. In A. Cumming (Ed.), Alternatives in TESOL research: Descriptive, interpretive, and ideological orientations. *TESOL Quarterly, 28,* 685–688.

Spence, P., & Liu, G. Z. (2013). Engineering English and the high-tech industry: A case study of an English needs analysis of process integration engineers at a semiconductor manufacturing company in Taiwan. *English for Specific Purposes, 32*(2), 97–109.

Spencer-Oatey, H. (Ed.) (2004). *Culturally speaking: Managing rapport through talk across cultures.* London: Continuum.

Spinner, P., & Gass, S. M. (2019). *Using judgments in second language acquisition research.* London: Routledge.

Stake, R. (1995). *The art of case study research.* Thousand Oaks, CA: Sage.

Staples, S., Kang, O., & Wittner, E. (2014). Considering interlocutors in university discourse communities: Impacting US undergraduates' perceptions of ITAs through a structured contact program. *English for Specific Purposes, 35,* 54–65.

Stewart, D. W., Shamdasani, P. N., & Rook, D. W. (2007). *Focus groups: Theory and practice* (2nd edn., vol. *20*). Newbury Park, CA: Sage.

Stickler, U., & Shi, L. (2017). Eyetracking methodology in SCMC: A tool for empowering learning and teaching. *ReCALL, 29*(2), 160–177.

Sturges, J. E., & Hanrahan, K. J. (2004). Comparing telephone and face-to-face qualitative interviewing: A research note. *Qualitative research, 4*(1), 107–118.

Swain, M., & Wesche, M. (1973). Linguistic interaction: Case study of a bilingual child. *Working Papers on Bilingualism, 1,* 10–34.

Sweeney, E., & Zhu Hua (2016). Discourse completion tasks. In Zhu Hua (Ed.), *Research methods in intercultural communication: A practical guide* (pp. 212–222). Oxford: Wiley-Blackwell.

Tabachnick, B. G., & Fidell, L. S. (2014). *Using Multivariate Statistics* (6th edn.). Harlow: Pearson Education.

Talmy, S. (2010a). Qualitative interviews in applied linguistics: From research instrument to social practice. *Annual Review of Applied Linguistics, 30,* 128–148.

Talmy, S. (2010b). The interview as collaborative achievement: Interaction, identity, and ideology in a speech event. *Applied Linguistics, 32*(1), 25–42.

Talmy, S., & Richards, K. (2011). Theorizing qualitative research interviews in applied linguistics. *Applied Linguistics, 32*(1), 1–5.

Teng, L. S., & Zhang, L. J. (2016). A questionnaire-based validation of multidimensional models of self-regulated learning strategies. *The Modern Language Journal, 100*(3), 674–701.

Thomas, J. (1993). Doing critical ethnography. In *Qualitative Research Methods* (Vol. *26*). Thousand Oaks, CA: Sage.

Thompson, P. (2004). Spoken language corpora. In M. Wynne (Ed.), *Developing linguistic corpora: A guide to good practice*. Oxford: Oxbow Books.

Timmermans, S., & Tavory, I. (2012). Theory construction in qualitative research: From grounded theory to abductive analysis. *Sociological Theory, 30*(3), 167–186.

Timms, W., & Eccott, A. (1972). *International picture stories*. London: Hodder & Stoughton.

Ting-Toomey, S., & Dorjee, T. (2019). *Communicating across cultures* (2nd edn.). New York: Guilford.

Towell, R., Hawkins, R., & Bazergui, N. (1996). The development of fluency in advanced learners of French. *Applied Linguistics, 17*(1), 84–119.

Ullman, R., & Geva, E. (1984). Approaches to observation in second language classes. In P. Allen, & M. Swain (Eds.), *Language issues and educational policies: Exploring Canada's multilingual resources* (pp. 113–128). Oxford: Pergamon Press.

van der Slik, F. W. P., van Hout, R. W. N. M., & Schepens, J. J. (2015). The gender gap in second language acquisition: Gender differences in the acquisition of Dutch among immigrants from 88 countries with 49 mother tongues. *PLoS ONE, 10*(11): e0142056. https://journals.plos.org/plosone/article?id=10.1371/journal.pone.0142056 [Last accessed 1 January 2019].

Van Praag, B., & Sanchez, H. S. (2015). Mobile technology in second language classrooms: Insights into its uses, pedagogical implications, and teacher beliefs. *ReCALL, 27*(3), 288–303.

Vandergrift, L. (2003). Orchestrating strategy use: Toward a model of the skilled second language listener. *Language Learning, 53*(3), 463–496.

Vandergrift, L. (2010). Researching listening in applied linguistics. In B. Paltridge & A. Phakiti (Eds.), *Continuum companion to research methods in applied linguistics* (pp. 301–317). London: Continuum.

Vandergrift, L., & Baker, S. C. (2018). Learner variables important for success in L2 listening comprehension in French immersion classrooms. *The Canadian Modern Language Review, 74*(1), 79–100.

Venuti, L. (2012). *The translation studies reader*. London: Routledge.

Viberg, O., & Grönlund, Å. (2017). Understanding students' learning practices: Challenges for design and integration of mobile technology into distance education. *Learning, Media and Technology, 42*(3), 357–377.

Vyatkina, N. (2012). The development of second language writing complexity in groups and individuals: A longitudinal learner corpus study. *The Modern Language Journal, 96*(4), 576–598.

Wagner, E. (2015). Survey research in applied linguistics. In B. Paltridge & A. Phakiti (Eds.), *Research methods in applied linguistics* (pp. 83–99). London: Bloomsbury.

Wang, W. (2020). Text analysis. In J. McKinley & H. Rose (Eds.), *The Routledge handbook of research methods in applied linguistics* (in press). Abingdon: Routledge.

Weitz, M., Pahl, S., Flyman Mattsson, A., Buyl, A., & Kalbe, E. (2010). The Input Quality Observation Scheme (IQOS): The nature of L2 input and its influence on L2 development in bilingual preschools. *Bilingual Preschools, 1*, 5–44.

Weninger, C., & Kiss, T. (2013). Culture in English as a foreign language (EFL) textbooks: A semiotic approach. *TESOL Quarterly, 47*(4), 694–715.

Wheeler, L., & Reis, H. T. (1991). Self-recording of everyday life events: Origins, types, and uses. *Journal of personality, 59*(3), 339–354.

Wilkinson, S. (2004). Focus group research. In D. Silverman (Ed.), *Qualitative research: Theory, method, and practice* (pp. 177–199). Thousand Oaks, CA: Sage.

Witzel, A., & Reiter, H. (2012). *The problem-centred interview*. Los Angeles: Sage.

Wolter, B., & Yamashita, J. (2015). Processing collocations in a second language: A case of first language activation? *Applied Psycholinguistics, 36*(5), 1193–1221.

Wray, A., Trott, K., & Bloomer, A. (1998). *Projects in linguistics: A practical guide to researching language*. London: Arnold.

Wynne, M. (Ed.) (2005). *Developing linguistic corpora: A guide to good practice*. Oxford: Oxbow Books.

Yan, J. X., & Horwitz, E. K. (2008). Learners' perceptions of how anxiety interacts with personal and instructional factors to influence their achievement in English: A qualitative analysis of EFL learners in China. *Language learning, 58*(1), 151–183.

Yang, C., Hu, G., & Zhang, L. J. (2014). Reactivity of concurrent verbal reporting in second language writing. *Journal of Second Language Writing, 24*, 51–70.

Yin, R. K. (2009). *Case study research and applications: Design and methods* (4th edn.). Thousand Oaks, CA: Sage.

Yin, R. K. (2018). *Case study research and applications: Design and methods* (6th edn.). Thousand Oaks, CA: Sage.

Zhang, L. & Zhang, D. (2020). Think aloud protocols. In J. McKinley & H. Rose (Eds.), *The Routledge handbook of research methods in applied linguistics* (in press). Abingdon: Routledge.

Index